Teen

Diet and Nutrition
SOURCEBOOK

Fourth Edition

Health Reference Series

Fourth Edition

Diet and Nutrition SOURCEBOOK

Basic Consumer Health Information about Dietary Guidelines, Servings and Portions, Recommended Daily Nutrient Intakes and Meal Plans, Vitamins and Supplements, Weight Loss and Maintenance, Nutrition for Different Life Stages and Medical Conditions, and Healthy Food Choices

Along with Details about Government Nutrition Support Programs, a Glossary of Nutrition and Dietary Terms, and a Directory of Resources for More Information

Edited by
Laura Larsen

Omnigraphics

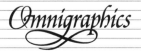

155 W. Congress, Suite 200, Detroit, MI 48226

Bibliographic Note
Because this page cannot legibly accommodate all the copyright notices, the Bibliographic
Note portion of the Preface constitutes an extension of the copyright notice.

Edited by Laura Larsen

Health Reference Series

Karen Bellenir, *Managing Editor*
David A. Cooke, MD, FACP, *Medical Consultant*
Elizabeth Collins, *Research and Permissions Coordinator*
Cherry Edwards, *Permissions Assistant*
EdIndex, Services for Publishers, *Indexers*

* * *

Omnigraphics, Inc.
Matthew P. Barbour, *Senior Vice President*
Kevin M. Hayes, *Operations Manager*

* * *

Peter E. Ruffner, *Publisher*

Copyright © 2011 Omnigraphics, Inc.
ISBN 978-0-7808-1152-2

Library of Congress Cataloging-in-Publication Data

Diet and nutrition sourcebook : basic consumer health information about
dietary guidelines, servings and portions, recommended daily nutrient
intakes and meal plans, vitamins and supplements, weight loss and
maintenance, nutrition for different life stages and medical conditions, and
healthy food choices ... / edited by Laura Larsen. -- 4th ed.
    p. cm.
  Includes bibliographical references and index.
  Summary: "Provides basic consumer health information about nutrition
through the lifespan including facts about dietary guidelines and eating
plans, weight control, and related medical concerns. Includes index,
glossary of related terms, and other resources"-- Provided by publisher.
  ISBN 978-0-7808-1152-2 (hardcover : alk. paper) 1. Nutrition--Popular
works. 2. Diet--Popular works. 3. Health--Popular works. 4. Consumer
education. I. Larsen, Laura.
  RA784.D542 2011
  613.2'5--dc23
                                                              2011034798

Table of Contents

Visit www.healthreferenceseries.com to view *A Contents Guide to the Health Reference Series*, a listing of more than 16,000 topics and the volumes in which they are covered.

Part II: The Elements of Good Nutrition

Part III: Nutrition Through the Life Span

Part IV: Lifestyle and Nutrition

Part V: Nutrition-Related Health Concerns

Part VII: Nutrition for People with Other Medical Concerns

Part VIII: Additional Help and Information

Preface

About This Book

Nutrition affects health, well-being, quality of life, and longevity, yet according to the U.S. Department of Health and Human Services, many Americans consume more calories than they need without meeting the recommended intakes for a number of important nutrients. This, along with increasingly sedentary lifestyles and busy schedules, can lead to obesity, heart disease, certain cancers, and diabetes. According to a report in the *New England Journal of Medicine*, unless Americans make healthy changes to their diets and physical activity levels, today's children comprise the first generation that may not live as long as their parents.

Diet and Nutrition Sourcebook, Fourth Edition provides up-to-date data on nutrition and health, including information from the recently updated *Dietary Guidelines for Americans* and facts about the new MyPlate food guidance system. It details how children, seniors, vegetarians, athletes, and others can benefit from good nutrition. It offers tips for smart grocery shopping, healthy food preparation, and the consumption of a varied, balanced, and nutritious diet. It also discusses strategies for maintaining healthy eating patterns in restaurants, fast food establishments, and other places where meals are consumed away from home. People with certain medical concerns will learn how dietary choices play a role in disease management practices, and a special section discusses the link between nutrition and weight loss and weight maintenance. The book concludes with a glossary, information about government nutrition programs, and a directory of related organizations.

How to Use This Book

This book is divided into parts and chapters. Parts focus on broad areas of interest. Chapters are devoted to single topics within a part.

Part I: Guidelines for Healthy Food Consumption introduces basic concepts from the recently updated *Dietary Guidelines for Americans* and the new MyPlate food guidance system. It also discusses portions and serving sizes, food labeling information, and dietary supplements.

Part II: The Elements of Good Nutrition presents details about basic food groups, fluids, vitamins, minerals, and functional foods. Individual chapters describe the importance of protein, carbohydrates, fats, fruits and vegetables, dairy products, and grains. Other chapters explain why vitamins, minerals, phytochemicals, and antioxidants are important dietary components.

Part III: Nutrition through the Life Span provides dietary information for people in different age groups. These include infants and toddlers, children and tweens, teens and college students, pregnant and menopausal women, and older persons.

Part IV: Lifestyle and Nutrition presents nutrition statistics and explores ways for Americans to make healthy food choices when shopping for food, when cooking at home, or when eating out. It also provides tips about vegetarian eating patterns, sports nutrition, and alcohol use.

Part V: Nutrition-Related Health Concerns describes the most common dietary issues facing Americans, such as the link between the typical Western diet and metabolic syndrome and other concerns about added sugars, food additives, excess sodium, and high-calorie beverage consumption.

Part VI: Nutrition and Weight Control focuses on the health risks faced by those who are overweight, and a special chapter addresses weight concerns in children. Other chapters provide tips for healthy weight loss and evaluate popular diet plans, diet medications and supplements, and low-fat foods.

Part VII: Nutrition for People with Other Medical Concerns discusses healthy eating patterns for people with diabetes, heart disease, lactose intolerance, food allergies, celiac disease, eating disorders, and cancer. It also describes the role nutrition plays in oral health.

Part VIII: Additional Help and Information includes a glossary of nutrition terms and details about government-sponsored nutrition programs for people who lack access to affordable food, including programs for women and infants, school-aged children, and seniors. It concludes with a directory of sources for more information.

Bibliographic Note

This volume contains documents and excerpts from publications issued by the following U.S. government agencies: Administration on Aging (AoA); Centers for Disease Control and Prevention (CDC); National Cancer Institute (NCI); National Center for Complementary and Alternative Medicine (NCCAM); National Diabetes Education Program (NDEP); National Heart, Lung, and Blood Institute (NHLBI); National Institute of Allergy and Infectious Diseases (NIAID); National Institute of Child Health and Human Development (NICHD); National Institute of Diabetes and Digestive and Kidney Diseases (NIDDK); National Institute of Mental Health (NIMH); Navy and Marine Corps Public Health Center; Office of Dietary Supplements (ODS); Office on Women's Health; U.S. Department of Agriculture (USDA); U.S. Department of Health and Human Services (HHS); U.S. Environmental Protection Agency (EPA); and U.S. Food and Drug Administration (FDA).

In addition, this volume contains copyrighted documents from the following organizations: A.D.A.M., Inc.; American College of Sports Medicine (ACSM); American Dietetic Association (ADA); American Heart Association (AHA); American Psychological Association (APA); Calorie Control Council; Center for Science in the Public Interest (CSPI); Cincinnati Children's Hospital Medical Center; Cleveland Clinic; Helpguide.org; International Food Information Council; Iowa State University Extension Service; Natural Standard; Nemours Foundation; Obesity Action Coalition; A Place for Mom; University of Florida Cooperative Extension, Institute of Food and Agriculture Sciences; University of California San Diego News Center; and University of Wisconsin.

Full citation information is provided on the first page of each chapter or section. Every effort has been made to secure all necessary rights to reprint the copyrighted material. If any omissions have been made, please contact Omnigraphics to make corrections for future editions.

Acknowledgements

Thanks go to the many organizations, agencies, and individuals who have contributed materials for this *Sourcebook* and to medical consultant Dr. David Cooke and prepress services provider WhimsyInk. Special thanks go to managing editor Karen Bellenir and research and permissions coordinator Liz Collins for their help and support.

About the Health Reference Series

The *Health Reference Series* is designed to provide basic medical information for patients, families, caregivers, and the general public. Each volume takes a particular topic and provides comprehensive coverage. This is especially important for people who may be dealing with a newly diagnosed disease or a chronic disorder in themselves or in a family member. People looking for preventive guidance, information about disease warning signs, medical statistics, and risk factors for health problems will also find answers to their questions in the *Health Reference Series*. The *Series*, however, is not intended to serve as a tool for diagnosing illness, in prescribing treatments, or as a substitute for the physician/patient relationship. All people concerned about medical symptoms or the possibility of disease are encouraged to seek professional care from an appropriate health care provider.

A Note about Spelling and Style

Health Reference Series editors use *Stedman's Medical Dictionary* as an authority for questions related to the spelling of medical terms and the *Chicago Manual of Style* for questions related to grammatical structures, punctuation, and other editorial concerns. Consistent adherence is not always possible, however, because the individual volumes within the Series include many documents from a wide variety of different producers and copyright holders, and the editor's primary goal is to present material from each source as accurately as is possible following the terms specified by each document's producer. This sometimes means that information in different chapters or sections may follow other guidelines and alternate spelling authorities. For example, occasionally a copyright holder may require that eponymous terms be shown in possessive forms (Crohn's disease *vs.* Crohn disease) or that British spelling norms be retained (leukaemia *vs.* leukemia).

Locating Information within the Health Reference Series

The *Health Reference Series* contains a wealth of information about a wide variety of medical topics. Ensuring easy access to all the fact sheets, research reports, in-depth discussions, and other material contained within the individual books of the *Series* remains one of our highest priorities. As the *Series* continues to grow in size and scope, however, locating the precise information needed by a reader may become more challenging.

A Contents Guide to the Health Reference Series was developed to direct readers to the specific volumes that address their concerns. It presents an extensive list of diseases, treatments, and other topics of general interest compiled from the Tables of Contents and major index headings. To access *A Contents Guide to the Health Reference Series*, visit www.healthreferenceseries.com.

Medical Consultant

Medical consultation services are provided to the *Health Reference Series* editors by David A. Cooke, MD, FACP. Dr. Cooke is a graduate of Brandeis University, and he received his M.D. degree from the University of Michigan. He completed residency training at the University of Wisconsin Hospital and Clinics. He is board-certified in Internal Medicine. Dr. Cooke currently works as part of the University of Michigan Health System and practices in Ann Arbor, MI. In his free time, he enjoys writing, science fiction, and spending time with his family.

Our Advisory Board

We would like to thank the following board members for providing guidance to the development of this *Series*:

- Dr. Lynda Baker, Associate Professor of Library and Information Science, Wayne State University, Detroit, MI

- Nancy Bulgarelli, William Beaumont Hospital Library, Royal Oak, MI

- Karen Imarisio, Bloomfield Township Public Library, Bloomfield Township, MI

- Karen Morgan, Mardigian Library, University of Michigan-Dearborn, Dearborn, MI

- Rosemary Orlando, St. Clair Shores Public Library, St. Clair Shores, MI

Health Reference Series Update Policy

The inaugural book in the *Health Reference Series* was the first edition of *Cancer Sourcebook* published in 1989. Since then, the *Series* has been enthusiastically received by librarians and in the medical community. In order to maintain the standard of providing high-quality health information for the layperson the editorial staff at Omnigraphics felt it was necessary to implement a policy of updating volumes when warranted.

Medical researchers have been making tremendous strides, and it is the purpose of the *Health Reference Series* to stay current with the most recent advances. Each decision to update a volume is made on an individual basis. Some of the considerations include how much new information is available and the feedback we receive from people who use the books. If there is a topic you would like to see added to the update list, or an area of medical concern you feel has not been adequately addressed, please write to:

Editor
Health Reference Series
Omnigraphics, Inc.
155 W. Congress, Suite 200
Detroit, MI 48226
E-mail: editorial@omnigraphics.com

Part One

Guidelines for
Healthy Food Consumption

Chapter 1

Federal Dietary Guidelines and Food Guidance System

Chapter Contents

Section 1.1

Dietary Guidelines for Americans

This section excerpted from "Dietary Guidelines for Americans 2010: Executive Summary," U.S. Department of Health and Human Services (www.hhs.gov), January 31, 2011.

Eating and physical activity patterns that are focused on consuming fewer calories, making informed food choices, and being physically active can help people attain and maintain a healthy weight, reduce their risk of chronic disease, and promote overall health. The *Dietary Guidelines for Americans, 2010* exemplifies these strategies through recommendations that accommodate the food preferences, cultural traditions, and customs of the many and diverse groups who live in the United States.

By law, *Dietary Guidelines for Americans* is reviewed, updated if necessary, and published every five years. The U.S. Department of Agriculture (USDA) and the U.S. Department of Health and Human Services (HHS) jointly create each edition.

Dietary Guidelines recommendations traditionally have been intended for healthy Americans ages two years and older. However, *Dietary Guidelines for Americans, 2010* is being released at a time of rising concern about the health of the American population. Poor diet and physical inactivity are the most important factors contributing to an epidemic of overweight and obesity affecting men, women, and children in all segments of our society. Even in the absence of overweight, poor diet and physical inactivity are associated with major causes of morbidity and mortality in the United States. Therefore, the *Dietary Guidelines for Americans, 2010* is intended for Americans ages two years and older, including those at increased risk of chronic disease.

Dietary Guidelines for Americans, 2010 also recognizes that in recent years nearly 15% of American households have been unable to acquire adequate food to meet their needs. This dietary guidance can help them maximize the nutritional content of their meals. Many other Americans consume less than optimal intake of certain nutrients even though they have adequate resources for a healthy diet. This dietary guidance and nutrition information can help them choose a healthy, nutritionally adequate diet.

The intent of the Dietary Guidelines is to summarize and synthesize knowledge about individual nutrients and food components into an interrelated set of recommendations for healthy eating that can be adopted by the public. Taken together, the Dietary Guidelines recommendations encompass two over-arching concepts:

- Maintain calorie balance over time to achieve and sustain a healthy weight. People who are most successful at achieving and maintaining a healthy weight do so through continued attention to consuming only enough calories from foods and beverages to meet their needs and by being physically active. To curb the obesity epidemic and improve their health, many Americans must decrease the calories they consume and increase the calories they expend through physical activity.

- Focus on consuming nutrient-dense foods and beverages. Americans currently consume too much sodium and too many calories from solid fats, added sugars, and refined grains. These replace nutrient-dense foods and beverages and make it difficult for people to achieve recommended nutrient intake while controlling calorie and sodium intake. A healthy eating pattern limits intake of sodium, solid fats, added sugars, and refined grains and emphasizes nutrient-dense foods and beverages—vegetables, fruits, whole grains, fat-free or low-fat milk and milk products, seafood, lean meats and poultry, eggs, beans and peas, and nuts and seeds.

A basic premise of the Dietary Guidelines is that nutrient needs should be met primarily through consuming foods. In certain cases, fortified foods and dietary supplements may be useful in providing one or more nutrients that otherwise might be consumed in less than recommended amounts. Two eating patterns that embody the Dietary Guidelines are the USDA Food Patterns and their vegetarian adaptations and the DASH (Dietary Approaches to Stop Hypertension) Eating Plan.

A healthy eating pattern needs not only to promote health and help to decrease the risk of chronic diseases, but it also should prevent foodborne illness. Four basic food safety principles (Clean, Separate, Cook, and Chill) work together to reduce the risk of foodborne illnesses. In addition, some foods (such as milks, cheeses, and juices that have not been pasteurized, and undercooked animal foods) pose high risk for foodborne illness and should be avoided.

The information in the *Dietary Guidelines for Americans* is used in developing educational materials and aiding policymakers in designing and carrying out nutrition-related programs, including federal food, nutrition education, and information programs.

The following are the *Dietary Guidelines for Americans, 2010* Key Recommendations. These Key Recommendations are the most important in terms of their implications for improving public health. To get the full benefit, individuals should carry out the Dietary Guidelines recommendations in their entirety as part of an overall healthy eating pattern.

Key Recommendations

Balancing Calories to Manage Weight

- Prevent and/or reduce overweight and obesity through improved eating and physical activity behaviors.

- Control total calorie intake to manage body weight. For people who are overweight or obese, this will mean consuming fewer calories from foods and beverages.

- Increase physical activity and reduce time spent in sedentary behaviors.

- Maintain appropriate calorie balance during each stage of life— childhood, adolescence, adulthood, pregnancy and breastfeeding, and older age.

Foods and Food Components to Reduce

- Reduce daily sodium intake to less than 2,300 milligrams (mg) and further reduce intake to 1,500 mg among persons who are 51 and older and those of any age who are African American or have hypertension, diabetes, or chronic kidney disease. The 1,500 mg recommendation applies to about half of the U.S. population, including children, and the majority of adults.

- Consume less than 10% of calories from saturated fatty acids by replacing them with monounsaturated and polyunsaturated fatty acids.

- Consume less than 300 mg per day of dietary cholesterol.

- Keep trans fatty acid consumption as low as possible by limiting foods that contain synthetic sources of trans fats, such as partially hydrogenated oils, and by limiting other solid fats.

- Reduce the intake of calories from solid fats and added sugars.

- Limit the consumption of foods that contain refined grains, especially refined grain foods that contain solid fats, added sugars, and sodium.

- If alcohol is consumed, it should be consumed in moderation—up to one drink per day for women and two drinks per day for men—and only by adults of legal drinking age.

Foods and Nutrients to Increase

Individuals should meet the following recommendations as part of a healthy eating pattern while staying within their calorie needs.

- Increase vegetable and fruit intake.

- Eat a variety of vegetables, especially dark-green and red and orange vegetables and beans and peas.

- Consume at least half of all grains as whole grains. Increase whole-grain intake by replacing refined grains with whole grains.

- Increase intake of fat-free or low-fat milk and milk products, such as milk, yogurt, cheese, or fortified soy beverages.

- Choose a variety of protein foods, which include seafood, lean meat and poultry, eggs, beans and peas, soy products, and unsalted nuts and seeds.

- Increase the amount and variety of seafood consumed by choosing seafood in place of some meat and poultry.

- Replace protein foods that are higher in solid fats with choices that are lower in solid fats and calories and/or are sources of oils.

- Use oils to replace solid fats where possible.

- Choose foods that provide more potassium, dietary fiber, calcium, and vitamin D, which are nutrients of concern in American diets. These foods include vegetables, fruits, whole grains, and milk and milk products.

Recommendations for Specific Population Groups

Women capable of becoming pregnant should follow these guidelines:

- Choose foods that supply heme iron, which is more readily absorbed by the body, additional iron sources, and enhancers of iron absorption such as vitamin C–rich foods.

- Consume 400 micrograms (mcg) per day of synthetic folic acid (from fortified foods and/or supplements) in addition to food forms of folate from a varied diet.

Women who are pregnant or breastfeeding should follow these guidelines:

- Consume 8 to 12 ounces of seafood per week from a variety of seafood types.

- Due to their high methyl mercury content, limit white (albacore) tuna to 6 ounces per week and do not eat the following four types of fish: tilefish, shark, swordfish, and king mackerel.

- If pregnant, take an iron supplement, as recommended by an obstetrician or other health care provider.

Individuals ages 50 years and older should follow this recommendation:

- Consume foods fortified with vitamin B12, such as fortified cereals, or dietary supplements.

Building Healthy Eating Patterns

- Select an eating pattern that meets nutrient needs over time at an appropriate calorie level.

- Account for all foods and beverages consumed and assess how they fit within a total healthy eating pattern.

- Follow food safety recommendations when preparing and eating foods to reduce the risk of foodborne illnesses.

Section 1.2

Introduction to the MyPlate Food Guidance System

"First Lady, Agriculture Secretary Launch MyPlate Icon as a New Reminder to Help Consumers to Make Healthier Food Choices," press release, U.S. Department of Agriculture (www.usda.gov), June 2, 2011.

On June 2, 2011, First Lady Michelle Obama and Agriculture Secretary Tom Vilsack unveiled the federal government's new food icon, MyPlate, to serve as a reminder to help consumers make healthier food choices. MyPlate is a new generation icon with the intent to prompt consumers to think about building a healthy plate at meal times and to seek more information to help them do that by going to www.Choose MyPlate.gov. The new MyPlate icon emphasizes the fruit, vegetable, grains, protein, and dairy food groups.

"This is a quick, simple reminder for all of us to be more mindful of the foods that we're eating and as a mom, I can already tell how much this is going to help parents across the country," said First Lady Michelle Obama. "When mom or dad comes home from a long day of work, we're already asked to be a chef, a referee, a cleaning crew. So it's tough to be a nutritionist, too. But we do have time to take a look at our kids' plates. As long as they're half full of fruits and vegetables, and paired with lean proteins, whole grains and low-fat dairy, we're golden. That's how easy it is."

"With so many food options available to consumers, it is often difficult to determine the best foods to put on our plates when building a healthy meal," said Secretary Vilsack. "MyPlate is an uncomplicated symbol to help remind people to think about their food choices in order to lead healthier lifestyles. This effort is about more than just giving information, it is a matter of making people understand there are options and practical ways to apply them to their daily lives."

Originally identified in the Child Obesity Task Force report which noted that simple, actionable advice for consumers is needed, MyPlate will replace the MyPyramid image as the government's primary food group symbol as an easy-to-understand visual cue to help consumers adopt healthy eating habits consistent with the *2010 Dietary Guidelines for*

Americans. MyPyramid will remain available to interested health professionals and nutrition educators in a special section of the new website.

ChooseMyPlate.gov provides practical information to individuals, health professionals, nutrition educators, and the food industry to help consumers build healthier diets with resources and tools for dietary assessment, nutrition education, and other user-friendly nutrition information. As Americans are experiencing epidemic rates of overweight and obesity, the online resources and tools can empower people to make healthier food choices for themselves, their families, and their children. Later this year, USDA will unveil an exciting "go-to" online tool that consumers can use to personalize and manage their dietary and physical activity choices.

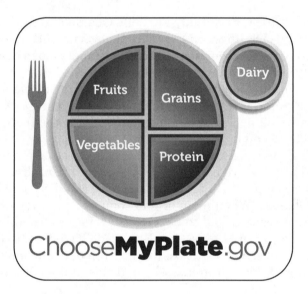

Figure 1.1. *MyPlate Icon*

Over the next several years, USDA will work with First Lady Michelle Obama's Let's Move! initiative and public and private partners to promote MyPlate and ChooseMyPlate.gov as well as the supporting nutrition messages and "how-to" resources.

The *2010 Dietary Guidelines for Americans*, launched in January of this year, form the basis of the federal government's nutrition education programs, federal nutrition assistance programs, and dietary advice provided by health and nutrition professionals. The *Guidelines* messages include the following advice:

Balance Calories

- Enjoy your food, but eat less.
- Avoid oversized portions.

Foods to Increase

- Make half your plate fruits and vegetables.
- Switch to fat-free or low-fat (1%) milk.
- Make at least half your grains whole grains.

Foods to Reduce

- Compare sodium (salt) in foods like soup, bread, and frozen meals, and choose foods with lower numbers.
- Drink water instead of sugary drinks.

Coupled with these tested, actionable messages will be the "how-tos" for consumer behavior change. A multi-year campaign calendar will focus on one action-prompting message at a time starting with "Make Half Your Plate Fruits and Vegetables."

"What we have learned over the years is that consumers are bombarded by so many nutrition messages that it makes it difficult to focus on changes that are necessary to improve their diet," said Secretary Vilsack. "This new campaign calendar will help unify the public and private sectors to coordinate efforts and highlight one desired change for consumers at a time."

As part of this new initiative, USDA wants to see how consumers are putting MyPlate in to action by encouraging consumers to take a photo of their plates and share on Twitter with the hash-tag #MyPlate. USDA also wants to see where and when consumers think about healthy eating. Take the Plate (available at http://www.choosemyplate .gov/images/MyPlateImages/JPG/myplate_green.jpg) and snap a photograph with MyPlate to share with our USDA Flickr Photo Group (http://www.flickr.com/people/usdagov/).

For more information, visit www.ChooseMyPlate.gov. Additional resources include: www.DietaryGuidelines.gov and www.LetsMove.gov.

Chapter 2

Portion Sizes and Servings

Chapter Contents

13

Section 2.1

Healthy Portions

This section includes "Portion Distortion and Serving Size," National Heart, Lung, and Blood Institute (www.nhlbi.nih.gov), 2010, and excerpts from "Just Enough for You: About Food Portions," Weight-Control Information Network, National Institute of Diabetes and Digestive Diseases (win.niddk.nih.gov), June 2009.

Portion Distortion and Serving Size

Portions and Servings: What's the Difference?

A portion is the amount of food that you choose to eat for a meal or snack. It can be big or small—you decide.

A serving is a measured amount of food or drink, such as one slice of bread or one cup (eight ounces) of milk.

Many foods that come as a single portion actually contain multiple servings. The Nutrition Facts label on packaged foods—on the backs of cans, sides of boxes, etc.—tells you the number of servings in the container.

For example, look at the label of a 20-ounce soda (typically consumed as one portion), and you'll see that it has 2.5 servings in it. A 3-ounce bag of chips—which some would consider a single portion—contains 3 servings.

Portion Distortion

Average portion sizes have grown so much over the past 20 years that sometimes the plate arrives and there's enough food for two or even three people on it. These growing portion sizes are changing what Americans think of as a "normal" portion at home, too. We call it portion distortion. Growing portions lead to increased calories.

For more eye-opening examples, check out the National Heart, Lung, and Blood Institute (NHLBI's) Portion Distortion website (hp2010 .nhlbihin.net/portion/index.htm).

Table 2.1. Comparison of Portions and Calories 20 Years Ago to Present Day

	20 Years Ago		Today	
	Portion	**Calories**	**Portion**	**Calories**
Bagel	3" diameter	140	6" diameter	350
Cheeseburger	1	333	1	590
Spaghetti w/ meatballs	1 cup sauce, 3 small meatballs	500	2 cups sauce, 3 large meatballs	1,020
Soda	6.5 oz	82	20 oz	250
Blueberry muffin	1.5 oz	210	5 oz	500

Just Enough for You: About Food Portions

How do I know how big my portions are?

The portion size that you are used to eating may be equal to two or three standard servings. Take a look at the Nutrition Facts for macaroni and cheese. The serving size is one cup, but the package actually has two cups of this food product. If you eat the entire package, you are eating two servings of macaroni and cheese—and double the calories, fat, and other nutrients in a standard serving.

To see how many servings a package has, check the "servings per container" listed on its Nutrition Facts. You may be surprised to find that small containers often have more than one serving inside.

Learning to recognize standard serving sizes can help you judge how much you are eating. When cooking at home, look at the serving sizes listed on the Nutrition Facts for the packaged food products you eat. Use measuring cups and spoons to put the suggested serving size on your plate before you start eating. This will help you see what one standard serving of that food looks like compared to how much you normally eat.

It may also help to compare serving sizes to everyday objects. For example, 1/4 cup of raisins is about the size of a large egg. Three ounces of meat or poultry is about the size of a deck of cards. See other serving size comparisons in the following. (Keep in mind that these size comparisons are approximations.)

- 1 cup of cereal = a fist
- 1/2 cup of cooked rice, pasta, or potato = 1/2 baseball

15

- 1 baked potato = a fist
- 1 medium fruit = a baseball
- 1/2 cup of fresh fruit = 1/2 baseball
- 1 1/2 ounces of low-fat or fat-free cheese = 4 stacked dice
- 1/2 cup of ice cream = 1/2 baseball
- 2 tablespoons of peanut butter = a ping-pong ball

How can I control portions at home?

You do not need to measure and count everything you eat for the rest of your life—just do this long enough to recognize typical serving sizes. Try the ideas listed here to help you control portions at home.

- Take the amount of food that is equal to one serving, according to the Nutrition Facts, and eat it off a plate instead of eating straight out of a large box or bag.

- Avoid eating in front of the TV or while busy with other activities. Pay attention to what you are eating, chew your food well, and fully enjoy the smell and taste of your foods.

- Eat slowly so your brain can get the message that your stomach is full.

- Try using smaller dishes, bowls, and glasses. This way, when you fill up your plate or glass, you will be eating and drinking less.

- To control your intake of the higher-fat, higher-calorie parts of a meal, take seconds of vegetables and salads (watch the toppings) instead of desserts and dishes with heavy sauces.

- When cooking in large batches, freeze food that you will not serve right away. This way, you will not be tempted to finish eating the whole batch before the food goes bad. And you will have ready-made food for another day. Freeze leftovers in amounts that you can use for a single serving or for a family meal another day.

- Try to eat meals at regular intervals. Skipping meals or leaving large gaps of time between meals may lead you to eat larger amounts of food the next time that you eat.

- When buying snacks, go for single-serving prepackaged items and foods that are lower-calorie options. If you buy larger bags or boxes of snacks, divide the items into single-serve packages.

- Make snacks count. Eating many high-calorie snacks throughout the day may lead to weight gain. Replace snacks like chips and soda with snacks such as low-fat or fat-free yogurt, smoothies, fruit, or whole-grain crackers.

- When you do have a treat like chips or ice cream, measure out 1/2 cup of ice cream or one ounce of chips, as indicated by the Nutrition Facts, eat it slowly, and enjoy it!

Is getting more food for your money always a good value?

Have you noticed that it only costs a few cents more to get larger sizes of fries or soft drinks at restaurants? Getting a larger portion of food for just a little extra money may seem like a good value, but you end up with more food and calories than you need.

Before you buy your next "value combo," be sure you are making the best choice for your wallet and your health. If you are with someone else, share the large-size meal. If you are eating alone, skip the special deal and just order what you need.

How can I control portions when eating out?

Research shows that the more often a person eats out, the more body fat he or she has. Try to prepare more meals at home. Eat out and get take-out foods less often. When you do eat away from home, try these tips to help you control portions:

- Share your meal, order a half-portion, or order an appetizer as a main meal. Examples of healthier appetizers include tuna or chicken salad, minestrone soup, and tomato or corn salsas.

- Take at least half of your meal home. Ask for a portion of your meal to be boxed up when it is served so you will not be tempted to eat more than you need.

- Stop eating when you begin to feel full. Focus on enjoying the setting and your friends or family for the rest of the meal.

- Avoid large beverages such as "supersize" sugar-sweetened soft drinks. They have a large number of calories. Instead, try drinking water with a slice of lemon. If you want to drink soda, choose a calorie-free beverage or a small sugar-sweetened soft drink.

- When traveling, pack a small cooler of foods that are hard to find on the road, such as fresh fruit, sliced raw vegetables, and fat-free or low-fat yogurt. Also, pack a few bottles of water instead of sugar-sweetened soda or juice. You can also bring dried fruit, nuts, and seeds to snack on. Since these foods can be high in calories, measure and pack small portions (1/4 cup) in advance. If you stop at a restaurant, try to choose one that serves a variety of foods such as salads, grilled or steamed entrees, or a plain baked potato. Consider drinking water or low-fat or fat-free milk instead of sugar-sweetened soft drinks with your meal. If you choose a higher-fat option like french fries or pizza, order the small size, or ask for a single slice of pizza with vegetable toppings such as mushrooms, peppers, or olives.

How can I control portions when money is tight?

Eating well does not have to cost a lot of money. Here are some ways you can keep track of your portions without adding extra costs to your grocery bill.

- Buy meats in bulk. When you get home, divide the meats into single-serving packages and freeze for later use.

- Buy fruits and vegetables when they are in season. Buy only as much as you will use, so they will not go bad. Check out your local farmers market, as it may be less expensive than a grocery store.

- Watch your portion sizes. Try to stick to the serving sizes listed on the Nutrition Facts label of prepackaged foods. Doing so can help you get the most out of the money you spend on that food. In addition, you can better control the fat and calories you eat.

Remember ... The amount of calories you eat affects your weight and health. In addition to selecting a healthy variety of foods, look at the size of the portions you eat. Choosing nutritious foods and keeping portion sizes sensible may help you reach and stay at a healthy weight.

Section 2.2

Food Servings and Food Exchange Lists

"Food Exchange Lists," National Heart, Lung, and Blood
Institute (www.nhlbi.nih.gov), August 2005. Reviewed by
David A. Cooke, MD, FACP, January 2011.

You can use the American Dietetic Association food exchange lists
to check out serving sizes for each group of foods and to see what other
food choices are available for each group of foods.

Vegetables contain 25 calories and 5 grams of carbohydrate. One
serving equals the following:

- 1/2 cup cooked vegetables (carrots, broccoli, zucchini, cabbage, etc.)
- 1 cup raw vegetables or salad greens
- 1/2 cup vegetable juice

If you're hungry, eat more fresh or steamed vegetables.

Fat-free and very low-fat milk contain 90 calories per serving.
One serving equals the following:

- 1 cup milk, fat-free or 1% fat
- 3/4 cup yogurt, plain nonfat or low-fat
- 1 cup yogurt, artificially sweetened

Very lean protein choices have 35 calories and 1 gram of fat per
serving. One serving equals the following:

- 1 oz turkey breast or chicken breast, skin removed
- 1 oz fish fillet (flounder, sole, scrod, cod, etc.)
- 1 oz canned tuna in water
- 1 oz shellfish (clams, lobster, scallops, shrimp)
- 3/4 cup cottage cheese, nonfat or low-fat
- 2 egg whites

- 1/4 cup egg substitute
- 1 oz fat-free cheese
- 1/2 cup beans, cooked (black beans, kidney beans, chickpeas, or lentils): count as one starch/bread and one very lean protein

Fruits contain 15 grams of carbohydrate and 60 calories. One serving equals the following:

- 1 small apple, banana, orange, nectarine
- 1 med. fresh peach
- 1 kiwi
- 1/2 grapefruit
- 1/2 mango
- 1 cup fresh berries (strawberries, raspberries, or blueberries)
- 1 cup fresh melon cubes
- 1/8 honeydew melon
- 4 oz unsweetened juice
- 4 tsp jelly or jam

Lean protein choices have 55 calories and 2–3 grams of fat per serving. One serving equals the following:

- 1 oz chicken—dark meat, skin removed
- 1 oz turkey—dark meat, skin removed
- 1 oz salmon, swordfish, herring
- 1 oz lean beef (flank steak, London broil, tenderloin, roast beef)*
- 1 oz veal, roast or lean chop*
- 1 oz lamb, roast or lean chop*
- 1 oz pork, tenderloin or fresh ham*
- 1 oz low-fat cheese (with 3 g or less of fat per ounce)
- 1 oz low-fat luncheon meats (with 3 g or less of fat per ounce)
- 1/4 cup 4.5% cottage cheese
- 2 med. sardines

* Limit to 1–2 times per week.

Medium-fat proteins have 75 calories and 5 grams of fat per serving. One serving equals the following:

- 1 oz beef (any prime cut), corned beef, ground beef**
- 1 oz pork chop
- 1 whole egg (medium)**
- 1 oz mozzarella cheese
- 1/4 cup ricotta cheese
- 4 oz tofu (this is a heart-healthy choice)

** Choose these very infrequently.

Starches contain 15 grams of carbohydrate and 80 calories per serving. One serving equals the following:

- 1 slice bread (white, pumpernickel, whole wheat, rye)
- 2 slices reduced-calorie or "lite" bread
- 1/4 (1 oz) bagel (varies)
- 1/2 English muffin
- 1/2 hamburger bun
- 3/4 cup cold cereal
- 1/3 cup rice, brown or white, cooked
- 1/3 cup barley or couscous, cooked
- 1/3 cup legumes (dried beans, peas, or lentils), cooked
- 1/2 cup pasta, cooked
- 1/2 cup bulgur, cooked
- 1/2 cup corn, sweet potato, or green peas
- 3 oz baked sweet or white potato
- 3/4 oz pretzels
- 3 cup popcorn, hot air popped or microwave (80% light)

Fats contain 45 calories and 5 grams of fat per serving. One serving equals the following:

- 1 tsp oil (vegetable, corn, canola, olive, etc.)
- 1 tsp butter
- 1 tsp stick margarine

- 1 tsp mayonnaise
- 1 Tbsp reduced-fat margarine or mayonnaise
- 1 Tbsp salad dressing
- 1 Tbsp cream cheese
- 2 Tbsp lite cream cheese
- 1/8 avocado
- 8 large black olives
- 10 large stuffed green olives
- 1 slice bacon

Source: Based on American Dietetic Association Exchange Lists.

Section 2.3

Calories and Energy Balance

"Balance Food and Activity," National Heart, Lung, and Blood
Institute (www.nhlbi.nih.gov), 2010.

What Is Energy Balance?

Energy is another word for "calories." Your energy balance is the balance of calories consumed through eating and drinking compared to calories burned through physical activity. What you eat and drink is ENERGY IN. What you burn through physical activity is ENERGY OUT.

You burn a certain number of calories just by breathing air and digesting food. You also burn a certain number of calories (ENERGY OUT) through your daily routine. For example, children burn calories just being students—walking to their lockers, carrying books, etc.—and adults burn calories walking to the bus stop, going shopping, etc.

An important part of maintaining energy balance is the amount of ENERGY OUT (physical activity) that you do. People who are more physically active burn more calories than those who are not as physically active.

- The same amount of ENERGY IN (calories consumed) and EN-ERGY OUT (calories burned) over time = weight stays the same

- More IN than OUT over time = weight gain

- More OUT than IN over time = weight loss

Your ENERGY IN and OUT don't have to balance every day. It's having a balance over time that will help you stay at a healthy weight for the long term. Children need to balance their energy, too, but they're also growing and that should be considered as well. Energy balance in children happens when the amount of ENERGY IN and ENERGY OUT supports natural growth without promoting excess weight gain.

Estimated Calorie Requirements

The calorie requirement chart in Table 2.2 presents estimated amounts of calories needed to maintain energy balance (and a healthy body weight) for various gender and age groups at three different levels of physical activity. The estimates are rounded to the nearest 200 calories and were determined using an equation from the Institute of Medicine (IOM).

- These levels are based on Estimated Energy Requirements (EER) from the IOM Dietary Reference Intakes macronutrients report, 2002, calculated by gender, age, and activity level for reference-sized individuals. "Reference size," as determined by IOM, is based on median height and weight for ages up to age 18 years of age and median height and weight for that height to give a BMI of 21.5 for adult females and 22.5 for adult males.

- Sedentary means a lifestyle that includes only the light physical activity associated with typical day-to-day life.

- Moderately active means a lifestyle that includes physical activity equivalent to walking about 1.5 to 3 miles per day at three to four miles per hour, in addition to the light physical activity associated with typical day-to-day life.

- Active means a lifestyle that includes physical activity equivalent to walking more than 3 miles per day at three to four miles per hour, in addition to the light physical activity associated with typical day-to-day life.

- The calorie ranges shown are to accommodate needs of different ages within the group. For children and adolescents, more calories are needed at older ages. For adults, fewer calories are needed at older ages.

Table 2.2. Estimated Calorie Requirements (in Kilocalories) for Each Gender and Age Group at Three Levels of Physical Activity

			Activity Level	
Gender	**Age (years)**	Sedentary	Moderately Active	Active
Child	2–3	1,000	1,000–1,400	1,000–1,400
Female	4–8	1,200	1,400–1,600	1,400–1,800
Female	9–13	1,600	1,600–2,000	1,800–2,000
Female	14–18	1,800	2,000	2,400
Female	19–30	2,000	2,000–2,200	2,400
Female	31–50	1,800	2,000	2,200
Female	51+	1,600	1,800	2,000–2,200
Male	4–8	1,400	1,400–1,600	1,600–2,000
Male	9–13	1,800	1,800–2,200	2,000–2,600
Male	14–18	2,200	2,400–2,800	2,800–3,200
Male	19–30	2,400	2,600–2,800	3,000
Male	31–50	2,200	2,400–2,600	2,800–3,000
Male	51+	2,000	2,200–2,400	2,400–2,800

Source: HHS/USDA Dietary Guidelines for Americans, 2005

Energy Balance in Real Life

Think of it as balancing your "lifestyle budget." For example, if you know you and your family will be going to a party and may eat more high-calorie foods than normal, then you may wish to eat fewer calories for a few days before so that it balances out. Or, you can increase your physical activity level for the few days before or after the party so you can burn off the extra energy.

The same applies to your kids. If they'll be going to a birthday party and eating cake and ice cream—or other foods high in fat and added sugar—help them balance their calories the day before and/or after by providing ways for them to be more physically active.

Here's another way of looking at energy balance in real life. Eating just 150 calories more a day than you burn can lead to an extra 5 pounds over six months. That's a gain of 10 pounds a year. If you don't want this weight gain to happen, or you want to lose the extra weight, you can either reduce your ENERGY IN or increase your ENERGY OUT. Doing both is the best way to achieve and maintain a healthy body weight.

Here are some ways to cut 150 calories (ENERGY IN):

- Drink water instead of a 12-ounce regular soda.

- Order a small serving of french fries instead of a medium, or order a salad with dressing on the side instead.

- Eat an egg-white omelet (with three eggs), instead of whole eggs.

- Use tuna canned in water (6-ounce can), instead of oil.

Here are some ways to burn 150 calories (ENERGY OUT) in just 30 minutes (for a 150-pound person):

- Shoot hoops.

- Walk two miles.

- Do yard work (gardening, raking leaves, etc.).

- Go for a bike ride.

- Dance with your family or friends.

Chapter 3

The Health Benefits of Eating Breakfast

Research shows that many of us believe that it's the most important meal of the day—and there is plenty of science to support it. Still, more than half of us do not eat breakfast every day. Learn about the long-standing and latest reasons to enjoy the morning meal.

Breakfast Fuels Your Empty Tank

Do you bypass breakfast to save time in the morning? This tactic often backfires, because running on empty can leave you feeling fatigued and out-of-sorts—not on top of your game like you need to be. So, stoke your energy engine! Break for breakfast—it takes just a few minutes to fuel up.

Your kids are more likely to eat breakfast if you do, too. Eating breakfast together is even a better bonus—it helps instill more healthful eating habits in kids as they grow up.

Breakfast Boosts Brain Power

How totally cool that breakfast fuels kids' brains for school! Several studies suggest that eating breakfast may help children do better in school by improving memory, alertness, concentration, problem-solving ability, test scores, school attendance, and mood. Adult breakfast skippers, take a lesson—eating breakfast may help boost your brain power, too.

"Wake Up to the Benefits of Breakfast," © 2009 International Food Information Council (www.foodinsight.org). Reprinted with permission.

Breakfast Is Just Plain Good for You

Breakfast-eating kids and adults get more fiber, calcium, vitamins A and C, riboflavin, zinc, and iron in their diets than breakfast skippers. It's no wonder when you consider that nutrient-rich foods such as whole-grain hot and ready-to-eat cereals, fat-free and low-fat milk and yogurt, and fruit and 100% fruit juice are popular breakfast picks.

Breakfast Is the "Weigh" to Go

The first meal of the day can help keep weight gain away, so don't skip breakfast to manage your weight. Research suggests that adult breakfast skippers are at greater risk for obesity and weight gain, while breakfast eaters tend to have healthier weights. Kids and teens who eat breakfast are less likely to be overweight, too. And, according to findings from the National Weight Control Registry, almost 8 in 10 adults who maintain a 30-plus pound weight loss for at least a year eat breakfast every day.

Why the breakfast benefit? Research shows a link between healthier body weights and eating foods such as hot and ready-to-eat cereal and fat-free or low-fat milk and milk products. Breakfast foods like oatmeal and high-protein milk products and eggs also may help you feel full.

Breakfast Builds Better Bodies

Eating breakfast may help your heart, digestion, bones, and more to meet dietary guidelines!

- **A healthier heart:** Adults and kids who skip breakfast tend to have higher blood cholesterol levels—a risk factor for heart disease—than do breakfast eaters. Why? Breakfast-eating adults tend to get less fat and more fiber in their diets. Kids and teens who eat breakfast get more fiber, too.

Common breakfast foods may promote heart health. For instance, the soluble fiber in oatmeal may help reduce cholesterol and the whole grains and fiber in some cereals and breads may help reduce heart disease risk. Morning foods like fat-free or low-fat milk and yogurt, fruit, 100% fruit juices, and whole-grain cereals can be part of an eating plan that helps control blood pressure and reduce LDL (bad [low-density lipoprotein]) cholesterol levels.

- **Better digestion:** The insoluble fiber in many breakfast cereals and in other breakfast foods like whole-wheat breads, bagels, and English muffins and fruits may help keep you regular. Some research suggests that fiber may reduce the risk of colon cancer. "Friendly" bacteria that may promote digestive health and the components that help them thrive are found in some yogurts, yogurt drinks, and cereals.

- **Stronger bones:** A wholesome breakfast serves up nutrients important for healthy bones. For instance, milk—the most commonly consumed breakfast food—provides calcium, vitamin D, and protein to name a few. Adults, teens, and kids who regularly eat breakfast consume more calcium and other nutrients each day. And people who start the day with the traditional cereal and milk combo get seven times more calcium at breakfast than those who eat cereal without milk.

- **Improved metabolism:** Newer, emerging research suggests that eating a nutritious breakfast of whole-grain cereal and milk may help the body better regulate insulin levels. Studies also suggest that popular breakfast foods such as whole-grain cereals and breads, milk products, and fruit may help reduce risk for metabolic syndrome. This condition is linked to being overweight and increases the risk for heart disease and type 2 diabetes.

Invest Time to Save Time

Invest in a little planning time to gain the big benefits of breakfast.

- Sit down with the family to plan nutritious breakfasts for the week. Post the plan in plain sight in the kitchen. Getting kids involved encourages them to eat the morning meal.

- Add breakfast items to your shopping list so your kitchen is well stocked.

- Each evening, set the table for breakfast and put out nonperishables such as cereal boxes, oatmeal containers, whole-grain bread, peanut butter, and fruit.

- Store milk, yogurt, hard-cooked eggs, 100% fruit juice, and other perishable breakfast foods in the front of the fridge so they're quick to grab.

- If the family is brown-bagging breakfast, pack and label each person's bag the night before and store them in the fridge. Better yet, get everyone to assemble their own breakfast bag.

- On weekends, take time for a fun and healthful family breakfast to share the details of your busy week.

Chapter 4

Food Labels

Chapter Contents

Section 4.1

How to Use Nutrition Labels

"A Key to Choosing Healthful Foods: Using the Nutrition
Facts on the Food Label," Food and Drug Administration
(www.fda.gov), January 27, 2011.

Have you ever read the Nutrition Facts label on food packages and
wondered: serving sizes, percentages, daily values—what do they all
mean? Well, you're not alone. Many consumers would like to know how
to use the Nutrition Facts label more easily and effectively. Use this
information to make quick, informed food choices that contribute to
healthy lifelong eating habits for you and your family.

Product Info and "Daily Values"

The Nutrition Facts label is divided into two main areas:

- Sections 1–5 provide product-specific information (serving size,
  calories, and nutrient information). These vary with each food
  product.

- Section 6 is a footnote with Daily Values (DVs). The footnote provides information about the DVs for important nutrients, including fats, sodium, and fiber. The DVs are listed for people who eat
  2,000 or 2,500 calories each day.

  - The amounts for total fat, saturated fat, cholesterol, and so-
    dium are maximum amounts. That means you should try to
    stay below the amounts listed.

  - The DVs for total carbohydrate and dietary fiber daily repre-
    sent the minimum amounts recommended for a 2,000-calorie
    diet. This means you should consume at least this amount
    per day for each of these nutrients.

  - The footnote is only found on larger labels and does not
    change from product to product.

Details on the Daily Value: Three Easy Ways to Use the % Daily Value

1. Look at highs and lows.

The %DV gives you a framework for deciding if a food is high or low in a nutrient. Use this quick guide to %DV: 5% or less is low, and 20% or more is high.

Compare products. Use the %DV to compare one food product or brand to a similar product. Make sure the servings sizes are similar, especially the weight (e.g., gram, milligram, ounces) of each product so you can see which foods are higher or lower in nutrients.

2. Evaluate claims.

So you don't have to memorize definitions, use the %DV to help you quickly distinguish one claim from another, such as "reduced fat" vs. "light" or "nonfat." Just compare the %DVs for Total Fat in each food product to see which one is higher or lower in that nutrient. There is no need to memorize definitions. This works when comparing all nutrient content claims—e.g., less, light, low, free, more, high, etc.

3. Make dietary trade-offs.

Make dietary trade-offs using the %DV. For example, when a food you like is high in saturated fat, select foods that are low in saturated fat at other times of the day.

What's on the Label?

The Nutrition Label is divided into six sections.

1. Serving Size

This section is the basis for determining number of calories, amount of each nutrient, and %DVs of a food. Use it to compare a serving size to how much you actually eat. Serving sizes are given in familiar units, such as cups or pieces, followed by the metric amount—e.g., number of grams.

2. Amount of Calories

If you want to manage your weight (lose, gain, or maintain), this section is especially helpful. The amount of calories is listed on the left side. The right side shows how many calories in one serving come from fat. The key is to balance how many calories you eat with how many calories your body uses. Tip: Remember that a product that's fat free isn't necessarily calorie free.

3. Nutrients to Limit

Eating too much total fat (including saturated fat and trans fat), cholesterol, or sodium may increase your risk of certain chronic diseases, such as heart disease, some cancers, or high blood pressure. The goal is to stay below 100%DV for each of these nutrients per day.

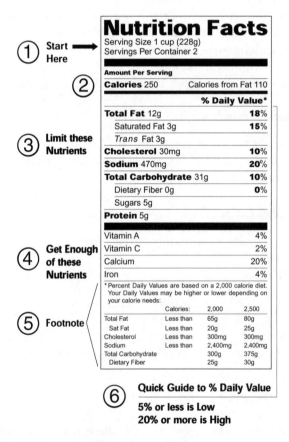

Figure 4.1. Nutrition Facts label

34

4. Nutrients to Emphasize

Americans often don't get enough dietary fiber, vitamin A, vitamin C, calcium, and iron in their diets. Eating enough of these nutrients may improve your health and help reduce the risk of some diseases and conditions.

5. Percent (%) Daily Value

This section tells you whether the nutrients (total fat, sodium, dietary fiber, etc.) in one serving of food contribute a little or a lot to your total daily diet.

The %DVs are based on a 2,000-calorie diet. Each listed nutrient is based on 100% of the recommended amounts for that nutrient. For example, 18% for total fat means that one serving furnishes 18% of the total amount of fat that you could eat in a day and stay within public health recommendations.

6. Footnote with %DVs

The footnote provides information about the DVs for important nutrients, including fats, sodium, and fiber. The DVs are listed for people who eat 2,000 or 2,500 calories each day.

The amounts for total fat, saturated fat, cholesterol, and sodium are maximum amounts. That means you should try to stay below the amounts listed.

Section 4.2

Understanding Claims on Food Labels

This section excerpted from "Food Label Helps Consumers Make Healthier Choices," Food and Drug Administration (www.fda.gov), March 27, 2008, and "Food Labels and More," National Women's Health Information Center, Department of Health and Human Services (www.womenshealth.gov), June 17, 2008.

Food Label Helps Consumers Make Healthier Choices

Consumers often compare prices of food items in the grocery store to choose the best value for their money. But comparing items using the food label can help them choose the best value for their health.

For example, someone with high blood pressure who needs to watch salt (sodium) intake may be faced with five different types of tomato soup on the shelf. You can quickly and easily compare the sodium content of each product by looking at the part of the label that lists nutrition information (Nutrition Facts label) to choose the one with the lowest sodium content.

Food and Drug Administration (FDA) regulations require nutrition information to appear on most foods, and any claims on food products must be truthful and not misleading. In addition, "low sodium," "reduced fat," and "high fiber" must meet strict government definitions. FDA has defined other terms used to describe the content of a nutrient, such as "low," "reduced," "high," "free," "lean," "extra lean," "good source," "less," "light," and "more." So a consumer who wants to reduce sodium intake can be assured that the manufacturer of a product claiming to be "low sodium" or "reduced in sodium" has met these definitions.

But you don't have to memorize the definitions. Just look at the Nutrition Facts label to compare the claims of different products with similar serving sizes.

The terms "natural," "healthy," and "organic" often cause confusion. "Consumers seem to think that 'natural' and 'organic' imply 'healthy,'" says Barbara Schneeman, PhD, director of the FDA's Office of Nutrition, Labeling, and Dietary Supplements. "But these terms have different meanings from a regulatory point of view."

According to FDA policy, "natural" means the product does not contain synthetic or artificial ingredients. "Healthy," which is defined by regulation, means the product must meet certain criteria that limit the amounts of fat, saturated fat, cholesterol, and sodium and require specific minimum amounts of vitamins, minerals, or other beneficial nutrients.

Food labeled "organic" must meet the standards set by the Department of Agriculture (USDA). Organic food differs from conventionally produced food in the way it is grown or produced. But USDA makes no claims that organically produced food is safer or more nutritious than conventionally produced food.

For example, says Schneeman, "A premium ice cream could be 'natural' or 'organic' and still be high in fat or saturated fat so would not meet the criteria for 'healthy.' "

Food Labels and More: Other Labels on Foods You Eat

Some foods have labels such as "fat free," "reduced calorie," or "light." The following are some useful definitions for you.

Calorie Terms

- Low calorie: 40 calories or less per serving

- Reduced calorie: At least 25% fewer calories per serving when compared with a similar food

- Light or lite: One-third fewer calories; if more than half the calories are from fat, fat content must be reduced by 50% or more

Sugar Terms

- Sugar free: Less than 1/2 gram sugar per serving

- Reduced sugar: At least 25% less sugar per serving when compared with a similar food

Fat Terms

- Fat free or 100% fat free: Less than 1/2 gram fat per serving

- Low fat: 3 grams or less per serving

- Reduced fat: At least 25% less fat when compared with a similar food

It's important to remember that fat free doesn't mean calorie free. People tend to think they can eat as much as they want of fat-free foods.

Even if you cut fat from your diet but consume more calories than you use, you will gain weight. Also, fat-free or low-fat foods may contain high amounts of added sugars or sodium to make up for the loss of flavor when fat is removed. For example, a fat-free muffin may be just as high in calories as a regular muffin. So, remember, it is important to read your food labels and compare products.

Chapter 5

Healthy Use of Dietary Supplements

Chapter Contents

Section 5.1

Information about Dietary Supplements

This section excerpted from "Using Dietary Supplements Wisely," National Center for Complementary and Alternative Medicine (nccam.nih.gov), March 2010, and "Dietary Supplements: Background Information," Office of Dietary Supplements (ods.od.nih.gov), July 9, 2009.

Using Dietary Supplements Wisely

Many people take dietary supplements, products that contains vitamins, minerals, herbs or other botanicals, amino acids, enzymes, and/or other ingredients intended to supplement the diet, in an effort to be well and stay healthy. With so many dietary supplements available and so many claims made about their health benefits, how can a consumer decide what's safe and effective?

About Dietary Supplements

Dietary supplements were defined in a law passed by Congress in 1994 called the Dietary Supplement Health and Education Act (DSHEA). According to DSHEA, a dietary supplement is a product with the following characteristics:

- Is intended to supplement the diet

- Contains one or more dietary ingredients (including vitamins, minerals, herbs or other botanicals, amino acids, and certain other substances) or their constituents

- Is intended to be taken by mouth, in forms such as tablet, capsule, powder, softgel, gelcap, or liquid

- Is labeled as being a dietary supplement

Herbal supplements are one type of dietary supplement. An herb is a plant or plant part (such as leaves, flowers, or seeds) that is used for its flavor, scent, and/or therapeutic properties. "Botanical" is often used as a synonym for "herb." An herbal supplement may contain a single herb or mixtures of herbs.

Research has shown that some uses of dietary supplements are effective in preventing or treating diseases. For example, scientists have found that folic acid (a vitamin) prevents certain birth defects, and a regimen of vitamins and zinc can slow the progression of the age-related eye disease macular degeneration. Also, calcium and vitamin D supplements can be helpful in preventing and treating bone loss and osteoporosis (thinning of bone tissue).

Research has also produced some promising results suggesting that other dietary supplements may be helpful for other health conditions (e.g., omega-3 fatty acids for coronary disease), but in most cases, additional research is needed before firm conclusions can be drawn.

Dietary Supplement Use in the United States

A national survey conducted in 2007 found that 17.7% of American adults had used "natural products" (i.e., dietary supplements other than vitamins and minerals) in the past 12 months. The most popular products used by adults for health reasons in the past 30 days were fish oil/omega 3/DHA (37.4%); glucosamine, a substance found in the fluid around joints and used by the body to make and repair cartilage (19.9%); echinacea (19.8%); flaxseed oil or pills (15.9%); and ginseng (14.1%). In another earlier national survey covering all types of dietary supplements, approximately 52% of adult respondents said they had used some type of supplement in the last 30 days; the most commonly reported were multivitamins/multiminerals (35%), vitamins E and C (12–13%), calcium (10%), and B-complex vitamins (5%).

Federal Regulation of Dietary Supplements

The federal government regulates dietary supplements through the U.S. Food and Drug Administration (FDA). The regulations for dietary supplements are not the same as those for prescription or over-the-counter drugs. In general, the regulations for dietary supplements are less strict.

- A manufacturer does not have to prove the safety and effectiveness of a dietary supplement before it is marketed. A manufacturer is permitted to say that a dietary supplement addresses a nutrient deficiency, supports health, or is linked to a particular body function (e.g., immunity) if there is research to support the claim. Such a claim must be followed by the words "This statement has not been evaluated by the U.S. Food and Drug Administration (FDA). This product is not intended to diagnose, treat, cure, or prevent any disease."

- Manufacturers are expected to follow certain "good manufacturing practices" (GMPs) to ensure that dietary supplements are processed consistently and meet quality standards. Requirements for GMPs went into effect in 2008 for large manufacturers and are being phased in for small manufacturers through 2010.

- Once a dietary supplement is on the market, the FDA monitors safety. If it finds a product to be unsafe, it can take action against the manufacturer and/or distributor and may issue a warning or require that the product be removed from the marketplace.

Also, once a dietary supplement is on the market, the FDA monitors product information, such as label claims and package inserts. The Federal Trade Commission (FTC) is responsible for regulating product advertising; it requires that all information be truthful and not misleading.

The federal government has taken legal action against a number of dietary supplement promoters or websites that promote or sell dietary supplements because they have made false or deceptive statements about their products or because marketed products have proven to be unsafe.

Sources of Science-Based Information for Dietary Supplements

It's important to look for reliable sources of information on dietary supplements so you can evaluate the claims that are made about them. The most reliable information on dietary supplements is based on the results of rigorous scientific testing.

Follow these methods to get reliable information on a particular dietary supplement:

- Ask your health care providers. Even if they do not know about a specific dietary supplement, they may be able to access the latest medical guidance about its uses and risks.

- Look for scientific research findings on the dietary supplement. The National Center for Complementary and Alternative Medicine (NCCAM) and the National Institutes of Health (NIH) Office of Dietary Supplements (ODS), as well as other federal agencies, have free publications, clearinghouses, and information on their websites.

Safety Considerations of Dietary Supplements

If you are thinking about or are using a dietary supplement, here are some points to keep in mind.

Tell your health care providers about any complementary and alternative practices you use, including dietary supplements. Give them a full picture of what you do to manage your health. This will help ensure coordinated and safe care. (For tips about talking with your health care providers about complementary and alternative medicine, see NCCAM's Time to Talk campaign at nccam.nih.gov/timetotalk.) It is especially important to talk to your health care provider if you are considering the following:

- Thinking about replacing your regular medication with one or more dietary supplements

- Taking any medications (whether prescription or over-the-counter), as some dietary supplements have been found to interact with medications

- Planning to have surgery; certain dietary supplements may increase the risk of bleeding or affect the response to anesthesia

- Pregnant or nursing a baby, or are considering giving a child a dietary supplement; most dietary supplements have not been tested in pregnant women, nursing mothers, or children

If you are taking a dietary supplement, read the label instructions. Talk to your health care provider if you have any questions, particularly about the best dosage for you to take. If you experience any side effects that concern you, stop taking the dietary supplement and contact your health care provider. You can also report your experience to the FDA's MedWatch program. Consumer safety reports on dietary supplements are an important source of information for the FDA.

Keep in mind that although many dietary supplements (and some prescription drugs) come from natural sources, "natural" does not always mean "safe." For example, the herbs comfrey and kava can cause serious harm to the liver. Also, a manufacturer's use of the term "standardized" (or "verified" or "certified") does not necessarily guarantee product quality or consistency.

Be aware that an herbal supplement may contain dozens of compounds and that its active ingredients may not be known. Researchers are studying many of these products in an effort to identify active ingredients and understand their effects in the body. Also consider the possibility that what's on the label may not be what's in the bottle. Analyses of dietary supplements sometimes find differences between labeled and actual ingredients.

- An herbal supplement may not contain the correct plant species.

- The amount of the active ingredient may be lower or higher than the label states. That means you may be taking less—or more—of the dietary supplement than you realize.

- The dietary supplement may be contaminated with other herbs, pesticides, or metals or even adulterated with unlabeled ingredients such as prescription drugs.

For current information from the federal government on the safety of particular dietary supplements, check the "Dietary Supplement and Safety Information" section of the FDA website at www.fda.gov/Food/DietarySupplements/Alerts/ or the "Alerts and Advisories" section of the NCCAM website at nccam.nih.gov/news/alerts.

Dietary Supplement Background Information

What claims can manufacturers make for dietary supplements and drugs?

The types of claims that can be made on the labels of dietary supplements and drugs differ. Drug manufacturers may claim that their product will diagnose, cure, mitigate, treat, or prevent a disease. Such claims may not legally be made for dietary supplements.

The label of a dietary supplement or food product may contain one of three types of claims: a health claim, nutrient content claim, or structure/function claim. Health claims describe a relationship between a food, food component, or dietary supplement ingredient and reducing risk of a disease or health-related condition. Nutrient content claims describe the relative amount of a nutrient or dietary substance in a product. A structure/function claim is a statement describing how a product may affect the organs or systems of the body, and it cannot mention any specific disease. Structure/function claims do not require FDA approval, but the manufacturer must provide FDA with the text of the claim within 30 days of putting the product on the market. Product labels containing such claims must also include a disclaimer that reads, "This statement has not been evaluated by the FDA. This product is not intended to diagnose, treat, cure, or prevent any disease."

What information is required on a dietary supplement label?

FDA requires that certain information appear on the dietary supplement label:

General Information

- Name of product (including the word "supplement" or a statement that the product is a supplement)
- Net quantity of contents
- Name and place of business of manufacturer, packer, or distributor
- Directions for use

Supplement Facts Panel

- Serving size, list of dietary ingredients, amount per serving size (by weight), percent of Daily Value (%DV), if established
- If the dietary ingredient is a botanical, the scientific name of the plant or the common or usual name standardized in the reference *Herbs of Commerce, 2nd Edition* (2000 edition) and the name of the plant part used
- If the dietary ingredient is a proprietary blend (i.e., a blend exclusive to the manufacturer), the total weight of the blend and the components of the blend in order of predominance by weight

Other Ingredients

- Nondietary ingredients such as fillers, artificial colors, sweeteners, flavors, or binders; listed by weight in descending order of predominance and by common name or proprietary blend

The label of the supplement may contain a cautionary statement, but the lack of a cautionary statement does not mean that no adverse effects are associated with the product.

Are dietary supplements standardized?

Standardization is a process that manufacturers may use to ensure batch-to-batch consistency of their products. In some cases, standardization involves identifying specific chemicals (known as markers) that can be used to manufacture a consistent product. The standardization process can also provide a measure of quality control.

Dietary supplements are not required to be standardized in the United States. In fact, no legal or regulatory definition exists in the United States for standardization as it applies to dietary supplements. Because of this, the term "standardization" may mean many different things. Some manufacturers use the term "standardization" incorrectly to refer to uniform manufacturing practices; following a recipe is not sufficient for a product to be called standardized. Therefore, the presence of the word "standardized" on a supplement label does not necessarily indicate product quality.

Section 5.2

Safety Tips for Dietary Supplement Users

This section excerpted from "Tips for Older Dietary Supplement Users," Food and Drug Administration (www.fda.gov), May 7, 2009.

Even if you eat a wide variety of foods, how can you be sure that you are getting all the vitamins, minerals, and other nutrients you need? Especially if you are over 50, your nutritional needs may change. Informed food choices are the first place to start, making sure you get a variety of foods while watching your calorie intake. Supplements and fortified foods may also help you get appropriate amounts of nutrients. To help you make informed decisions, talk to your doctor and/or registered dietitian. They can work together with you to determine if your intake of a specific nutrient might be too low or too high and then decide how you can achieve a balance between the foods and nutrients you personally need.

While certain products may be helpful to some individuals, there may be circumstances when these products may not benefit your health or when they may create unexpected risks. Many supplements contain active ingredients that have strong biological effects in the body. This could make them unsafe in some situations and hurt or complicate your health, as in these examples:

- **Are you taking both medicines and supplements?** Are you substituting one for the other? Taking a combination of supplements, using these products together with medications (whether prescription or over-the-counter), or substituting them in place of medicines your doctor prescribes could lead to harmful, even life-threatening, results. Be alert to any advisories about these products. Coumadin (a prescription medicine), *Ginkgo biloba* (an herbal supplement), aspirin (an over-the-counter drug), and vitamin E (a vitamin supplement) can each thin the blood. Taking any of these products alone or together can increase the potential for internal bleeding or stroke. Another example is St. John's wort, which may reduce the effectiveness of prescription drugs for heart disease, depression, seizures, certain cancers, or HIV.

- **Are you planning surgery?** Some supplements can have unwanted effects before, during, and after surgery. It is important to fully inform your health care professional, including your pharmacist, about the vitamins, minerals, herbals, and any other supplements you are taking, especially before surgery. You may be asked to stop taking these products at least two to three weeks ahead of the procedure to avoid potentially dangerous supplement/drug interactions, such as changes in heart rate, blood pressure, or bleeding risk that could adversely affect the outcome of your surgery.

- **Is taking more of a good thing better?** Some people might think that if a little is good, taking a lot is even better. But taking too much of some nutrients, even vitamins and minerals, can also cause problems. Depending on the supplement, your age, and the status of your health, taking more than 100% of the Daily Value (see the Supplements Facts panel) of certain vitamins and minerals—e.g., vitamin A, vitamin D, and iron (from supplements and food sources like vitamin-fortified cereals and drinks)—may actually harm your health. Large amounts can also interfere with how your medicines work. Your combined intake from all supplements (including multivitamins, single supplements, and combination products) plus fortified foods, like some cereals and drinks, could cause health problems.

Why Speak to My Health Care Provider about Dietary Supplements?

You and your health professionals (doctors, nurses, registered dietitians, pharmacists, and other caregivers) are a team working toward a common goal—to develop a personalized health plan for you.

Your doctor and other members of the health team can help monitor your medical condition and overall health, especially if any problems develop. Although they may not immediately have answers to your questions, these health professionals have access to the most current research on dietary supplements.

There are numerous resources that provide information about dietary supplements. These include TV, radio, newspapers, magazines, store clerks, friends, family, or the internet. It is important to question recommendations from people who have no formal training in nutrition, botanicals, or medicine. While some of these sources may seem to offer a wealth of accurate information, these same sources may contain misinformation that may not be obvious. Given the abundance and conflicting nature of information now available about supplements, it is more important than ever to partner with your health care team to sort the reliable information from the questionable.

Websites with Information on Dietary Supplements and Nutrition from Government Agencies and Others

Federal Government Agencies

- Administration on Aging (www.aoa.gov)
- FDA, Center for Food Safety and Applied Nutrition, Dietary Supplements (www.fda.gov/Food/DietarySupplements/default.htm)
- Federal Trade Commission (www.ftc.gov)
- NCCAM (nccam.nih.gov)
- Office of Dietary Supplements (ods.od.nih.gov)
- U.S. Department of Agriculture, Food and Nutrition Information Center (www.nal.usda.gov/fnic)

Others

- American Dietetic Association (www.eatright.org)
- American Pharmacists Association (www.pharmacyandyou.org)
- Food Marketing Institute (www.fmi.org)
- International Food Information Council Foundation (www.ific.org)
- National Council on Patient Information and Education (www .talkaboutrx.org)
- AARP (www.aarp.org)

How Will I Be Able to Spot False Claims?

Be savvy! Although the benefits of some dietary supplements have been documented, the claims of others may be unproven. If something sounds too good to be true, it usually is. Here are some signs of a false claim:

- Statements that the product is a quick and effective "cure-all" (For example: "Extremely beneficial in treatment of rheumatism, arthritis, infections, prostate problems, ulcers, cancer, heart trouble, hardening of the arteries, and more.")

- Statements that suggest the product can treat or cure diseases (For example: "shrinks tumors" or "cures impotency." Actually, these are drug claims and should not be made for dietary supplements.)

- Statements that claim the product is "totally safe," "all natural," or has "definitely no side effects"

- Promotions that use words like "scientific breakthrough," "miraculous cure," "exclusive product," "secret ingredient," or "ancient remedy" (For example: "A scientific breakthrough formulated by using proven principles of natural health-based medical science.")

- Text that uses overly impressive-sounding terms, like those for a weight-loss product: "hunger stimulation point" and "thermogenesis"

- Personal testimonials by consumers or doctors claiming amazing results (For example: "My husband has Alzheimer's. He began eating a teaspoonful of this product each day. And now in just 22 days, he mowed the grass, cleaned out the garage, and weeded the flower beds; we take our morning walk together again.")

- Limited availability and advance payment required (For example: "Hurry. This offer will not last. Send us a check now to reserve your supply.")

- Promises of no-risk "money-back guarantees" (For example: "If after 30 days you have not lost at least four pounds each week, your uncashed check will be returned to you.")

What Are the Key "Points to Ponder" Before I Buy?

- Think twice about chasing the latest headline. Sound health advice is generally based on research over time, not a single study. Be wary of results claiming a "quick fix" that depart from scientific research and established dietary guidance. Keep in mind that science does not generally proceed by dramatic breakthroughs, but rather by taking many small steps, slowly building toward scientific agreement.

- We may think, "Even if a product may not help me, it at least won't hurt me." It's best not to assume that this will always be true. Some product ingredients, including nutrients and plant components, can be toxic based on their activity in your body. Some products may become harmful when consumed in high enough amounts, for a long enough time, or in combination with certain other substances.

- The term "natural" does not always mean safe. Do not assume this term assures wholesomeness or that these products have milder effects, making them safer to use than prescribed drugs. For example, many weight-loss products claim to be "natural" or "herbal," but this doesn't necessarily make them safe. The ingredients may interact with drugs or may be dangerous for people with certain medical conditions.

- Spend your money wisely. Some supplement products may be expensive and may not work, given your specific condition. Be wary of substituting a product or therapy for prescription medicines. Be sure to talk with your health care team to help you determine what is best for your overall health.

- Remember: Safety first. Resist the pressure to decide "on the spot" about trying an untested product or treatment. Ask for more information and consult your doctor, nurse, dietitian, pharmacist, and/or caregiver about whether the product is right for you and safe for you to use.

Who Is Responsible for Ensuring the Safety and Efficacy of Dietary Supplements?

Unlike prescription and over-the-counter medicines, dietary supplement products are not reviewed by the government before they are marketed. Under the law, manufacturers of dietary supplements are responsible for making sure their products are safe before they go to market. If you want to know more about the product you are purchasing, check with the manufacturer:

- Can the firm supply information to support the claims for their products?

- Can the company share information on the safety or efficacy of the ingredients in the product?

- Has the manufacturer received any adverse event reports from consumers using their products?

What Is FDA's Responsibility?

FDA has the responsibility to take action against unsafe dietary supplement products after they reach the market. The agency may also take legal action against dietary supplement manufacturers if FDA can prove that claims on marketed dietary supplements are false and misleading.

What If I Think I Have Had a Reaction to a Dietary Supplement?

Adverse effects from the use of dietary supplements should be reported to the FDA's MedWatch Program. You, your health care provider, or anyone should report a serious adverse event or illness directly to FDA if you believe it is related to the use of any dietary supplement product by calling FDA at 800-FDA-1088, by fax at 800-FDA-0178, or reporting online. FDA would like to know whenever you think a product caused you a serious problem, even if you are not sure that the product was the cause, and even if you do not visit a doctor or clinic.

What's the Bottom Line?

- Dietary supplements are intended to supplement the diet, not to cure, prevent, or treat diseases or replace the variety of foods important to a healthful diet.

- Supplements can help you meet daily requirements for certain nutrients, but when you combine drugs and foods, too much of some nutrients can also cause problems.

- Many factors play a role in deciding if a supplement is right for you, including possible drug interactions and side effects.

- Do not self-diagnose any health condition. Together, you and your health care team can make the best decision for optimal health.

Use the following questions to talk to your doctor, nurse, dietitian, pharmacist, and/or caregiver about dietary supplements.

- Is taking a dietary supplement an important part of my total diet?

- Are there any precautions or warnings I should know about (e.g., is there an amount or "upper limit" I should not go above)?

- Are there any known side effects (e.g., loss of appetite, nausea, headaches, etc.)? Do they apply to me?

- Are there any foods, medicines (prescription or over-the counter), or other supplements I should avoid while taking this product?

- If I am scheduled for surgery, should I be concerned about the dietary supplements I am taking?

- What is this product for? What are its intended benefits? How, when, and for how long should I take it?

Savvy Consumers Share Information with Their Health Care Team

If you take dietary supplements, you may find it helpful to answer the following questions and share the information with your health care team, who need this information to help develop a personalized plan for you.

To have as accurate a record as possible, list the supplements you take and how often. Include multiple, single, or combination vitamins; minerals (like calcium and iron); or any herbal or botanical supplements you may have on your kitchen or medicine cabinet shelf. Because supplements come in so many forms that resemble other food and drug products, check to see if there is a Supplement Facts label on the product to be certain it is a dietary supplement.

1. What supplements do you take, how often, how much, and for what reasons?

2. Are you currently taking or have you recently taken any over-the-counter medications (e.g., aspirin, cold medicine, stool softener, pain reliever, etc.)?

3. What prescription medication(s) are you currently taking, if any?

Section 5.3

An Introduction to Probiotics

This section excerpted from "An Introduction to Probiotics," National Center for Complementary and Alternative Medicine (nccam.nih.gov), August 2008.

Probiotics are live microorganisms (in most cases, bacteria) that are similar to beneficial microorganisms found in the human gut. They are also called "friendly bacteria" or "good bacteria." Probiotics are available to consumers mainly in the form of dietary supplements and foods.

Experts have debated how to define probiotics. One widely used definition, developed by the World Health Organization and the Food and Agriculture Organization of the United Nations, is that probiotics are "live microorganisms, which, when administered in adequate amounts, confer a health benefit on the host." (Microorganisms are tiny living organisms—such as bacteria, viruses, and yeasts—that can be seen only under a microscope.)

Probiotics are not the same thing as prebiotics—nondigestible food ingredients that selectively stimulate the growth and/or activity of beneficial microorganisms already in people's colons. When probiotics and prebiotics are mixed together, they form a symbiotic.

Probiotics are available in foods and dietary supplements (for example, capsules, tablets, and powders) and in some other forms as well. Examples of foods containing probiotics are yogurt, fermented and unfermented milk, miso, tempeh, and some juices and soy beverages. In probiotic foods and supplements, the bacteria may have been present originally or added during preparation.

Most probiotics are bacteria similar to those naturally found in people's guts, especially in those of breast-fed infants (who have natural protection against many diseases). Most often, the bacteria come from two groups, *Lactobacillus* or *Bifidobacterium*. Within each group, there are different species (i.e., *Lactobacillus acidophilus* and *Bifidobacterium bifidus*), and within each species, different strains (or varieties). A few common probiotics, such *as Saccharomyces boulardii*, are yeasts, which are different from bacteria.

Some probiotic foods date back to ancient times, such as fermented foods and cultured milk products. Interest in probiotics in general has been growing; Americans' spending on probiotic supplements, for example, nearly tripled from 1994 to 2003.

Uses for Health Purposes

There are several reasons that people are interested in probiotics for health purposes. First, the world is full of microorganisms (including bacteria), and so are people's bodies—in and on the skin, in the gut, and in other orifices. Friendly bacteria are vital to proper development of the immune system, to protection against microorganisms that could cause disease, and to the digestion and absorption of food and nutrients. Each person's mix of bacteria varies. Interactions between a person and the microorganisms in his body, and among the microorganisms themselves, can be crucial to the person's health and well-being.

This bacterial "balancing act" can be thrown off in two major ways:

1. By antibiotics, when they kill friendly bacteria in the gut along with unfriendly bacteria. Some people use probiotics to try to offset side effects from antibiotics like gas, cramping, or diarrhea. Similarly, some use them to ease symptoms of lactose intolerance—a condition in which the gut lacks the enzyme needed to digest significant amounts of the major sugar in milk, and which also causes gastrointestinal symptoms.

2. "Unfriendly" microorganisms such as disease-causing bacteria, yeasts, fungi, and parasites can also upset the balance. Researchers are exploring whether probiotics could halt these unfriendly agents in the first place and/or suppress their growth and activity in conditions like the following:

   - Infectious diarrhea
   - Irritable bowel syndrome
   - Inflammatory bowel disease (e.g., ulcerative colitis and Crohn disease)
   - Infection with *Helicobacter pylori* (*H. pylori*), a bacterium that causes most ulcers and many types of chronic stomach inflammation
   - Tooth decay and periodontal disease
   - Vaginal infections
   - Stomach and respiratory infections that children acquire in day care
   - Skin infections

Another part of the interest in probiotics stems from the fact there are cells in the digestive tract connected with the immune system. One theory is that if you alter the microorganisms in a person's intestinal tract (as by introducing probiotic bacteria), you can affect the immune system's defenses.

What the Science Says

Scientific understanding of probiotics and their potential for preventing and treating health conditions is at an early stage but moving ahead. In November 2005, a conference that was co-funded by NCCAM and convened by the American Society for Microbiology explored this topic.

According to the conference report, some uses of probiotics for which there is some encouraging evidence from the study of specific probiotic formulations are as follows:

- To treat diarrhea (this is the strongest area of evidence, especially for diarrhea from rotavirus)

- To prevent and treat infections of the urinary tract or female genital tract

- To treat irritable bowel syndrome

- To reduce recurrence of bladder cancer

- To shorten the duration of an intestinal infection that is caused by a bacterium called *Clostridium difficile*

- To prevent and treat pouchitis (a condition that can follow surgery to remove the colon)

- To prevent and manage atopic dermatitis (eczema) in children

The conference panel also noted that in studies of probiotics as cures, any beneficial effect was usually low; a strong placebo effect often occurs; and more research (especially in the form of large, carefully designed clinical trials) is needed in order to draw firmer conclusions.

Some other areas of interest to researchers on probiotics are the following:

- What is going on at the molecular level with the bacteria themselves and how they may interact with the body (such as the gut and its bacteria) to prevent and treat diseases

- Issues of quality (i.e., what happens when probiotic bacteria are treated or are added to foods—is their ability to survive, grow, and have a therapeutic effect altered?)

- The best ways to administer probiotics for therapeutic purposes, as well as the best doses and schedules

- Probiotics' potential to help with the problem of antibiotic-resistant bacteria in the gut

- Whether they can prevent unfriendly bacteria from getting through the skin or mucous membranes and traveling through the body (e.g., which can happen with burns, shock, trauma, or suppressed immunity)

Side Effects and Risks

Some live microorganisms have a long history of use as probiotics without causing illness in people. Probiotics' safety has not been thoroughly studied scientifically, however. More information is especially needed on how safe they are for young children, elderly people, and people with compromised immune systems.

Probiotics' side effects, if they occur, tend to be mild and digestive (such as gas or bloating). More serious effects have been seen in some people. Probiotics might theoretically cause infections that need to be treated with antibiotics, especially in people with underlying health conditions. They could also cause unhealthy metabolic activities, too much stimulation of the immune system, or gene transfer (insertion of genetic material into a cell).

Probiotic products taken by mouth as a dietary supplement are manufactured and regulated as foods, not drugs.

Some Other Points to Consider

- If you are thinking about using a probiotic product as complementary and alternative medicine (CAM), consult your health care provider first. No CAM therapy should be used in place of conventional medical care or to delay seeking that care.

- Effects from one species or strain of probiotics do not necessarily hold true for others, or even for different preparations of the same species or strain.

- If you use a probiotic product and experience an effect that concerns you, contact your health care provider.

- You can locate research reports in peer-reviewed journals on probiotics' effectiveness and safety through the resources PubMed (www.ncbi.nlm.nih.gov/pubmed) and CAM on PubMed® (nccam.nih.gov/research/camonpubmed).

Part Two

The Elements of
Good Nutrition

Chapter 6

Protein

What do you think about when you hear the word *protein*? Maybe it's an ad for some protein shake that promises massive muscles? Or is it the last high-protein diet craze you read about? With all this talk about protein, you might think Americans were at risk for not eating enough. In fact, most of us eat more protein than we need. Protein is in many foods that we eat on a regular basis.

What is protein?

Proteins are part of every cell, tissue, and organ in our bodies. These body proteins are constantly being broken down and replaced. The protein in the foods we eat is digested into amino acids that are later used to replace these proteins in our bodies.

Protein is found in the following foods:

- Meats, poultry, and fish
- Legumes (dry beans and peas)
- Tofu
- Eggs
- Nuts and seeds
- Milk and milk products

"Protein," Centers for Disease Control and Prevention (www.cdc.gov), November 9, 2009.

- Grains, some vegetables, and some fruits (provide only small amounts of protein relative to other sources)

Most adults in the United States get more than enough protein to meet their needs. It's rare for someone who is healthy and eating a varied diet to not get enough protein.

What are the types of protein?

Proteins are made up of amino acids. Think of amino acids as the building blocks. There are 20 different amino acids that join together to make all types of protein. Some of these amino acids can't be made by our bodies, so these are known as *essential* amino acids. It's *essential* that our diet provide these.

In the diet, protein sources are labeled according to how many of the essential amino acids they provide:

- A *complete* protein source is one that provides all of the essential amino acids. You may also hear these sources called *high-quality proteins*. Animal-based foods—for example, meat, poultry, fish, milk, eggs, and cheese—are considered complete protein sources.

- An *incomplete* protein source is one that is low in one or more of the essential amino acids. *Complementary* proteins are two or more incomplete protein sources that together provide adequate amounts of all the essential amino acids.

For example, rice contains low amounts of certain essential amino acids; however, these same essential amino acids are found in greater amounts in dry beans. Similarly, dry beans contain lower amounts of other essential amino acids that can be found in larger amounts in rice. Together, these two foods can provide adequate amounts of all the essential amino acids the body needs.

In the past, it was thought that these complementary proteins needed to be eaten at the same meal for your body to use them together. Now studies show that your body can combine complementary proteins that are eaten within the same day.[1]

How much protein do I need?

Maybe you've wondered how much protein you need each day. In general, it's recommended that 10%–35% of your daily calories come from protein. The following are the Recommended Dietary Allowances (RDA) for different age groups.[2]

Recommended Dietary Allowance for Protein (Grams Needed Each Day)

- Children ages 1–3: 13 g
- Children ages 4–8: 19 g
- Children ages 9–13: 34 g
- Girls ages 14–18: 46 g
- Boys ages 14–18: 52 g
- Women ages 19–70+: 46 g
- Men ages 19–70+: 56 g

Here are examples of amounts of protein in food:

- 1 cup of milk has 8 grams of protein.
- A 3-ounce piece of meat has about 21 grams of protein.
- 1 cup of dry beans has about 16 grams of protein.
- An 8-ounce container of yogurt has about 11 grams of protein.

Added together, just these four sources would meet the protein needs of an adult male (56 grams). This doesn't count all the other foods that add smaller amounts of protein to his diet.

Rather than just focusing on your protein needs, choose an overall healthy eating plan that provides the protein you need as well as other nutrients.

Follow these guidelines to help you get the amounts of protein you need:

- Compare the amount of meat, poultry, fish, eggs, legumes, nuts, and seeds you are eating per day to what is recommended. As an example, if you refer to ChooseMyPlate.gov, a 48-year-old female who is active less than 30 minutes a day only needs about five ounces each day from the meat and beans group. Some precut slices of meat and poultry, such as a pork chop or chicken breast, can be four to five ounces each. You can see how it would be easy to eat too much.

- Save your money and don't buy protein supplements. If you're healthy, you probably get all the protein you need from your diet.

Follow these guidelines to help you make lower-fat protein choices:

- Choose meats that are leaner cuts and trim away any fat you can see. For chicken and turkey, remove the skin to reduce fat.

- Substitute pinto or black beans for meat in chili and tacos.

- Choose low-fat or fat-free milk and yogurt.

- Choose egg whites or pasteurized egg white products.

Is there any harm in getting more protein than I need?

Most people eat more protein than they need without harmful effects. However, protein contributes to calorie intake, so if you eat more protein than you need, your overall calorie intake could be greater than your calorie needs and contribute to weight gain.

Besides that, animal sources of protein can be sources of saturated fat, which has been linked to elevated low-density lipoprotein (LDL) cholesterol, a risk factor for heart disease.

In addition, for people with certain kidney diseases, a lower-protein diet may be recommended to help prevent an impairment in kidney function.

What if I am a vegetarian?

Because some vegetarians avoid eating all (or most) animal foods, they must rely on plant-based sources of protein to meet their protein needs. With some planning, a vegetarian diet can easily meet the recommended protein needs of adults and children.

ChooseMyPlate.gov includes meal planning resources for vegetarians. See "Vegetarian Choices" (www.choosemyplate.gov/foodgroups/vegetarian.html) and "Vegetarian Diets" (www.choosemyplate.gov/tipsresources/vegetarian_diets.html) for more information.

Sources

1. Position of the American Dietetic Association and Dietitians of Canada: Vegetarian diets. *JADA*, 2003; 103(6) 748–765.

2. Source for Acceptable Macronutrient Distribution Range (AMDR) reference and RDAs: Institute of Medicine (IOM) Dietary Reference Intakes for Energy, Carbohydrate, Fiber, Fat, Fatty Acids, Cholesterol, Protein, and Amino Acids. This report may be accessed via www.nap.edu.

Chapter 7

Carbohydrates

Not sure what to think about carbohydrates these days? Here are the facts to separate the hype from the truth about carbohydrates.

What Are Carbohydrates?

Your body uses carbohydrates (carbs) to make glucose, the fuel that gives you energy and helps keep everything going. Your body can use glucose immediately or store it in your liver and muscles for when it is needed.

You can find carbohydrates in fruits; vegetables; breads, cereals, and other grains; milk and milk products; and foods containing added sugars (e.g., cakes, cookies, and sugar-sweetened beverages).

Healthier foods higher in carbohydrates include ones that provide dietary fiber and whole grains as well as those without added sugars.

What about foods higher in carbohydrates such as sodas and candies that also contain added sugars? Those are the ones that add extra calories but not many nutrients to your diet.

What Is the Difference between "Good" Carbs and "Bad" Carbs?

Some diet books use "bad" carbs to talk about foods with refined carbohydrates (i.e., meaning they're made from white flour and added

"Carbohydrates," Centers for Disease Control and Prevention (www.cdc.gov), December 3, 2008.

sugars). Examples include white bread, cakes, and cookies. "Good" carbs is used to describe foods that have more fiber and complex carbohydrates. Complex carbohydrates are carbohydrates that take longer to break down into glucose. These terms aren't used in the *Dietary Guidelines for Americans 2005*. Instead, the guidelines recommend choosing fiber-rich carbohydrate choices from the vegetable, fruit, and grain groups and avoiding added sugars. It is also recommended that at least half of your daily grain choices are whole grains.

What Are the Types of Carbohydrates?

There are two main types of carbohydrates, complex carbohydrates and simple carbohydrates.

Complex Carbohydrates

Starch and dietary fiber are the two types of complex carbohydrates. Starch must be broken down through digestion before your body can use it as a glucose source.

Quite a few foods contain starch and dietary fiber:

- Starch is in certain vegetables (i.e., potatoes, dry beans, peas, and corn).
- Starch is also found in breads, cereals, and grains.
- Dietary fiber is in vegetables, fruits, and whole grains.

Dietary fiber: You may have seen dietary fiber on the label listed as soluble fiber or insoluble fiber. Soluble fiber is found in the following:

- Oatmeal
- Oat bran
- Nuts and seeds
- Most fruits (e.g., strawberries, blueberries, pears, and apples)
- Dry beans and peas

Insoluble fiber is found in the following:

- Whole wheat bread
- Barley
- Brown rice
- Couscous

- Bulgur or whole grain cereals

- Wheat bran

- Seeds

- Most vegetables

- Fruits

Which type is best? Both! Each has important health benefits, so eat a variety of these foods to get enough of both. You're also more likely to get other nutrients that you might miss if you just chose one or two high-fiber foods.

How much dietary fiber do I need each day? It's recommended that you get 14 grams of dietary fiber for every 1,000 calories that you consume each day. If you need 2,000 calories each day, you should try to include 28 grams of dietary fiber.

To find out how many calories you need each day, visit ChooseMyPlate.gov and enter your age, sex, height, weight, and activity level in the MyPlate Daily Food Plan tool. Then refer to Table 7.1 to find how many grams you need.

Table 7.1. Easy Dietary Fiber Estimator

Daily Calorie Needs	Daily Dietary Fiber Needs (grams)
1,000	14 g
1,200	17 g
1,400	20 g
1,600	22 g
1,800	25 g
2,000	28 g
2,200	31 g
2,400	34 g
2,600	36 g
2,800	39 g
3,000	42 g

At first, you may find it challenging to eat all of your daily fiber grams. Just take it slowly and try to choose higher-fiber foods more often. Over time, you'll gradually be eating more fiber!

Try these tips to jumpstart your intake of dietary fiber:

- Choose whole fruits more often than fruit juice. Fresh, frozen, or canned—it doesn't matter— they all count!

- Try to eat two vegetables with your evening meal.

- Keep a bowl of veggies already washed and prepared in your refrigerator—try carrots, cucumbers, or celery for a quick snack.

- Make a meal around dried beans or peas (also called legumes) instead of meat. Check www.fruitsandveggiesmatter.gov for some new ideas.

- Choose whole-grain foods more often. Take a look at the following "whole grains buzz words" list to help you decide. A good guide is to make at least half of your grain choices whole grains.

- Start your day with a whole-grain breakfast cereal low in added sugar. Top your cereal with fruit for even more fiber. While bananas may come to your mind first, you can add even more variety by trying sliced peaches or berries. You can often find these fruits year-round in the frozen foods section of your grocery store.

Whole grains: Whole grains are a good source of fiber and nutrients. Whole grains refer to grains that have all of the parts of the grain seed (sometimes called the kernel). These parts of the kernel are called the bran, the germ, and the endosperm.

If the whole grain has been cracked, crushed, or flaked (as in cracked whole-grain bread or flake cereal), then the whole grain must still have about the same proportions of bran, germ, and endosperm to be called a whole grain.

When whole grains are processed, some of the dietary fiber and other important nutrients are removed. A processed grain is called a "refined" grain.

Some refined grain products have key nutrients, such as folic acid and iron, which were removed during the initial processing and added back. These are called enriched grains. White rice and white bread are enriched grain products.

Some enriched grain foods have extra nutrients added. These are called fortified grains.

Whole grain buzz words: The *Dietary Guidelines for Americans* recommend that you try to make at least half of your daily grain choices whole grains.

You can find out if the food you are eating is made of whole grains by looking at the ingredients list of the food label. The whole grain should be the first ingredient listed. The following are some examples of how whole grains could be listed:

- Brown rice
- Buckwheat

- Bulgur (cracked wheat)
- Wild rice
- Quinoa
- Whole-grain barley
- Whole oats/oatmeal
- Whole wheat
- Millet
- Popcorn*
- Triticale
- Whole-grain corn
- Whole rye

* Popcorn is a whole grain that can have added fat and salt. Try air-popping your popcorn to avoid these extras. If you're buying microwave popcorn, look for a lower-fat variety. You may also want to try the snack size bag to help with portion control.

Grains galore: Here are some explanations of less-familiar grains:

- **Bulgur:** A staple of Middle Eastern dishes. Bulgur wheat consists of kernels that have been steamed, dried, and crushed. It has a tender and chewy texture.

- **Millet:** A staple grain in parts of Africa and Asia. Millet comes in several varieties and has a bland flavor that is a background to other seasonings.

- **Quinoa:** A grain that has been traditionally used in South American cuisine. Its texture has been compared to that of couscous.

- **Triticale:** A grain that is a hybrid of wheat and rye. It comes in several varieties including whole berry, flakes, and flour.

Simple Carbohydrates

Simple carbohydrates include sugars found naturally in foods such as fruits, vegetables, milk, and milk products. Simple carbohydrates also include sugars added during food processing and refining. What's the difference? In general, foods with added sugars have fewer nutrients than foods with naturally occurring sugars.

How can I avoid added sugars? One way to avoid these sugars is to read the ingredient lists on food labels. Look for these ingredients as added sugars:

- Brown sugar
- Corn syrup
- Corn sweetener
- Dextrose

- Fructose
- Glucose
- Honey
- Lactose
- Malt syrup
- Raw sugar
- Sugar

- Fruit juice concentrates
- High-fructose corn syrup
- Invert sugar
- Maltose
- Molasses
- Sucrose
- Syrup

If you see any of these in the ingredient list, you know the food has added sugars. The closer to the top of the list, the more of that sugar is in the food.

Tips for avoiding added sugars include the following:

- Choose water instead of sugar-sweetened sodas.

- Choose four fluid ounces (1/2 cup) of 100% fruit juice rather than a fruit drink.

- Have a piece of fruit for dessert and skip desserts with added sugar.

- Choose breakfast cereals that contain less or no added sugars.

How Much Carbohydrate Do I Need?

Your best approach is to follow a meal plan that gives you 45% to 65% of your calories as carbohydrates. How do you do this? Check out the following meal plans, which can give you the calories you need and the right amounts of carbohydrate.

- ChooseMyPlate.gov lets you enter your age, sex, height, weight, and activity level to get a meal plan specific to your calorie needs.

- DASH (Dietary Approaches to Stop Hypertension) Eating Plan (www.nhlbi.nih.gov/health/public/heart/hbp/dash/new_dash.pdf) provides a healthy eating plan with menu examples and recipes to get you started.

Chapter 8

Dietary Fats: An Overview

Dietary Fat

What counts as fat? Are some fats better than other fats? While fats are essential for normal body function, some fats are better for you than others. Trans fats, saturated fats, and cholesterol are less healthy than polyunsaturated and monounsaturated fats.

How Much Total Dietary Fat Do I Need?

The *Dietary Guidelines for Americans 2005* recommend that Americans keep their total fat intake within certain limits. This limit is defined as a percentage of your total calorie needs.

Table 8.1. Fat Intake per Total Calories

Age Group	Total Fat Limits
Children ages 2 to 3	30% to 35% of total calories
Children and adolescents ages 4 to 18	25% to 35% of total calories
Adults, ages 19 and older	20% to 35% of total calories

You can meet this recommendation by following a healthy meal plan that meets your calorie needs and is designed to provide 20% to 35% of calories from total fat. The ChooseMyPlate.gov and DASH eating plans are examples of healthy meal plans that can meet your calorie needs and provide the right amounts of fat.

"Dietary Fat," "Saturated Fat," and "Dietary Cholesterol," February 23, 2011, and "Trans Fat," April 14, 2010, Centers for Disease Control and Prevention (www.cdc.gov).

- ChooseMyPlate.gov lets you enter your age, sex, height, weight, and activity level to get a meal plan specific to your calorie needs.

- DASH (Dietary Approaches to Stop Hypertension) Eating Plan (www.nhlbi.nih.gov/health/public/heart/hbp/dash/new_dash.pdf) provides a healthy eating plan with menu examples and recipes to get you started.

If you have children, you may be concerned about whether they should watch their fat intake. For proper growth, children and teens need healthy diets that provide the recommended fat intakes. Children less than two years of age need more calories due to rapid growth and development. For this reason, nonfat and low-fat milks are not recommended for children two years and under.

Trans Fat

You may have heard about trans fats recently in the news. These fats made headlines when food manufacturers were required to list them on the Nutrition Facts Label by 2006. The *Dietary Guidelines for Americans 2005* recommend keeping the amount of trans fat you consume as low as possible.

So what's the story with trans fats? These fats are created during food processing when liquid oils are converted into semisolid fats—a process called hydrogenation. This creates partially hydrogenated oils that tend to keep food fresh longer while on grocery shelves. The problem is that these partially hydrogenated oils contain trans fats, which can also increase low-density lipoprotein (LDL) cholesterol and decrease high-density lipoprotein (HDL) cholesterol—risk factors for heart disease.

Though some fried foods and commercially baked goods may contain trans fats, the good news is that some manufacturers have changed how they process foods to reduce the amounts of trans fats in their products. Be on the lookout for foods that contain trans fats, such as commercially baked cookies, crackers, and pies. Some commercial restaurants may also use partially hydrogenated oils when frying their entrees and side items or preparing baking goods and spreads.

How Do I Control My Trans Fat Intake?

Here are some ideas on how to reduce the trans fat in your diet:

- Look for the trans fat listing on the Nutrition Facts label. Compare brands and choose the one lowest in trans fat, preferably with no trans fat.

- Replace margarine containing trans fat with unsaturated vegetable oil.

- If you use margarine, choose a soft margarine spread instead of stick margarine. Check your labels to be sure the soft margarine does contain less trans fat. If possible, find one that says zero grams of trans fat.

Saturated Fat

Diets high in saturated fat have been linked to chronic disease, specifically, coronary heart disease. The *Dietary Guidelines for Americans 2005* recommend consuming less than 10% of daily calories as saturated fat.

You may have heard that saturated fats are the "solid" fats in your diet. For the most part, this is true. For example, if you open a container of meat stew, you will probably find some fat floating on top. This fat is saturated fat.

But other saturated fats can be more difficult to see in your diet. In general, saturated fat can be found in the following foods:

- High-fat cheeses
- Whole-fat milk and cream
- Ice cream and ice cream products
- High-fat cuts of meat
- Butter
- Palm and coconut oils

It's important to note that lower-fat versions of these foods usually will contain saturated fats, but typically in smaller quantities than the regular versions.

As you look at this list, notice two things. First, animal fats are a primary source of saturated fat. Secondly, certain plant oils are another source of saturated fats: palm oils, coconut oils, and cocoa butter. You may think you don't use palm or coconut oils, but they are often added to commercially prepared foods, such as cookies, cakes, doughnuts, and pies. Solid vegetable shortening often contains palm oils and some whipped dessert toppings contain coconut oil.

How Do I Control My Saturated Fat Intake?

In general, saturated fat can be found in the following foods:

- High-fat cheeses
- High-fat cuts of meat
- Whole-fat milk and cream

- Butter
- Ice cream and ice cream products

So how can you cut back on your intake of saturated fats? Try these tips:

- Choose leaner cuts of meat that do not have a marbled appearance (where the fat appears embedded in the meat). Leaner cuts include round cuts and sirloin cuts. Trim all visible fat off meats before eating.

- Remove the skin from chicken, turkey, and other poultry before cooking.

- When reheating soups or stews, skim the solid fats from the top before heating.

- Drink low-fat (1%) or fat-free (skim) milk rather than whole or 2% milk.

- Buy low-fat or non-fat versions of your favorite cheeses and other milk or dairy products.

- When you want a sweet treat, reach for a low-fat or fat-free version of your favorite ice cream or frozen dessert. These versions usually contain less saturated fat.

- Use low-fat spreads instead of butter. Most margarine spreads contain less saturated fat than butter. Look for a spread that is low in saturated fat and doesn't contain trans fats.

- Choose baked goods, breads, and desserts that are low in saturated fat. You can find this information on the Nutrition Facts label.

- Pay attention at snack time. Some convenience snacks such as sandwich crackers contain saturated fat. Choose instead to have non-fat or low-fat yogurt and a piece of fruit.

What should I choose—butter or margarine? Should I choose a stick, tub, or liquid? With such a variety of products available, it can be a difficult decision. Here are some general rules of thumb to help you compare products:

Look at the Nutrition Facts label to compare both the trans fat and the saturated fat content. Choose the one that has the fewest grams of trans fat and the fewest grams of saturated fat and dietary cholesterol. If possible, find one that says zero grams of trans fat.

When looking at the Daily Value for saturated fat and cholesterol remember that 5% is low and 20% is high.

If you are also trying to reduce calories, you may want to look for a version that says "light." These products contain fewer calories and can help you stay within your calorie goals.

If you find two products that seem comparable, try them both and choose the one that tastes better!

Dietary Cholesterol

Cholesterol is a fatty substance that's found in animal-based foods such as meats, poultry, egg yolks, and whole milks. Saturated fat is the other type of fat that is found in animal-based products.

So, when you follow the tips to reduce your saturated fat intake, in most cases, you will be reducing your dietary cholesterol intake at the same time. For example, if you switch to low-fat and fat-free dairy products, you will reduce your intake of both saturated fat and cholesterol.

The *Dietary Guidelines for Americans 2005* recommend that individuals consume less than 300 milligrams (mg) of cholesterol each day.

I've heard that some people have high blood cholesterol because of the foods they eat but that other people have high cholesterol because of genetics. What's the difference? Not only do you get cholesterol from the foods you eat (your diet), but your body also makes cholesterol to use in normal body functions. The cholesterol made by your body is partly influenced by your genes, which are shared by your family members. Even though genetics play a role, families often also share the same eating and lifestyle habits. Some health problems that seem to run in families may be worsened by these unhealthful habits. If you have a genetic tendency to produce more cholesterol, you may still obtain additional benefits from reducing the cholesterol in your diet.

Cholesterol in Your Blood

- **Total cholesterol:** This is the total measured cholesterol in your blood. This number includes all other types of cholesterol, such as HDL and LDL, as defined in the following. High blood cholesterol can increase your risk of heart disease.

- **It is important to know your numbers:** You can't tell if the cholesterol in your blood is high by how you feel. You'll need a blood test from your health care provider to know. If you don't know what your blood cholesterol level is, talk to your health care provider.

- **HDL:** HDL stands for high-density lipoprotein cholesterol. The HDL cholesterol is often called "good" cholesterol because it helps carry cholesterol away from your body's organs and to your liver, where it can be removed. To help you remember that HDL is the "good" cholesterol, recall that the *H* stands for high and higher HDL cholesterol is good.

- **LDL:** LDL stands low-density lipoprotein cholesterol. The LDL cholesterol is sometimes called "bad" cholesterol because it's the type of cholesterol that is linked with a higher chance of heart disease. Remember that *L* stands for "low" and you want to keep LDL lower in your blood.

What Is High Blood Cholesterol?

Too much cholesterol in the blood, or high blood cholesterol, can be serious. People with high blood cholesterol have a greater chance of getting heart disease. Cholesterol can build up on the walls of your arteries (blood vessels that carry blood from the heart to other parts of the body). This buildup of cholesterol is called plaque. Over time, plaque can cause narrowing of the arteries.

If you've already been diagnosed with high blood cholesterol or want more information about how to prevent it, read these documents from the National Heart, Lung, and Blood Institute (NHLBI):

- "High Blood Cholesterol" (www.nhlbi.nih.gov/health/dci/Diseases/Hbc/HBC_WhatIs.html): This site explains what high blood cholesterol is, its signs and symptoms, and how it is diagnosed and treated.

- "High Blood Cholesterol: What You Need to Know" (www.nhlbi.nih.gov/health/public/heart/chol/wyntk.pdf): This document explains what your cholesterol numbers mean, how to calculate your heart disease risk, and how to treat high levels of cholesterol using the Therapeutic Lifestyle Changes (TLC) diet.

Please note that these websites are intended for adults who have been diagnosed with high cholesterol. For information about cholesterol and children, please visit the American Heart Association's "Cholesterol and Atherosclerosis in Children" (www.americanheart.org/presenter.jhtml?identifier=4499).

Chapter 9

Polyunsaturated and Monounsaturated Fats and Fatty Acids

Chapter Contents

Section 9.1

The Health Benefits of Some Fats

"Polyunsaturated Fats and Monounsaturated Fats," Centers for Disease
Control and Prevention (www.cdc.gov), February 23, 2011.

Examples of Fats

Most of the fat that you eat should come from unsaturated sources:
polyunsaturated fats and monounsaturated fats. In general, nuts, vegetable oils, and fish are sources of unsaturated fats. The following are
examples of specific types of unsaturated fats.

Monounsaturated Fat Sources

- Nuts
- Canola oil
- High oleic safflower oil
- Avocado
- Vegetable oils
- Olive oil
- Sunflower oil

Omega-6 Polyunsaturated Fat Sources

- Soybean oil
- Safflower oil
- Corn oil

Omega-3 Polyunsaturated Fat Sources

- Soybean oil
- Walnuts
- Fish: trout, herring, and salmon
- Canola oil
- Flaxseed

Types of Polyunsaturated Fats

Polyunsaturated fats can also be broken down into two types:

- **Omega-6 polyunsaturated fats:** These fats provide an essential fatty acid that our bodies need, but can't make.

- **Omega-3 polyunsaturated fats:** These fats also provide an essential fatty acid that our bodies need. In addition, omega-3 fatty acids, particularly from fish sources, may have potential health benefits.

Follow these tips for including appropriate amounts of unsaturated fats in your diet:

- Replace solid fats used in cooking with liquid oils. Visit ChooseMyPlate.gov "What's My Allowance?" (www.choosemyplate.gov/foodgroups/oils_allowance.aspx) to learn more about your daily recommendations.

- Remember, any type of fat is high in calories. To avoid additional calories, substitute polyunsaturated and monounsaturated fats for saturated fats and trans fats rather than adding these fats to your diet.

- Have an ounce of dry-roasted nuts as a snack. Nuts and seeds count as part of your meat and beans allowance on the MyPlate plan.

Section 9.2

Omega 3 Fatty Acids in Food and Fish Oil Supplements

The information in this section is excerpted from "Omega-3 Fatty Acids, Fish Oil, Alpha-Linolenic Acid," © 2010 Natural Standard (www.natural standard.com). All rights reserved. Reprinted with permission.

Background

Dietary sources of omega-3 fatty acids include fish oil and certain plant/nut oils. Fish oil contains both docosahexaenoic acid (DHA) and eicosapentaenoic acid (EPA), while some nuts (English walnuts) and vegetable oils (canola, soybean, flaxseed/linseed, olive) contain alpha-linolenic acid (ALA).

There is evidence from multiple studies supporting that intake of recommended amounts of DHA and EPA in the form of dietary fish or fish oil supplements lowers triglycerides; reduces the risk of death, heart attack, dangerous abnormal heart rhythms, and strokes in people with known cardiovascular disease; slows the buildup of atherosclerotic plaques ("hardening of the arteries"); and lowers blood pressure slightly. However, high doses may have harmful effects, such as an increased risk of bleeding. Although similar benefits are proposed for alpha-linolenic acid, scientific evidence is less compelling, and beneficial effects may be less pronounced.

Some species of fish carry a higher risk of environmental contamination, such as with methylmercury.

Evidence

These uses have been tested in humans or animals. Safety and effectiveness have not always been proven. Some of these conditions are potentially serious and should be evaluated by a qualified health care provider.

Uses Based on Scientific Evidence

High blood pressure (grade: A): Multiple human trials report small reductions in blood pressure with intake of omega-3 fatty acid. DHA may have greater benefits than EPA. However, high intakes of omega-3 fatty acids per day may be necessary to obtain clinically relevant effects, and at this dose level, there is an increased risk of bleeding. Therefore, a qualified health care provider should be consulted prior to starting treatment with supplements.

Hypertriglyceridemia (fish oil/EPA plus DHA) (grade: A): There is strong scientific evidence from human trials that omega-3 fatty acids from fish or fish oil supplements (EPA + DHA) significantly reduce blood triglyceride levels. Benefits appear to be dose-dependent. Fish oil supplements also appear to cause small improvements in high-density lipoprotein ("good cholesterol"); however, increases (worsening) in low-density lipoprotein levels (LDL/"bad cholesterol") are also observed. It is not clear if alpha-linolenic acid significantly affects triglyceride levels, and there is conflicting evidence in this area. The American Heart Association has published recommendations for EPA + DHA. Because of the risk of bleeding from omega-3 fatty acids, a qualified health care provider should be consulted prior to starting treatment with supplements.

Secondary cardiovascular disease prevention (fish oil/EPA plus DHA) (grade: A): Several well-conducted randomized controlled trials report that in people with a history of heart attack, regular consumption of oily fish or fish oil/omega-3 supplements reduces the risk of nonfatal heart attack, fatal heart attack, sudden death, and all-cause mortality (death due to any cause). Most patients in these studies were also using conventional heart drugs, suggesting that the benefits of fish oils may add to the effects of other therapies.

Primary cardiovascular disease prevention (fish intake) (grade: B): Several large studies of populations ("epidemiologic" studies) report a significantly lower rate of death from heart disease in men and women who regularly eat fish. Other epidemiologic research reports no such benefits. It is not clear if reported benefits only occur in certain groups of people, such as those at risk of developing heart disease. Overall, the evidence suggests benefits of regular consumption of fish oil. However, well-designed randomized controlled trials which classify people by their risk of developing heart disease are necessary before a firm conclusion can be drawn.

Rheumatoid arthritis (fish oil) (grade: B): Multiple randomized controlled trials report improvements in morning stiffness and joint tenderness with the regular intake of fish oil supplements for up to three months. Benefits have been reported as additive with anti-inflammatory medications such as NSAIDs (like ibuprofen or aspirin). However, because of weaknesses in study designs and reporting, better research is necessary before a strong favorable recommendation can be made. Effects beyond three months of treatment have not been well evaluated.

Asthma (grade: C): Several studies in this area do not provide enough reliable evidence to form a clear conclusion, with some studies reporting no effects, and others finding benefits. Because most studies have been small without clear descriptions of design or results, the results cannot be considered conclusive.

Atherosclerosis (grade: C): Some research reports that regular intake of fish or fish oil supplements reduces the risk of developing atherosclerotic plaques in the arteries of the heart, while other research reports no effects. Additional evidence is necessary before a firm conclusion can be drawn in this area.

Cancer prevention (grade: C): Several population (epidemiologic) studies report that dietary omega-3 fatty acids or fish oil may reduce the risk of developing breast, colon, or prostate cancer. Randomized controlled trials are necessary before a clear conclusion can be drawn.

Cardiac arrhythmias (abnormal heart rhythms) (grade: C):
There is promising evidence that omega-3 fatty acids may decrease the
risk of cardiac arrhythmias. This is one proposed mechanism behind
the reduced number of heart attacks in people who regularly ingest
fish oil or EPA + DHA. Additional research is needed in this area specifically before a firm conclusion can be reached.

Colon cancer (grade: C): Omega-3 fatty acids are commonly
taken by cancer patients. Although preliminary studies report that
growth of colon cancer cells may be reduced by taking fish oil, effects
on survival or remission have not been measured adequately.

Crohn's disease (grade: C): It has been suggested that effects of
omega-3 fatty acids on inflammation may be beneficial in patients with
Crohn's disease when added to standard therapy, and several studies
have been conducted in this area. Results are conflicting, and no clear
conclusion can be drawn at this time.

Depression (grade: C): Several studies on the use of omega-3
fatty acids in depression, including positive results in postpartum
depression, do not provide enough reliable evidence to form a clear
conclusion or replace standard treatments. However, based on one
recent study, omega-3 fatty acids may have therapeutic benefits in
childhood depression. Promising initial evidence requires confirmation
with larger, well-designed trials.

Dysmenorrhea (painful menstruation) (grade: C): There is
preliminary evidence suggesting possible benefits of fish oil/omega-3
fatty acids in patients with dysmenorrhea. Additional research is necessary before a firm conclusion can be reached.

Infant eye/brain development (grade: C): Well-designed research is necessary before a clear conclusion can be reached.

**Secondary cardiovascular disease prevention (ALA) (grade:
C):** Several randomized controlled trials have examined the effects of
alpha-linolenic acid in people with a history of heart attack. Although
some studies suggest benefits, others do not. Additional research is
necessary before a conclusion can be drawn in this area.

Stroke prevention (grade: C): Several large studies of populations ("epidemiologic" studies) have examined the effects of omega-3
fatty acid intake on stroke risk. Some studies suggest benefits, while
others do not. Effects are likely on ischemic or thrombotic stroke risk,

and very large intakes of omega-3 fatty acids ("Eskimo" amounts) may actually increase the risk of hemorrhagic (bleeding) stroke. At this time, it is unclear if there are benefits in people with or without a history of stroke, or if effects of fish oil are comparable to other treatment strategies.

Hypercholesterolemia (grade: D): Although fish oil is able to reduce triglycerides, beneficial effects on blood cholesterol levels have not been demonstrated. Fish oil supplements appear to cause small improvements in high-density lipoprotein ("good cholesterol"); however, increases (worsening) in low-density lipoprotein levels ("bad cholesterol") are also observed. Fish oil does not appear to affect C-reactive protein (CRP) levels.

Key to Grades

A: Strong scientific evidence for this use
B: Good scientific evidence for this use
C: Unclear scientific evidence for this use
D: Fair scientific evidence against this use

Dosing

The following doses are based on scientific research, publications, traditional use, or expert opinion. Many herbs and supplements have not been thoroughly tested, and safety and effectiveness may not be proven. Brands may be made differently, with variable ingredients, even within the same brand. These doses may not apply to all products. You should read product labels and discuss doses with a qualified health care provider before starting therapy.

Adults (18 Years and Older)

Average dietary intake of omega-3/omega-6 fatty acids: Average Americans consume approximately 1.6 grams of omega-3 fatty acids each day, of which about 1.4 grams (~90%) comes from alpha-linolenic acid, and only 0.1–0.2 grams (~10%) from EPA and DHA. In Western diets, people consume roughly 10 times more omega-6 fatty acids than omega-3 fatty acids. These large amounts of omega-6 fatty acids come from the common use of vegetable oils containing linoleic acid (for example: corn oil, evening primrose oil, pumpkin oil, safflower oil, sesame oil, soybean oil, sunflower oil, walnut oil, wheat germ oil). Because omega-6 and omega-3 fatty acids compete with each other to be converted to active metabolites in the body, benefits can be reached either by decreasing intake of omega-6 fatty acids or by increasing omega-3 fatty acids.

Recommended daily intake of omega-3 fatty acids (healthy adults): For healthy adults with no history of heart disease, the American Heart Association recommends eating fish at least two times per week. In particular, fatty fish are recommended, such as anchovies, bluefish, carp, catfish, halibut, herring, lake trout, mackerel, pompano, salmon, striped sea bass, tuna (albacore), and whitefish. It is also recommended to consume plant-derived sources of alpha-linolenic acid, such as tofu/soybeans, walnuts, flaxseed oil, and canola oil. The World Health Organization and governmental health agencies of several countries recommend consuming 0.3–0.5 grams of daily EPA + DHA and 0.8–1.1 grams of daily alpha-linolenic acid. A doctor and pharmacist should be consulted for dosing for other conditions.

Children (Younger Than 18 Years)

Omega-3 fatty acids are used in some infant formulas, although effective doses are not clearly established. Ingestion of fresh fish should be limited in young children due to the presence of potentially harmful environmental contaminants. Fish oil capsules should not be used in children except under the direction of a physician.

Safety

The U.S. Food and Drug Administration does not strictly regulate herbs and supplements. There is no guarantee of strength, purity, or safety of products, and effects may vary. You should always read product labels. If you have a medical condition, or are taking other drugs, herbs, or supplements, you should speak with a qualified health care provider before starting a new therapy. Consult a health care provider immediately if you experience side effects.

Allergies

People with allergy or hypersensitivity to fish should avoid fish oil or omega-3 fatty acid products derived from fish. Skin rash has been reported rarely. People with allergy or hypersensitivity to nuts should avoid alpha-linolenic acid or omega-3 fatty acid products that are derived from the types of nuts to which they react.

Side Effects and Warnings

The U.S. Food and Drug Administration classifies intake of up to three grams per day of omega-3 fatty acids from fish as GRAS (generally regarded as safe). Caution may be warranted, however, in diabetic patients due to potential (albeit unlikely) increases in blood sugar levels, patients at risk of bleeding, or in those with high levels of low-density lipoprotein (LDL). Fish meat may contain methylmercury, and caution is warranted in young children and pregnant/breastfeeding women.

Omega-3 fatty acids may increase the risk of bleeding, although there is little evidence of significant bleeding risk at lower doses. Very large intakes of fish oil/omega-3 fatty acids ("Eskimo" amounts) may increase the risk of hemorrhagic (bleeding) stroke. High doses have also been associated with nosebleed and blood in the urine. Fish oils appear to decrease platelet aggregation and prolong bleeding time, increase fibrinolysis (breaking down of blood clots), and may reduce von Willebrand factor.

Potentially harmful contaminants such as dioxins, methylmercury, and polychlorinated biphenyls (PCBs) are found in some species of fish. Methylmercury accumulates in fish meat more than in fish oil, and fish oil supplements appear to contain almost no mercury. Therefore, safety concerns apply to eating fish but likely not to ingesting fish oil supplements. Heavy metals are most harmful in young children and pregnant/nursing women.

Gastrointestinal upset is common with the use of fish oil supplements. Diarrhea may also occur, with potentially severe diarrhea at very high doses. There are also reports of increased burping, acid reflux/heartburn/indigestion, abdominal bloating, and abdominal pain. Fishy aftertaste is a common effect. Gastrointestinal side effects can be minimized if fish oils are taken with meals and if doses are started low and gradually increased.

Multiple human trials report small reductions in blood pressure with intake of omega-3 fatty acids. Reductions of two to five mmHg [millimeters of mercury] have been observed, and effects appear to be dose responsive (higher doses have greater effects). DHA may have greater effects than EPA. Caution is warranted in patients with low blood pressure or in those taking blood-pressure-lowering medications.

Although slight increases in fasting blood glucose levels have been noted in patients with type 2 ("adult onset") diabetes, the available scientific evidence suggests that there are no significant long-term effects of fish oil in patients with diabetes, including no changes in hemoglobin A1c levels. Limited reports in the 1980s of increased insulin needs in diabetic patients taking long-term fish oils may be related to other dietary changes or weight gain.

Increases (worsening) in low-density lipoprotein levels ("bad cholesterol") by 5%–10% are observed with intake of omega-3 fatty acids. Effects are dose dependent.

Pregnancy and Breastfeeding

Potentially harmful contaminants such as dioxins, methylmercury, and polychlorinated biphenyls (PCBs) are found in some species of fish and may be harmful in pregnant/nursing women. Methylmercury accumulates in fish meat more than in fish oil, and fish oil supplements appear to contain almost no mercury. Therefore, these safety concerns apply to eating fish but likely not to ingesting fish oil supplements. However, unrefined fish oil preparations may contain pesticides.

It is not known if omega-3 fatty acid supplementation of women during pregnancy or breastfeeding is beneficial to infants. It has been suggested that high intake of omega-3 fatty acids during pregnancy, particularly DHA, may increase birth weight and gestational length. However, higher doses may not be advisable due to the potential risk of bleeding. Fatty acids are added to some infant formulas.

Interactions

Most herbs and supplements have not been thoroughly tested for interactions with other herbs, supplements, drugs, or foods. The interactions listed in this section are based on reports in scientific publications, laboratory experiments, or traditional use. You should always read product labels. If you have a medical condition, or are taking other drugs, herbs, or supplements, you should speak with a qualified health care provider before starting a new therapy.

Interactions with Drugs

In theory, omega-3 fatty acids may increase the risk of bleeding when taken with drugs that increase the risk of bleeding. Some examples include aspirin, anticoagulants ("blood thinners") such as warfarin (Coumadin®) or heparin, anti-platelet drugs such as clopidogrel (Plavix®), and non-steroidal anti-inflammatory drugs such as ibuprofen (Motrin®, Advil®) or naproxen (Naprosyn®, Aleve®).

Based on human studies, omega-3 fatty acids may lower blood pressure and add to the effects of drugs that may also affect blood pressure.

Fish oil supplements may lower blood sugar levels a small amount. Caution is advised when using medications that may also lower blood sugar. Patients taking drugs for diabetes by mouth or insulin should be monitored closely by a qualified health care provider. Medication adjustments may be necessary.

Omega-3 fatty acids lower triglyceride levels but can actually increase (worsen) low-density lipoprotein (LDL/"bad cholesterol") levels by a small amount. Therefore, omega-3 fatty acids may add to the triglyceride-lowering effects of agents like niacin/nicotinic acid, fibrates such as gemfibrozil (Lopid®), or resins such as cholestyramine (Questran®). However, omega-3 fatty acids may work against the LDL-lowering properties of "statin" drugs like atorvastatin (Lipitor®) and lovastatin (Mevacor®).

Interactions with Herbs and Dietary Supplements

In theory, omega-3 fatty acids may increase the risk of bleeding when taken with herbs and supplements that are believed to increase the risk of bleeding. Multiple cases of bleeding have been reported with the use of *Ginkgo biloba* and fewer cases with garlic and saw palmetto. Numerous other agents may theoretically increase the risk of bleeding, although this has not been proven in most cases.

Based on human studies, omega-3 fatty acids may lower blood pressure and theoretically may add to the effects of agents that may also affect blood pressure.

Fish oil supplements may lower blood sugar levels a small amount. Caution is advised when using herbs or supplements that may also lower blood sugar. Blood glucose levels may require monitoring, and doses may need adjustment.

Omega-3 fatty acids lower triglyceride levels but can actually increase (worsen) low-density lipoprotein (LDL/"bad cholesterol") levels by a small amount. Therefore, omega-3 fatty acids may add to the triglyceride-lowering effects of agents like niacin/nicotinic acid but may work against the potential LDL-lowering properties of agents like barley, garlic, guggul, psyllium, soy, or sweet almond.

Fish oil taken for many months may cause a deficiency of vitamin E, and therefore vitamin E is added to many commercial fish oil products. As a result, regular use of vitamin E–enriched products may lead to elevated levels of this fat-soluble vitamin. Fish liver oil contains the fat-soluble vitamins A and D, and therefore fish liver oil products (such as cod liver oil) may increase the risk of vitamin A or D toxicity. Since fat-soluble vitamins can build up in the body and cause toxicity, patients taking multiple vitamins regularly or in high doses should discuss this risk with their health care practitioners.

Section 9.3

Current Recommendations about the Role of Omega 6 Fatty Acids

"Omega-6 Fatty Acids: Make Them a Part of
Heart-Healthy Eating," reprinted with permission from
www.heart.org. © 2009 American Heart Association, Inc.

Omega-6 fatty acids—found in vegetable oils, nuts, and seeds—are a beneficial part of a heart-healthy eating plan, according to a science advisory published in *Circulation: Journal of the American Heart Association.*

View the full Omega-6 Advisory at circ.ahajournals.org/cgi/reprint/ CIRCULATIONAHA.108.191627.

The association recommends that people aim for at least 5% to 10% of calories from omega-6 fatty acids. Most Americans actually get enough of these oils in the foods they are currently eating, such as nuts, cooking oils, and salad dressings, the advisory reports. Recommended daily servings of omega-6 depend on physical activity level, age, and gender, but range from 12 to 22 grams per day.

Omega-6, and the similarly named omega-3 fatty acids (found in fattier fish such as tuna, mackerel, and salmon), are called polyunsaturated fatty acids (PUFA) and can have health benefits when consumed in the recommended amounts, especially when used to replace saturated fats or trans fats in the diet. Omega-6 and omega-3 PUFA play a crucial role in heart and brain function and in normal growth and development. PUFA are "essential" fats that your body needs but can't produce, so you must get them from food.

For more on good fats vs. bad fats, visit www.AmericanHeart.org/ FacetheFats.

"Of course, as with any news about a single nutrient, it's important to remember to focus on an overall healthy dietary pattern—one nutrient or one type of food isn't a cure-all," said William Harris, PhD, lead author of the advisory. "Our goal was simply to let Americans know that foods containing omega-6 fatty acids can be part of a healthy diet, and can even help improve your cardiovascular risk profile."

The American Heart Association's dietary recommendations suggest a broadly defined healthy eating pattern over time—with an emphasis on fruits, vegetables, high-fiber whole grains, lean meat, poultry, and fish twice a week. Diets rich in fruits, vegetables, and whole grains have been associated in a large number of studies with reduced cardiovascular risk.

Linoleic acid (LA) is the main omega-6 fatty acid in foods, accounting for 85% to 90% of the dietary omega-6 PUFA.

There has been some debate within the nutrition community regarding the benefits of omega-6 based on the belief that they may promote inflammation, thus increasing cardiovascular risk. "That idea is based more on assumptions and extrapolations than on hard data," said Harris, a research professor for the Sanford School of Medicine at the University of South Dakota [USD] and director of the Metabolism and Nutrition Research Center at Sanford Research/USD.

The linking of omega-6 intake to inflammation stems from the fact that arachidonic acid (AA), which can be formed from LA, is involved in the early stages of inflammation. However, the advisory explains that AA and LA also give rise to anti-inflammatory molecules.

For example, in the cells that form the lining of blood vessels, omega-6 PUFA have anti-inflammatory properties, suppressing the production of adhesion molecules, chemokines, and interleukins—all of which are key mediators of the atherosclerotic process. "Thus, it is incorrect to view the omega-6 fatty acids as 'pro-inflammatory,' " Harris explained. "Eating less LA will not lower tissue levels of AA (the usual rationale for reducing LA intakes) because the body tightly regulates the synthesis of AA from LA."

The advisory reviewed a meta-analysis of randomized, controlled trials, and more than two dozen observational, cohort, case/control, and ecological reports.

Observational studies showed that people who ate the most omega-6 fatty acids usually had the least heart disease. Other studies examined blood levels of omega-6 in heart patients compared with healthy people and found that patients with heart disease had lower levels of omega-6 in their blood.

In controlled trials in which researchers randomly assigned people to consume diets containing high versus low levels of omega-6 and then recorded the number of heart attacks over several years, those assigned to the higher omega-6 diets had less heart disease.

A meta-analysis of several trials indicated that replacing saturated fats with PUFA lowered risk for heart disease events by 24%. "When saturated fat in the diet is replaced by omega-6 PUFA, the blood cholesterol levels go down," Harris said. "This may be part of the reason why higher omega-6 diets are heart-healthy."

Co-authors are: Dariush Mozaffarian, MD; Eric Rimm, DSc.; Penny Kris-Etherton, PhD; Lawrence Rudel, PhD; Lawrence Appel, MD; Marguerite Engler, PhD; Mary Engler, PhD; and Frank Sacks, MD. Author disclosures are on the manuscript.

The American Heart Association receives funding primarily from individuals; foundations and corporations (including pharmaceutical, device manufacturers, and other companies) also make donations and fund specific association programs and events. The association has strict policies to prevent these relationships from influencing the science content. Revenues from pharmaceutical and device corporations are disclosed at www.americanheart.org/corporatefunding.

Chapter 10

Fruits and Vegetables

Chapter Contents

Section 10.1

Fruits

This section excerpted from "Food Groups: Fruits," ChoseMyPlate.gov, U.S. Department of Agriculture (www.choosemyplate.gov), May 31, 2011.

Key consumer message: Make half your plate fruits and vegetables.

What Foods Are in the Fruit Group?

Any fruit or 100% fruit juice counts as part of the fruit group. Fruits may be fresh, canned, frozen, or dried, and may be whole, cut up, or pureed. Some commonly eaten fruits are the following:

- Apples
- Apricots
- Bananas
- Berries
  - Strawberries
  - Blueberries
  - Raspberries
- Cherries
- Grapefruit
- Grapes
- Kiwi fruit
- Lemons
- Limes
- Mangoes
- Melons
  - Cantaloupe
  - Honeydew
  - Watermelon
- Mixed fruit cocktail
- Nectarines
- Oranges
- Peaches
- Pears
- Papaya
- Pineapple
- Plums
- Prunes
- Raisins
- Tangerines
- 100% fruit juice
  - Orange
  - Apple
  - Grape
  - Grapefruit

How Much Fruit Is Needed Daily?

The amount of fruit you need to eat depends on age, sex, and level of physical activity. Recommended amounts are shown in Table 10.1.

Table 10.1. Recommended Daily Fruit Servings

	Age	Daily Recommendation*
Children	2–3 years old	1 cup
	4–8 years old	1 to 1 1/2 cups
Girls	9–13 years old	1 1/2 cups
	14–18 years old	1 1/2 cups
Boys	9–13 years old	1 1/2 cups
	14–18 years old	2 cups
Women	19–30 years old	2 cups
	31–50 years old	1 1/2 cups
	51+ years old	1 1/2 cups
Men	19–30 years old	2 cups
	31–50 years old	2 cups
	51+ years old	2 cups

* These amounts are appropriate for individuals who get less than 30 minutes per day of moderate physical activity, beyond normal daily activities. Those who are more physically active may be able to consume more while staying within calorie needs.

What Counts as a Cup of Fruit?

In general, 1 cup of fruit or 100% fruit juice, or 1/2 cup of dried fruit, can be considered as 1 cup from the fruit group.

Why Is It Important to Eat Fruit?

Eating fruit provides health benefits—people who eat more fruits and vegetables as part of an overall healthy diet are likely to have a reduced risk of some chronic diseases. Fruits provide nutrients vital for health and maintenance of your body.

Health Benefits

- Eating a diet rich in some vegetables and fruits as part of an overall healthy diet may reduce risk for heart disease, including heart attack and stroke, and may protect against certain types of cancers.

- Diets rich in foods containing fiber, such as some vegetables and fruits, may reduce the risk of heart disease, obesity, and type 2 diabetes.

- Eating vegetables and fruits rich in potassium as part of an overall healthy diet may lower blood pressure, and may also reduce the risk of developing kidney stones and help to decrease bone loss.

Nutrients

- Most fruits are naturally low in fat, sodium, and calories. None have cholesterol.

- Fruits are sources of many essential nutrients that are under consumed, including potassium, dietary fiber, vitamin C, and folate (folic acid).

- Diets rich in potassium may help to maintain healthy blood pressure. Fruit sources of potassium include bananas, prunes and prune juice, dried peaches and apricots, cantaloupe, honeydew melon, and orange juice.

- Dietary fiber from fruits, as part of an overall healthy diet, helps reduce blood cholesterol levels and may lower risk of heart disease. Fiber is important for proper bowel function. Whole or cut-up fruits are sources of dietary fiber; fruit juices contain little or no fiber.

- Vitamin C is important for growth and repair of all body tissues, helps heal cuts and wounds, and keeps teeth and gums healthy.

Tips to Help You Eat Fruits

- Keep a bowl of whole fruit on the table, counter, or in the refrigerator.

- Refrigerate cut-up fruit to store for later.

- Buy fruits that are dried, frozen, and canned (in water or 100% juice) as well as fresh, so that you always have a supply on hand.

- Consider convenience when shopping. Try precut packages of fruit (such as melon or pineapple chunks) for a healthy snack in seconds. Choose packaged fruits that do not have added sugars.

For the Best Nutritional Value

- Make most of your choices whole or cut-up fruit rather than juice, for the benefits dietary fiber provides.

- Select fruits with more potassium often.

- When choosing canned fruits, select fruit canned in 100% fruit juice or water rather than syrup.
- Vary your fruit choices. Fruits differ in nutrient content.

At Meals

- At breakfast, top your cereal with bananas or peaches; add blueberries to pancakes; drink 100% orange or grapefruit juice. Or, mix fresh fruit with plain fat-free or low-fat yogurt.
- At lunch, pack a tangerine, banana, or grapes to eat, or choose fruits from a salad bar. Individual containers of fruits like peaches or applesauce are easy and convenient.
- At dinner, add crushed pineapple to coleslaw, or include orange sections or grapes in a tossed salad.
- Try meat dishes that incorporate fruit, such as chicken with apricots or mangoes.
- Add fruit like pineapple or peaches to kabobs as part of a barbecue meal.
- For dessert, have baked apples, pears, or a fruit salad.

As Snacks

- Cut-up fruit makes a great snack. Either cut them yourself, or buy precut packages of fruit pieces like pineapples or melons. Or, try whole fresh berries or grapes.
- Dried fruits also make a great snack. They are easy to carry and store well. Because they are dried, 1/4 cup is equivalent to 1/2 cup of other fruits.
- Frozen juice bars (100% juice) make healthy alternatives to high-fat snacks.

Make Fruit More Appealing

- Many fruits taste great with a low-fat dip or dressing.
- Make a fruit smoothie by blending fat-free or low-fat milk or yogurt with fresh or frozen fruit.
- Try unsweetened applesauce as a lower calorie substitute for some of the oil when baking cakes.

- For fresh fruit salads, mix apples, bananas, or pears with acidic fruits like oranges, pineapple, or lemon juice to keep them from turning brown.

Fruit Tips for Children

- Set a good example for children by eating fruit every day with meals or as snacks.

- Depending on their age, children can help shop for, clean, peel, or cut up fruits.

- Decorate plates or serving dishes with fruit slices.

- Pack a juice box (100% juice) in children's lunches instead of soda or other sugar-sweetened beverages.

- Look for and choose fruit options, such as sliced apples, mixed fruit cup, or 100% fruit juice, in fast food restaurants.

Section 10.2

Vegetables

This section excerpted from "Food Groups: Vegetables," ChoseMyPlate.gov, U.S. Department of Agriculture (www.choosemyplate.gov), June 8, 2011.

Key consumer message: Make half your plate fruits and vegetables.

What Foods Are in the Vegetable Group?

Any vegetable or 100% vegetable juice counts as a member of the vegetable group. Vegetables may be raw or cooked; fresh, frozen, canned, or dried/dehydrated; and may be whole, cut up, or mashed.

Vegetables are organized into five subgroups, based on their nutrient content. Some commonly eaten vegetables in each subgroup are listed here:

Dark Green Vegetables

- Bok choy
- Dark green leafy lettuce
- Mustard greens
- Turnip greens
- Broccoli
- Kale
- Romaine lettuce
- Watercress
- Collard greens
- Mesclun
- Spinach

Red and Orange Vegetables

- Acorn squash
- Pumpkin
- Tomatoes
- Butternut squash
- Red peppers
- Tomato juice
- Carrots
- Sweet potatoes

Beans and Peas

- Black beans
- Garbanzo beans (chickpeas)
- Lentils
- Navy beans
- Soy beans
- White beans
- Black-eyed peas
- Kidney beans
- Lima beans (mature)
- Pinto beans
- Split peas

Starchy Vegetables

- Corn
- Lima beans (green)
- Potatoes
- Green peas
- Plantains

Other Vegetables

- Artichokes
- Bean sprouts
- Cabbage
- Cucumbers
- Green peppers
- Okra
- Turnips
- Asparagus
- Beets
- Cauliflower
- Eggplant
- Iceberg (head) lettuce
- Onions
- Wax beans
- Avocado
- Brussels sprouts
- Celery
- Green beans
- Mushrooms
- Parsnips
- Zucchini

How Many Vegetables Are Needed Daily or Weekly?

Vegetable choices should be selected from among the vegetable subgroups. It is not necessary to eat vegetables from each subgroup daily. However, over a week, try to consume the amounts listed from each subgroup as a way to reach your daily intake recommendation.

The amount of vegetables you need to eat depends on your age, sex, and level of physical activity. Recommended total daily amounts are shown in Table 10.2. Recommended weekly amounts from each vegetable subgroup are shown in Table 10.3.

What Counts as a Cup of Vegetables?

In general, 1 cup of raw or cooked vegetables or vegetable juice, or 2 cups of raw leafy greens, can be considered as 1 cup from the vegetable group.

Why Is It Important to Eat Vegetables?

Eating vegetables provides health benefits—people who eat more vegetables and fruits as part of an overall healthy diet are likely to have a reduced risk of some chronic diseases. Vegetables provide nutrients vital for health and maintenance of your body.

Health Benefits

- Eating a diet rich in some vegetables and fruits as part of an overall healthy diet may reduce risk for heart disease, including heart attack and stroke, and may protect against certain types of cancers.

- Diets rich in foods containing fiber, such as some vegetables and fruits, may reduce the risk of heart disease, obesity, and type 2 diabetes.

- Eating vegetables and fruits rich in potassium as part of an overall healthy diet may lower blood pressure, and may also reduce the risk of developing kidney stones and help to decrease bone loss.

Nutrients

- Most vegetables are naturally low in fat and calories. None have cholesterol. (Sauces or seasonings may add fat, calories, or cholesterol.)

Table 10.2. Recommended Daily Vegetable Servings

	Age	Daily Recommendation*
Children	2–3 years old	1 cup
	4–8 years old	1 1/2 cups
Girls	9–13 years old	2 cups
	14–18 years old	2 1/2 cups
Boys	9–13 years old	2 1/2 cups
	14–18 years old	3 cups
Women	19–30 years old	2 1/2 cups
	31–50 years old	2 1/2 cups
	51+ years old	2 cups
Men	19–30 years old	3 cups
	31–50 years old	3 cups
	51+ years old	2 1/2 cups

* These amounts are appropriate for individuals who get less than 30 minutes per day of moderate physical activity, beyond normal daily activities. Those who are more physically active may be able to consume more while staying within calorie needs.

Table 10.3. Recommended Weekly Vegetable Servings by Subgroup

	Age	Dark Green Vegetables	Red & Orange Vegetables	Beans and Peas	Starchy Vegetables	Other Vegetables
Children	2–3 years old	1/2 cup	2 1/2 cups	1/2 cup	2 cups	1 1/2 cups
	4–8 years old	1 cup	3 cups	1/2 cup	3 1/2 cups	2 1/2 cups
Girls	9–13 years old	1 1/2 cups	4 cups	1 cup	4 cups	3 1/2 cups
	14–18 years old	1 1/2 cups	5 1/2 cups	1 1/2 cups	5 cups	4 cups
Boys	9–13 years old	1 1/2 cups	5 1/2 cups	1 1/2 cups	5 cups	4 cups
	14–18 yrs old	2 cups	6 cups	2 cups	6 cups	5 cups
Women	19–30 yrs old	1 1/2 cups	5 1/2 cups	1 1/2 cups	5 cups	4 cups
	31–50 yrs old	1 1/2 cups	5 1/2 cups	1 1/2 cups	5 cups	4 cups
	51+ yrs old	1 1/2 cups	4 cups	1 cup	4 cups	3 1/2 cups
Men	19–30 yrs old	2 cups	6 cups	2 cups	6 cups	5 cups
	31–50 yrs old	2 cups	6 cups	2 cups	6 cups	5 cups
	51+ yrs old	1 1/2 cups	5 1/2 cups	1 1/2 cups	5 cups	4 cups

- Vegetables are important sources of many nutrients, including potassium, dietary fiber, folate (folic acid), vitamin A, and vitamin C.

- Diets rich in potassium may help to maintain healthy blood pressure. Vegetable sources of potassium include sweet potatoes, white potatoes, white beans, tomato products (paste, sauce, and juice), beet greens, soybeans, lima beans, spinach, lentils, and kidney beans.

- Dietary fiber from vegetables, as part of an overall healthy diet, helps reduce blood cholesterol levels and may lower risk of heart disease. Fiber is important for proper bowel function.

- Vitamin A keeps eyes and skin healthy and helps to protect against infections.

- Vitamin C helps heal cuts and wounds and keeps teeth and gums healthy. Vitamin C aids in iron absorption.

Tips to Help You Eat Vegetables

- Buy fresh vegetables in season. They cost less and are likely to be at their peak flavor.

- Stock up on frozen vegetables for quick and easy cooking in the microwave.

- Buy vegetables that are easy to prepare. Pick up pre-washed bags of salad greens and add baby carrots or grape tomatoes for a salad. Buy packages of baby carrots or celery sticks for snacks.

For the Best Nutritional Value

- Select vegetables with more potassium often.

- Sauces or seasonings can add calories, saturated fat, and sodium to vegetables. Use the Nutrition Facts label to compare the calories and % Daily Value for saturated fat and sodium in plain and seasoned vegetables.

- Prepare more foods from fresh ingredients to lower sodium intake. Most sodium in the food supply comes from packaged or processed foods.

- Buy canned vegetables labeled "reduced sodium," "low sodium," or "no salt added."

At Meals

- Plan some meals around a vegetable main dish, such as a vegetable stir-fry or soup. Then add other foods to complement it.

- Try a main dish salad for lunch. Go light on the salad dressing.

- Include a green salad with your dinner every night.

- Shred carrots or zucchini into meatloaf, casseroles, quick breads, and muffins.

- Include chopped vegetables in pasta sauce or lasagna.

- Order a veggie pizza with toppings like mushrooms, green peppers, and onions, and ask for extra veggies.

- Use pureed, cooked vegetables such as potatoes to thicken stews, soups, and gravies. These add flavor, nutrients, and texture.

- Grill vegetable kabobs as part of a barbecue meal. Try tomatoes, mushrooms, green peppers, and onions.

Make Vegetables More Appealing

- Many vegetables taste great with a low-fat dip or dressing.

- Add color to salads by adding baby carrots, shredded red cabbage, or spinach leaves.

- Include beans or peas in flavorful mixed dishes, such as chili or minestrone soup.

- Keep a bowl of cut-up vegetables in a see-through container in the refrigerator.

Vegetable Tips for Children

- Set a good example for children by eating vegetables with meals and as snacks.

- Let children decide on the dinner vegetables or what goes into salads.

- Depending on their age, children can help shop for, clean, peel, or cut up vegetables.

- Use cut-up vegetables as part of afternoon snacks.

- Children often prefer foods served separately. So, rather than mixed vegetables try serving two vegetables separately.

Section 10.3

Fruits and Vegetables and Healthy Weight

"How to Use Fruits and Vegetables to Help Manage Your Weight," Centers for Disease Control and Prevention (www.cdc.gov), February 15, 2011.

Fruits and vegetables are part of a well-balanced and healthy eating plan. There are many different ways to lose or maintain a healthy weight. Using more fruits and vegetables along with whole grains and lean meats, nuts, and beans is a safe and healthy one. Helping control your weight is not the only benefit of eating more fruits and vegetables. Diets rich in fruits and vegetables may reduce the risk of some types of cancer and other chronic diseases. Fruits and vegetables also provide essential vitamins and minerals, fiber, and other substances that are important for good health.

To lose weight, you must eat fewer calories than your body uses. This doesn't necessarily mean that you have to eat less food. You can create lower-calorie versions of some of your favorite dishes by substituting low-calorie fruits and vegetables in place of higher-calorie ingredients. The water and fiber in fruits and vegetables will add volume to your dishes, so you can eat the same amount of food with fewer calories. Most fruits and vegetables are naturally low in fat and calories and are filling.

Here are some simple ways to cut calories and eat fruits and vegetables throughout your day:

Breakfast: Start the Day Right

- Substitute some spinach, onions, or mushrooms for one of the eggs or half of the cheese in your morning omelet. The vegetables will add volume and flavor to the dish with fewer calories than the egg or cheese.

- Cut back on the amount of cereal in your bowl to make room for some cut-up bananas, peaches, or strawberries. You can still eat a full bowl, but with fewer calories.

Lighten Up Your Lunch

- Substitute vegetables such as lettuce, tomatoes, cucumbers, or onions for two ounces of the cheese and two ounces of the meat in your sandwich, wrap, or burrito. The new version will fill you up with fewer calories than the original.

- Add a cup of chopped vegetables, such as broccoli, carrots, beans, or red peppers, in place of two ounces of the meat or one cup of noodles in your favorite broth-based soup. The vegetables will help fill you up, so you won't miss those extra calories.

Dinner

- Add in one cup of chopped vegetables such as broccoli, tomatoes, squash, onions, or peppers, while removing one cup of the rice or pasta in your favorite dish. The dish with the vegetables will be just as satisfying but have fewer calories than the same amount of the original version.

- Take a good look at your dinner plate. Vegetables, fruit, and whole grains should take up the largest portion of your plate. If they do not, replace some of the meat, cheese, white pasta, or rice with legumes, steamed broccoli, asparagus, greens, or another favorite vegetable. This will reduce the total calories in your meal without reducing the amount of food you eat. But re-member to use a normal- or small-size plate—not a platter. The total number of calories you eat counts, even if a good proportion of them come from fruits and vegetables.

Smart Snacks

- Most healthy eating plans allow for one or two small snacks a day. Choosing most fruits and vegetables will allow you to eat a snack with only 100 calories.

- Instead of a high-calorie snack from a vending machine, bring some cut-up vegetables or fruit from home. One snack-sized bag of corn chips (1 ounce) has the same number of calories as a small apple, 1 cup of whole strawberries, *and* 1 cup of carrots with 1/4 cup of low-calorie dip. Substitute one or two of these options for the chips, and you will have a satisfying snack with fewer calories.

Remember: Substitution is the key. It's true that fruits and vegetables are lower in calories than many other foods, but they do contain some calories. If you start eating fruits and vegetables in addition to what you usually eat, you are adding calories and may gain weight. The key is substitution. Eat fruits and vegetables instead of some other higher-calorie food.

More Tips for Making Fruits and Vegetables Part of Your Weight-Management Plan

Eat fruits and vegetables the way nature provided—or with fat-free or low-fat cooking techniques. Try steaming your vegetables, using low-calorie or low-fat dressings, and using herbs and spices to add flavor. Some cooking techniques, such as breading and frying, or using high-fat dressings or sauces, will greatly increase the calories and fat in the dish. And eat your fruit raw to enjoy its natural sweetness.

Canned or frozen fruits and vegetables are good options when fresh produce is not available. However, be careful to choose those without added sugar, syrup, cream sauces, or other ingredients that will add calories.

Choose whole fruit over fruit drinks and juices. Fruit juices have lost fiber from the fruit. It is better to eat the whole fruit because it contains the added fiber that helps you feel full. One 6-ounce serving of orange juice has 85 calories, compared to just 65 calories in a medium orange.

Whole fruit gives you a bigger size snack than the same fruit dried— for the same number of calories. A small box of raisins (1/4 cup) is about 100 calories. For the same number of calories, you can eat 1 cup of grapes.

Chapter 11

Milk and Dairy Products

Key consumer message: Switch to fat-free or low-fat (1%) milk.

What Foods Are Included in the Dairy Group?

All fluid milk products and many foods made from milk are considered part of this food group. Most dairy group choices should be fat free or low fat. Foods made from milk that retain their calcium content are part of the group. Foods made from milk that have little to no calcium, such as cream cheese, cream, and butter, are not. Calcium-fortified soymilk (soy beverage) is also part of the dairy group.

Some commonly eaten choices in the dairy group are the following:

Milk

- All fluid milk
  - Fat free (skim)
  - Low fat (1%)
  - Reduced fat (2%)
  - Whole milk
- Flavored milks
  - Chocolate
  - Strawberry
- Lactose-reduced milks
- Lactose-free milks

This section excerpted from "Food Groups: Dairy," ChoseMyPlate.gov, U.S. Department of Agriculture (www.choosemyplate.gov), May 31, 2011.

Milk-Based Desserts

- Puddings made with milk
- Frozen yogurt
- Ice milk
- Ice cream

Calcium-Fortified Soymilk

- Soy beverage

Cheese

- Hard natural cheeses
  - Cheddar
  - Mozzarella
  - Swiss
  - Parmesan
- Soft cheeses
  - Ricotta
  - Cottage cheese
- Processed cheeses
  - American

Yogurt

- All yogurt
  - Fat free
  - Reduced fat
- Low fat
- Whole-milk yogurt

Selection Tips

Choose fat-free or low-fat milk, yogurt, and cheese. If you choose milk or yogurt that is not fat free, or cheese that is not low fat, the fat in the product counts against your maximum limit for "empty calories" (calories from solid fats and added sugars).

If sweetened milk products are chosen (flavored milk, yogurt, drinkable yogurt, desserts), the added sugars also count against your maximum limit for "empty calories."

For those who are lactose intolerant, smaller portions (such as four fluid ounces of milk) may be well tolerated. Lactose-free and lower-lactose products are available. These include lactose-reduced or lactose-free milk, yogurt, and cheese, and calcium-fortified soymilk (soy beverage). Also, enzyme preparations can be added to milk to lower the lactose content. Calcium-fortified foods and beverages such as cereals, orange juice, rice milk, or almond milk may provide calcium, but may not provide the other nutrients found in dairy products.

How Much Food from the Dairy Group Is Needed Daily?

The amount of food from the dairy group you need to eat depends on age. Recommended daily amounts are shown in the following list of daily recommendations.

- Children 2–3 years old: 2 cups
- Children 4–8 years old: 2 1/2 cups
- Girls 9–18 years old: 3 cups
- Boys 9–18 years old: 3 cups
- Women 19+ years: 3 cups
- Men 19+ years: 3 cups

What Counts as 1 Cup in the Dairy Group?

In general, 1 cup of milk or yogurt, 1 1/2 ounces of natural cheese, or 2 ounces of processed cheese can be considered as 1 cup from the dairy group. Additionally, 1 cup of soymilk counts as 1 cup in the dairy group.

Health Benefits and Nutrients

Consuming dairy products provides health benefits—especially improved bone health. Foods in the dairy group provide nutrients that are vital for health and maintenance of your body. These nutrients include calcium, potassium, vitamin D, and protein.

Health Benefits

- Intake of dairy products is linked to improved bone health, and may reduce the risk of osteoporosis.
- The intake of dairy products is especially important to bone health during childhood and adolescence, when bone mass is being built.
- Intake of dairy products is also associated with a reduced risk of cardiovascular disease and type 2 diabetes, and with lower blood pressure in adults.

Nutrients

- Calcium is used for building bones and teeth and in maintaining bone mass. Dairy products are the primary source of calcium in American diets. Diets that provide three cups or the equivalent of dairy products per day can improve bone mass.
- Diets rich in potassium may help to maintain healthy blood pressure. Dairy products, especially yogurt, fluid milk, and soymilk (soy beverage), provide potassium.
- Vitamin D functions in the body to maintain proper levels of calcium and phosphorous, thereby helping to build and maintain

bones. Milk and soymilk (soy beverage) that are fortified with vitamin D are good sources of this nutrient.

Why is it important to make fat-free or low-fat choices from the Dairy Group? Choosing foods from the dairy group that are high in saturated fats and cholesterol can have health implications. Diets high in saturated fats raise "bad" cholesterol (low-density lipoprotein, or LDL) levels in the blood. High LDL cholesterol, in turn, increases the risk for coronary heart disease. Many cheeses, whole milk, and products made from them are high in saturated fat. To help keep blood cholesterol levels healthy, limit the amount of these foods you eat.

Tips for Making Wise Choices in the Dairy Group

- Include milk or calcium-fortified soymilk as a beverage at meals. Choose fat-free or low-fat milk.
- If you usually drink whole milk, switch gradually to fat-free milk, to lower saturated fat and calories.
- If you drink cappuccinos or lattes—ask for them with fat-free (skim) milk.
- Add fat-free or low-fat milk instead of water to oatmeal and hot cereals.
- Use fat-free or low-fat milk when making condensed cream soups (such as cream of tomato).
- Have fat-free or low-fat yogurt as a snack.
- Make a dip for fruits or vegetables from yogurt.
- Make fruit-yogurt smoothies in the blender.
- For dessert, make chocolate or butterscotch pudding with fat-free or low-fat milk.
- Top cut-up fruit with flavored yogurt for a quick dessert.
- Top casseroles, soups, stews, or vegetables with shredded reduced-fat or low-fat cheese.
- Top a baked potato with fat-free or low-fat yogurt.

For Those Who Choose Not to Consume Milk Products

- If you avoid milk because of lactose intolerance, the most reliable way to get the health benefits of dairy products is to choose lactose-free alternatives within the dairy group, such as cheese, yogurt, lactose-free milk, or calcium-fortified soymilk (soy beverage) or to consume the enzyme lactase before consuming milk.

Chapter 12

Dietary Fiber

Most of us know that fiber is one of those good-for-you nutrients. But you don't have to eat gravelly, tooth-breaking cereal to get it. Some of the best and most delicious foods have loads of fiber. Find out how to get your fill of fiber without sacrificing good taste—or tooth enamel!

Why Fiber Is Your Friend

So, what exactly is fiber? Why do you need it and what food should you eat to get it?

The term fiber refers to carbohydrates that cannot be digested. Fiber is found in the plants we eat for food—fruits, vegetables, grains, and legumes. Sometimes, a distinction is made between soluble fiber and insoluble fiber:

- Soluble fiber partially dissolves in water and has been shown to lower cholesterol.

- Insoluble fiber does not dissolve in water, but that's why it helps with constipation.

It's important to include both kinds of fiber as part of a healthy diet.

"Fiber," May 2007, reprinted with permission from www.kidshealth.org. Copyright © 2007 The Nemours Foundation. This information was provided by KidsHealth, one of the largest resources online for medically reviewed health information written for parents, kids, and teens. For more articles like this one, visit www.KidsHealth.org, or www.TeensHealth.org.

A diet that includes foods that are rich in fiber can help lower blood cholesterol and prevent diabetes and heart disease. When carbohydrates are combined with fiber, it slows the absorption of sugar and regulates insulin response. And foods with fiber make us feel full, which discourages overeating.

Also, fiber itself has no calories, and adequate amounts of fiber help move food through the digestive system, promoting healthy bowel function and protecting against constipation.

Figuring Out Fiber

Great sources of fiber include:

- whole-grain breads and cereals;
- fruits like apples, oranges, bananas, berries, prunes, and pears;
- green peas;
- legumes (split peas, soy, lentils, etc.);
- artichokes;
- almonds.

Look for the fiber content of foods on the nutrition labels—it's listed as part of the information given for "total carbohydrates." A high-fiber food has 5 grams or more of fiber per serving, and a good source of fiber is one that provides 2.5 to 4.9 grams per serving.

Here's how some fiber-friendly foods stack up:

- 1/2 cup (118 milliliters) cooked navy beans (9.5 grams of fiber)
- 1/2 cup (118 milliliters) cooked lima beans (6.6 grams)
- 1 medium baked sweet potato with peel (4.8 grams)
- 1 whole-wheat English muffin (4.4 grams)
- 1/2 cup (118 milliliters) of cooked green peas (4.4 grams)
- 1 medium pear with skin (4 grams)
- 1/2 cup (118 milliliters) raspberries (4 grams)
- 1 medium baked potato with peel left on (3.8 grams)
- 1/4 cup (59 milliliters) oat bran cereal (3.6 grams)
- 1 ounce (28 grams) almonds (3.3 grams)
- 1 medium apple with skin (3.3 grams)

- 1/2 cup (118 milliliters) raisins (3 grams)
- 1/4 cup (59 milliliters) baked beans (3 grams)
- 1 medium orange (3 grams)
- 1 medium banana (3 grams)
- 1/2 cup (118 milliliters) canned sauerkraut (3 grams)

Making Fiber Part of Your Diet

An easy way to figure out how much fiber you need is to follow the "age + 5" rule. For example, if you are 14 years old, you should try to eat at least 19 grams of fiber every day (14 + 5 = 19). The best sources are fresh fruits and vegetables, nuts and legumes, and whole-grain foods.

You probably eat some fiber every day without even realizing it, but here are some simple ways to make sure you're getting enough.

Breakfast

- Have a bowl of hot oatmeal.
- Opt for whole-grain cereals that list ingredients such as whole wheat or oats as one of the first few items on the ingredient list.
- Top fiber-rich cereal with apples, oranges, berries, or bananas. Add almonds to pack even more fiber punch.
- Try bran or whole-grain waffles or pancakes topped with apples, berries, or raisins.
- Enjoy whole-wheat bagels or English muffins instead of white toast.

Lunch and Dinner

- Make sandwiches with whole-grain breads (rye, oat, or wheat) instead of white.
- Make a fiber-rich sandwich with whole-grain bread, peanut butter, and bananas.
- Use whole-grain spaghetti and other pastas instead of white.
- Try wild or brown rice with meals instead of white rice. Add beans (kidney, black, navy, and pinto) to rice dishes for even more fiber.
- Spice up salads with berries and almonds, chickpeas, cooked artichokes, and beans (kidney, black, navy, or pinto).

- Use whole-grain (corn or whole wheat) soft-taco shells or tortillas to make burritos or wraps. Fill them with eggs and cheese for breakfast; turkey, cheese, lettuce, tomato, and light dressing for lunch; and beans, salsa, taco sauce, and cheese for dinner.

- Add lentils or whole-grain barley to your favorite soups.

- Create mini-pizzas by topping whole-wheat English muffins or bagels with pizza sauce, low-fat cheese, mushrooms, and chunks of grilled chicken.

- Add a little bran to meatloaf or burgers.

- Sweet potatoes, with the skins, are tasty side dishes.

- Top low-fat hot dogs or veggie dogs with sauerkraut and serve them on whole-wheat hot dog buns.

- Take fresh fruit when you pack lunch for school. Pears, apples, bananas, oranges, and berries are all high in fiber.

Snacks and Treats

- Bake cookies or muffins using whole-wheat flour instead of white. Add raisins, berries, bananas, or chopped or pureed apples to the mix for even more fiber.

- Add bran to baking items such as cookies and muffins.

- Top whole-wheat crackers with peanut butter or low-fat cheese.

- Go easy on the butter and salt and enjoy popcorn while watching TV or movies.

- Top ice cream, frozen yogurt, or regular yogurt with whole-grain cereal, berries, or almonds for some added nutrition and crunch.

- Try apples topped with peanut butter.

- Make fruit salad with pears, apples, bananas, oranges, and berries. Top with almonds for added crunch. Serve as a side dish with meals or alone as a snack.

- Make low-fat breads, muffins, or cookies with canned pumpkin.

- Leave the skins on fruits and veggies (but wash all produce before eating).

- Eat whole fruits instead of drinking fruit juices.

- Snack on raw vegetables instead of chips, crackers, or chocolate bars.

Chapter 13

Grains and Healthy Whole Grains

Key consumer message: Make at least half your grains whole.

What Foods Are in the Grain Group?

Any food made from wheat, rice, oats, cornmeal, barley, or another cereal grain is a grain product. Bread, pasta, oatmeal, breakfast cereals, tortillas, and grits are examples of grain products.

Grains are divided into two subgroups, *whole grains* and *refined grains*.

Whole grains contain the entire grain kernel—the bran, germ, and endosperm. Examples include the following:

- Whole-wheat flour
- Oatmeal
- Brown rice
- Bulgur (cracked wheat)
- Whole cornmeal

Refined grains have been milled, a process that removes the bran and germ. This is done to give grains a finer texture and improve their shelf life, but it also removes dietary fiber, iron, and many B vitamins. Some examples of refined grain products are these choices:

- White flour
- White bread
- Degermed cornmeal
- White rice

This section excerpted from "Food Groups: Grains," ChooseMyPlate.gov, U.S. Department of Agriculture (www.choosemyplate.gov), May 31, 2011.

Most refined grains are *enriched*. This means certain B vitamins (thiamin, riboflavin, niacin, folic acid) and iron are added back after processing. Fiber is not added back to enriched grains. Check the ingredient list on refined grain products to make sure that the word "enriched" is included in the grain name. Some food products are made from mixtures of whole grains and refined grains.

Some commonly eaten grain products are the following:

Whole Grains

- Amaranth
- Brown rice
- Buckwheat
- Bulgur (cracked wheat)
- Millet
- Oatmeal
- Popcorn
- Ready-to-eat breakfast cereals
  - Whole-wheat cereal flakes
  - Muesli
- Rolled oats
- Quinoa
- Whole-grain barley
- Whole-grain cornmeal
- Whole rye
- Whole-wheat bread
- Whole-wheat crackers
- Whole-wheat pasta
- Whole-wheat sandwich buns and rolls
- Whole-wheat tortillas
- Wild rice

Refined Grains

- Cornbread*
- Corn tortillas*
- Couscous*
- Crackers*
- Flour tortillas*
- Grits
- Noodles*
- Pasta*
  - Spaghetti
  - Macaroni
- Pitas*
- Pretzels
- Ready-to-eat breakfast cereals
  - Corn flakes
- White bread
- White sandwich buns and rolls
- White rice

* Most of these products are made from refined grains. Some are made from whole grains. Check the ingredient list for the words "whole grain" or "whole wheat" to decide if they are made from a whole grain. Some foods are made from a mixture of whole and refined grains.

Some grain products contain significant amounts of bran. Bran provides fiber, which is important for health. However, products with added bran or bran alone (e.g., oat bran) are not necessarily whole-grain products.

How Many Grain Foods Are Needed Daily?

The amount of grains you need to eat depends on your age, sex, and level of physical activity. See Table 13.1 for recommended daily amounts. Most Americans consume enough grains, but few are whole grains. At least half of all the grains eaten should be whole grains.

What Counts as an Ounce Equivalent of Grains?

In general, 1 slice of bread, 1 cup of ready-to-eat cereal, or 1/2 cup of cooked rice, cooked pasta, or cooked cereal can be considered as 1 ounce equivalent from the grains group.

Table 13.1. Recommended Daily Grain Servings

	Age	Daily Recommendation*	Daily Minimum Amount of Whole Grains
Children	2–3 years old	3 ounce equivalents	1 1/2 ounce equivalents
	4–8 years old	5 ounce equivalents	2 1/2 ounce equivalents
Girls	9–13 years old	5 ounce equivalents	3 ounce equivalents
	14–18 years old	6 ounce equivalents	3 ounce equivalents
Boys	9–13 years old	6 ounce equivalents	3 ounce equivalents
	14–18 years old	8 ounce equivalents	4 ounce equivalents
Women	19–30 years old	6 ounce equivalents	3 ounce equivalents
	31–50 years old	6 ounce equivalents	3 ounce equivalents
	51+ years old	5 ounce equivalents	3 ounce equivalents
Men	19–30 years old	8 ounce equivalents	4 ounce equivalents
	31–50 years old	7 ounce equivalents	3 1/2 ounce equivalents
	51+ years old	6 ounce equivalents	3 ounce equivalents

* These amounts are appropriate for individuals who get less than 30 minutes per day of moderate physical activity, beyond normal daily activities. Those who are more physically active may be able to consume more while staying within calorie needs.

Why Is It Important to Eat Grains, Especially Whole Grains?

Eating grains, especially whole grains, provides health benefits. People who eat whole grains as part of a healthy diet have a reduced risk of some chronic diseases. Grains provide many nutrients that are vital for the health and maintenance of our bodies.

Health Benefits

- Consuming whole grains as part of a healthy diet may reduce the risk of heart disease.

- Consuming foods containing fiber, such as whole grains, as part of a healthy diet, may reduce constipation.

- Eating whole grains may help with weight management.

- Eating grain products fortified with folate before and during pregnancy helps prevent neural tube defects during fetal development.

Nutrients

- Grains are important sources of many nutrients, including dietary fiber, several B vitamins (thiamin, riboflavin, niacin, and folate), and minerals (iron, magnesium, and selenium).

- Dietary fiber from whole grains or other foods may help reduce blood cholesterol levels and may lower risk of heart disease, obesity, and type 2 diabetes. Fiber is important for proper bowel function.

- The B vitamins thiamin, riboflavin, and niacin play a key role in metabolism. B vitamins are also essential for a healthy nervous system. Many refined grains are enriched with these B vitamins.

- Iron is used to carry oxygen in the blood. Many teenage girls and women in their childbearing years have iron-deficiency anemia. They should eat foods high in heme-iron (meats) or eat other iron-containing foods along with foods rich in vitamin C, which can improve absorption of non-heme iron. Whole and enriched refined grain products are major sources of non-heme iron in American diets.

- Whole grains are sources of magnesium and selenium. Magnesium is a mineral used in building bones and releasing energy from muscles. Selenium protects cells from oxidation. It is also important for a healthy immune system.

Tips to Help You Eat Whole Grains

At Meals

- To eat more whole grains, substitute a whole-grain product for a refined product—such as eating whole-wheat bread instead of white bread or brown rice instead of white rice. It's important to substitute the whole-grain product for the refined one, rather than adding the whole-grain product.

- For a change, try brown rice or whole-wheat pasta.

- Use whole grains in mixed dishes, such as barley in vegetable soup or stews and bulgur wheat in casserole or stir-fries.

- Create a whole-grain pilaf with a mixture of barley, wild rice, brown rice, broth, and spices. For a special touch, stir in toasted nuts or chopped dried fruit.

- Experiment by substituting whole-wheat or oat flour for up to half of the flour in pancake, waffle, muffin, or other flour-based recipes. They may need a bit more leavening.

- Use whole-grain bread or cracker crumbs in meatloaf.

- Try rolled oats or a crushed, unsweetened whole-grain cereal as breading for baked chicken, fish, veal cutlets, or eggplant parmesan.

- Freeze leftover cooked brown rice, bulgur, or barley. Heat and serve it later as a quick side dish.

As Snacks

- Snack on ready-to-eat, whole-grain cereals such as toasted oat cereal.

- Add whole-grain flour or oatmeal when making cookies or other baked treats.

- Try 100% whole-grain snack crackers.

- Popcorn, a whole grain, can be a healthy snack if made with little or no added salt and butter.

What to Look for on the Food Label

- Foods labeled with the words "multi-grain," "stone-ground," "100% wheat," "cracked wheat," "seven-grain," or "bran" are usually not whole-grain products.

- Color is not an indication of a whole grain. Bread can be brown because of molasses or other added ingredients. Read the ingredient list to see if it is a whole grain.

- Use the Nutrition Facts label and choose whole grain products with a higher % Daily Value (%DV) for fiber. Many, but not all, whole grain products are good or excellent sources of fiber.

- Read the food label's ingredient list. Look for terms that indicate added sugars (such as sucrose, high-fructose corn syrup, honey, malt syrup, maple syrup, molasses, or raw sugar) that add extra calories. Choose foods with fewer added sugars.

- Most sodium in the food supply comes from packaged foods. Similar packaged foods can vary widely in sodium content, including breads. Use the Nutrition Facts label to choose foods with a lower %DV for sodium. Foods with less than 140 mg sodium per serving can be labeled as low-sodium foods. Claims such as "low in sodium" or "very low in sodium" on the front of the food label can help you identify foods that contain less salt (or sodium).

Chapter 14

Empty Calories

Key Consumer Messages

- Enjoy your food, but eat less.
- Avoid oversized portions.
- Drink water instead of sugary drinks.

What Are Empty Calories?

Currently, many of the foods and beverages Americans eat and drink contain empty calories—calories from solid fats and/or added sugars. Solid fats and added sugars add calories to the food but few or no nutrients. For this reason, the calories from solid fats and added sugars in a food are often called empty calories.

Solid fats are fats that are solid at room temperature, like butter, beef fat, and shortening. Some solid fats are found naturally in foods. They can also be added when foods are processed by food companies or when they are prepared.

Added sugars are sugars and syrups that are added when foods or beverages are processed or prepared.

Solid fats and added sugars can make a food or beverage more appealing, but they also can add a lot of calories. The foods and beverages that provide the most empty calories for Americans are these choices:

This chapter excerpted from "Empty Calories," ChooseMyPlate.gov, U.S. Department of Agriculture (www.choosemyplate.gov), May 31, 2011.

117

- Cakes, cookies, pastries, and donuts (contain both solid fat and added sugars)

- Sodas, energy drinks, sports drinks, and fruit drinks (contain added sugars)

- Cheese (contains solid fat)

- Pizza (contains solid fat)

- Ice cream (contains both solid fat and added sugars)

- Sausages, hot dogs, bacon, and ribs (contain solid fat)

These foods and beverages are the major sources of empty calories, but many can be found in forms with less or no solid fat or added sugars. For example, low-fat cheese and low-fat hot dogs can be purchased. You can choose water, milk, or sugar-free soda instead of drinks with sugar. Check that the calories in these products are less than in the regular product.

In some foods, like most candies and sodas, all the calories are empty calories. These foods are often called "empty calorie foods." However, empty calories from solid fats and added sugars can also be found in some other foods that contain important nutrients. Some examples of foods that provide nutrients, shown in forms with and without empty calories, are the following:

- Sweetened applesauce (contains added sugars) vs. unsweetened applesauce

- Regular ground beef (75% lean) (contains solid fats) vs. extra lean ground beef (90% or more lean)

- Fried chicken (contains solid fats from frying and skin) vs. baked chicken breast without skin

- Sugar-sweetened cereals (contain added sugars) vs. unsweetened cereals

- Whole milk (contains solid fats) vs. fat-free milk

A small amount of empty calories is okay, but most people eat far more than is healthy. It is important to limit empty calories to the amount that fits your calorie and nutrient needs. You can lower your intake by eating and drinking foods and beverages containing empty calories less often or by decreasing the amount you eat or drink.

Chapter 15

Fluids and Hydration

Ever notice how lifeless a house plant looks when you forget to water it? Just a little water and it seems to perk back up. Water is just as essential for our bodies because it is in every cell, tissue, and organ in your body. That's why getting enough water every day is important for your health.

Healthy people meet their fluid needs by drinking when thirsty and drinking fluids with meals. But, if you're outside in hot weather for most of the day or doing vigorous physical activity, you'll need to make an effort to drink more fluids.

Where do I get the water I need?

Most of your water needs are met through the water and beverages you drink. You can get some fluid through the foods you eat. For example, broth soups and other foods that are 85% to 95% water such as celery, tomatoes, oranges, and melons.

What does water do in my body?

Water helps your body with the following:

- Keeps its temperature normal
- Lubricates and cushions your joints

"Water: Meeting Your Daily Fluid Needs," Centers for Disease Control and Prevention (www.cdc.gov), February 23, 2011.

- Protects your spinal cord and other sensitive tissues
- Gets rid of wastes through urination, perspiration, and bowel movements

Why do I need to drink enough water each day?

You need water to replace what your body loses through normal everyday functions. Of course, you lose water when you go to the bathroom or sweat, but you even lose small amounts of water when you exhale. You need to replace this lost water to prevent dehydration.

Your body also needs more water during the following conditions:

- In hot climates
- When you are more physically active
- When you are running a fever
- When you are having diarrhea or vomiting

To help you stay hydrated during prolonged physical activity or when it is hot outside, the *Dietary Guidelines for Americans 2005* recommend these two steps:

1. Drink fluid while doing the activity.
2. Drink several glasses of water or other fluid after the physical activity is completed.

Also, when you are participating in vigorous physical activity, it's important to drink before you even feel thirsty. Thirst is a signal that your body is on the way to dehydration.

Some people may have fluid restrictions because of a health problem, such as kidney disease. If your health care provider has told you to restrict your fluid intake, be sure to follow that advice.

How do I increase my fluid intake by drinking more water?

Under normal conditions, most people can drink enough fluids to meet their water needs. If you are outside in hot weather for most of the day or doing vigorous activity, you may need to increase your fluid intake.

If you think you're not getting enough water each day, the following tips may help:

- Carry a water bottle for easy access when you are at work or running errands.

- Freeze some freezer-safe water bottles. Take one with you for ice-cold water all day long.

- Choose water instead of sugar-sweetened beverages. This tip can also help with weight management. Substituting water for one 20-ounce sugar-sweetened soda will save you about 240 calories.

- Choose water instead of other beverages when eating out. Generally, you will save money and reduce calories.

- Give your water a little pizzazz by adding a wedge of lime or lemon. This may improve the taste, and you just might drink more water than you usually do.

Do sugar-sweetened beverages count? Although beverages that are sweetened with sugars do provide water, they usually have more calories than unsweetened beverages. To help with weight control, you should consume beverages and foods that don't have added sugars.

Examples of beverages with added sugars:

- Fruit drinks
- Some sports drinks
- Soft drinks and sodas (non-diet)

Chapter 16

Essential Vitamins

Chapter Contents

Section 16.1

Vitamin A

This section excerpted from "Vitamin A and Carotenoids,"
Office of Dietary Supplements (ods.od.nih.gov), April 23, 2006.
Reviewed by David A. Cooke, MD, FACP, January 2011.

Vitamin A: What is it?

Vitamin A is a group of compounds that play an important role in vision, bone growth, reproduction, cell division, and cell differentiation (in which a cell becomes part of the brain, muscle, lungs, blood, or other specialized tissue). Vitamin A helps regulate the immune system, which helps prevent or fight off infections by making white blood cells that destroy harmful bacteria and viruses. Vitamin A also may help lymphocytes (a type of white blood cell) fight infections more effectively.

Vitamin A promotes healthy surface linings of the eyes and the respiratory, urinary, and intestinal tracts. When those linings break down, it becomes easier for bacteria to enter the body and cause infection. Vitamin A also helps the skin and mucous membranes function as a barrier to bacteria and viruses.

In general, there are two categories of vitamin A, depending on whether the food source is an animal or a plant.

Vitamin A found in foods that come from animals is called preformed vitamin A. It is absorbed in the form of retinol, one of the most usable (active) forms of vitamin A. Sources include liver, whole milk, and some fortified food products. Retinol can be made into retinal and retinoic acid (other active forms of vitamin A) in the body.

Vitamin A that is found in colorful fruits and vegetables is called provitamin A carotenoid. They can be made into retinol in the body. In the United States, approximately 26% of vitamin A consumed by men and 34% of vitamin A consumed by women is in the form of provitamin A carotenoids. Common provitamin A carotenoids found in foods that come from plants are beta-carotene, alpha-carotene, and beta-cryptoxanthin. Among these, beta-carotene is most efficiently made into retinol. Alpha-carotene and beta-cryptoxanthin are also converted to vitamin A, but only half as efficiently as beta-carotene.

Of the 563 identified carotenoids, fewer than 10% can be made into vitamin A in the body. Lycopene, lutein, and zeaxanthin are carotenoids that do not have vitamin A activity but have other health-promoting properties. The Institute of Medicine (IOM) encourages consumption of all carotenoid-rich fruits and vegetables for their health-promoting benefits.

Some provitamin A carotenoids have been shown to function as antioxidants in laboratory studies; however, this role has not been consistently demonstrated in humans. Antioxidants protect cells from free radicals, which are potentially damaging by-products of oxygen metabolism that may contribute to the development of some chronic diseases.

What foods provide vitamin A?

Retinol is found in foods that come from animals such as whole eggs, milk, and liver. Most fat-free milk and dried nonfat milk solids sold in the United States are fortified with vitamin A to replace the amount lost when the fat is removed. Fortified foods such as fortified breakfast cereals also provide vitamin A. Provitamin A carotenoids are abundant in darkly colored fruits and vegetables. The 2000 National Health and Nutrition Examination Survey (NHANES) indicated that major dietary contributors of retinol are milk, margarine, eggs, beef liver, and fortified breakfast cereals, whereas major contributors of provitamin A carotenoids are carrots, cantaloupes, sweet potatoes, and spinach.

Vitamin A in foods that come from animals is well absorbed and used efficiently by the body. Vitamin A in foods that come from plants is not as well absorbed as animal sources of vitamin A.

What are recommended intakes of vitamin A?

Recommendations for vitamin A are provided in the Dietary Reference Intakes (DRIs) developed by the IOM. DRI is the general term for a set of reference values used for planning and assessing nutrient intake in healthy people. Three important types of reference values included in the DRIs are Recommended Dietary Allowances (RDA), Adequate Intakes (AI), and Tolerable Upper Intake Levels (UL). The RDA recommends the average daily dietary intake level that is sufficient to meet the nutrient requirements of nearly all (97% to 98%) healthy individuals in each age and gender group. An AI is set when there are insufficient scientific data to establish an RDA. AIs meet or exceed the amount needed to maintain nutritional adequacy in nearly all people. The UL, on the other hand, is the maximum daily intake unlikely to result in adverse health effects.

In Table 16.1, RDAs for vitamin A are listed as micrograms (mcg) of Retinol Activity Equivalents (RAE) to account for the different biological activities of retinol and provitamin A carotenoids. Table 16.1 also lists RDAs for vitamin A in International Units (IU), which are used on food and supplement labels (1 RAE = 3.3 IU).

Information is insufficient to establish an RDA for vitamin A for infants. AIs have been established based on the amount of vitamin A consumed by healthy infants fed breast milk (Table 16.2).

The NHANES III survey (1988–1994) found that most Americans consume recommended amounts of vitamin A. More recent NHANES data (1999–2000) show average adult intakes to be about 3,300 IU per day, which also suggests that most Americans get enough vitamin A.

There is no RDA for beta-carotene or other provitamin A carotenoids. The IOM states that consuming 3 mg [milligrams] to 6 mg of beta-carotene daily (equivalent to 833 IU to 1,667 IU vitamin A) will maintain blood levels of beta-carotene in the range associated with a lower risk of chronic diseases. A diet that provides five or more servings of fruits and vegetables per day and includes some dark green and leafy vegetables and deep yellow or orange fruits should provide sufficient beta-carotene and other carotenoids.

Table 16.1. Recommended Dietary Allowances for Vitamin A

Age (years)	Children (mcg RAE)	Males (mcg RAE)	Females (mcg RAE)	Pregnancy (mcg RAE)	Lactation (mcg RAE)
1–3	300 (1,000 IU)				
4–8	400 (1,320 IU)				
9–13	600 (2,000 IU)				
14–18		900 (3,000 IU)	700 (2,310 IU)	750 (2,500 IU)	1,200 (4,000 IU)
19+		900 (3,000 IU)	700 (2,310 IU)	770 (2,565 IU)	1,300 (4,300 IU)

Table 16.2. Adequate Intakes for Vitamin A for Infants

Age (months)	Males and Females (mcg RAE)
0–6	400 (1,320 IU)
7–12	500 (1,650 IU)

When can vitamin A deficiency occur?

Vitamin A deficiency is common in developing countries but rarely seen in the United States. Approximately 250,000 to 500,000 malnourished children in the developing world become blind each year from a deficiency of vitamin A. In the United States, vitamin A deficiency is most often associated with strict dietary restrictions and excess alcohol intake. Severe zinc deficiency, which is also associated with strict dietary limitations, often accompanies vitamin A deficiency. Zinc is required to make retinol binding protein (RBP), which transports vitamin A. Therefore, a deficiency in zinc limits the body's ability to move vitamin A stores from the liver to body tissues.

Night blindness is one of the first signs of vitamin A deficiency. In ancient Egypt, it was known that night blindness could be cured by eating liver, which was later found to be a rich source of the vitamin. Vitamin A deficiency contributes to blindness by making the cornea very dry and damaging the retina and cornea.

Vitamin A deficiency diminishes the ability to fight infections. In countries where such deficiency is common and immunization programs are limited, millions of children die each year from complications of infectious diseases such as measles. In vitamin A–deficient individuals, cells lining the lungs lose their ability to remove disease-causing microorganisms. This may contribute to the pneumonia associated with vitamin A deficiency.

There is increased interest in early forms of vitamin A deficiency, described as low storage levels of vitamin A that do not cause obvious deficiency symptoms. This mild degree of vitamin A deficiency may increase children's risk of developing respiratory and diarrheal infections, decrease growth rate, slow bone development, and decrease likelihood of survival from serious illness. Children in the United States who are considered to be at increased risk for subclinical vitamin A deficiency include the following:

- Toddlers and preschool age children
- Children living at or below the poverty level
- Children with inadequate health care or immunizations
- Children living in areas with known nutritional deficiencies
- Recent immigrants or refugees from developing countries with high incidence of vitamin A deficiency or measles
- Children with diseases of the pancreas, liver, or intestines, or with inadequate fat digestion or absorption

A deficiency can occur when vitamin A is lost through chronic diarrhea and through an overall inadequate intake, as is often seen with protein-energy malnutrition. Low blood retinol concentrations indicate depleted levels of vitamin A. This occurs with vitamin A deficiency but also can result from an inadequate intake of protein, calories, and zinc, since these nutrients are needed to make RBP. Iron deficiency can also affect vitamin A metabolism, and iron supplements provided to iron-deficient individuals may improve body stores of vitamin A and iron.

Excess alcohol intake depletes vitamin A stores. Also, diets high in alcohol often do not provide recommended amounts of vitamin A. It is very important for people who consume excessive amounts of alcohol to include good sources of vitamin A in their diets. Vitamin A supplements may not be recommended for individuals who abuse alcohol, however, because their livers may be more susceptible to potential toxicity from high doses of vitamin A. A medical doctor will need to evaluate this situation and determine the need for vitamin A supplements.

Who may need extra vitamin A to prevent a deficiency?

Vitamin A deficiency rarely occurs in the United States, but the World Health Organization (WHO) and the United Nations Children's Fund (UNICEF) recommend vitamin A administration for all children diagnosed with measles in communities where vitamin A deficiency is a serious problem and where death from measles is greater than 1%. In 1994, the American Academy of Pediatrics recommended vitamin A supplements for two subgroups of children likely to be at high risk for subclinical vitamin A deficiency: children aged 6 months to 24 months who are hospitalized with measles, and hospitalized children older than 6 months.

Fat malabsorption can result in diarrhea and prevent normal absorption of vitamin A. Over time this may result in vitamin A deficiency. Those conditions include the following:

- **Celiac disease:** Often referred to as sprue, celiac disease is a genetic disorder. People with celiac disease become sick when they eat a protein called gluten found in wheat and some other grains. In celiac disease, gluten can trigger damage to the small intestine, where most nutrient absorption occurs. Approximately 30% to 60% of people with celiac disease have gastrointestinal-motility disorders such as diarrhea. They must follow a gluten-free diet to avoid malabsorption and other symptoms.

- **Crohn disease:** This inflammatory bowel disease affects the small intestine. People with Crohn disease often experience diarrhea, fat malabsorption, and malnutrition.

- **Pancreatic disorders:** Because the pancreas secretes enzymes that are important for fat absorption, pancreatic disorders often result in fat malabsorption. Without these enzymes, it is difficult to absorb fat. Many people with pancreatic disease take pancreatic enzymes in pill form to prevent fat malabsorption and diarrhea.

Healthy adults usually have a reserve of vitamin A stored in their livers and should not be at risk of deficiency during periods of temporary or short-term fat malabsorption. Long-term problems absorbing fat, however, may result in deficiency. In these instances physicians may recommend additional vitamin A.

Vegetarians who do not consume eggs and dairy foods need provitamin A carotenoids to meet their need for vitamin A. They should include a minimum of five servings of fruits and vegetables in their daily diet and regularly choose dark green leafy vegetables and orange and yellow fruits to consume recommended amounts of vitamin A.

What are the health risks of too much vitamin A?

Hypervitaminosis A refers to high storage levels of vitamin A in the body that can lead to toxic symptoms. There are four major adverse effects of hypervitaminosis A: birth defects, liver abnormalities, reduced bone mineral density that may result in osteoporosis (see the previous section), and central nervous system disorders.

Toxic symptoms can also arise after consuming very large amounts of preformed vitamin A over a short period of time. Signs of acute toxicity include nausea and vomiting, headache, dizziness, blurred vision, and muscular uncoordination. Although hypervitaminosis A can occur when large amounts of liver are regularly consumed, most cases result from taking excess amounts of the nutrient in supplements.

What are the health risks of too many carotenoids?

Provitamin A carotenoids such as beta-carotene are generally considered safe because they are not associated with specific adverse health effects. Their conversion to vitamin A decreases when body stores are full. A high intake of provitamin A carotenoids can turn the skin yellow, but this is not considered dangerous to health.

Clinical trials that associated beta-carotene supplements with a greater incidence of lung cancer and death in current smokers raise concerns about the effects of beta-carotene supplements on long-term health; however, conflicting studies make it difficult to interpret the health risk. For example, the Physicians Health Study compared the effects of taking 50 mg beta-carotene every other day to a placebo in over 22,000 male physicians and found no adverse health effects. Also, a trial that tested the ability of four different nutrient combinations to help prevent the development of esophageal and gastric cancers in 30,000 men and women in China suggested that after five years those participants who took a combination of beta-carotene, selenium, and vitamin E had a 13% reduction in cancer deaths. In one lung cancer trial, men who consumed more than 11 grams/day of alcohol (approximately one drink per day) were more likely to show an adverse response to beta-carotene supplements, which may suggest a potential relationship between alcohol and beta-carotene.

The IOM did not set ULs for carotene or other carotenoids. Instead, it concluded that beta-carotene supplements are not advisable for the general population. As stated earlier, however, they may be appropriate as a provitamin A source for the prevention of vitamin A deficiency in specific populations.

Section 16.2

The Vitamin B Family

This section includes excerpts from documents from A.D.A.M., Inc; Office of Dietary Supplements; and the Institute of Food and Agriculture Sciences, University of Florida, all cited individually within the section.

Vitamin B1 (Thiamine)

"Vitamin B1 (Thiamine)," © 2011 A.D.A.M., Inc. Reprinted with permission.

Vitamin B1, also called thiamine or thiamin, is one of eight B vitamins. All B vitamins help the body convert food (carbohydrates) into fuel (glucose), which is "burned" to produce energy. These B vitamins, often referred to as B complex vitamins, also help the body metabolize fats and protein. B complex vitamins are necessary for healthy skin, hair, eyes, and liver. They also help the nervous system function properly, and are necessary for optimal brain function.

All B vitamins are water-soluble, meaning that the body does not store them.

Like other B complex vitamins, thiamine is considered an "antistress" vitamin because it may strengthen the immune system and improve the body's ability to withstand stressful conditions. It is named B1 because it was the first B vitamin discovered.

Thiamine is found in both plants and animals and plays a crucial role in certain metabolic reactions. For example, it is required for the body to form adenosine triphosphate (ATP), which every cell of the body uses for energy.

Thiamine deficiency is rare, but can occur in people who get most of their calories from sugar or alcohol. People who are deficient in thiamine may experience fatigue, irritability, depression, and abdominal discomfort. People with thiamine deficiency also have difficulty digesting carbohydrates. As a result, a substance called pyruvic acid builds up in their bloodstream, causing a loss of mental alertness, difficulty breathing, and heart damage (a disease known as beriberi).

Beriberi: The most important use of thiamine is to treat beriberi, which is caused by not getting enough thiamine in your diet. Symptoms include swelling, tingling, or burning sensation in the hands and feet, confusion, difficulty breathing (from fluid in the lungs), and uncontrolled eye movements (called nystagmus). Although people in the developed world generally do not have to worry about getting enough thiamine because foods such as cereals and breads are fortified with the vitamin, people can develop a deficiency fairly quickly, because the body does not store thiamine.

Wernicke-Korsakoff syndrome: Wernicke-Korsakoff syndrome is a brain disorder caused by thiamine deficiency; as with beriberi, it is treated by giving supplemental thiamine. Wernicke-Korsakoff is actually two disorders: Wernicke disease involves damage to nerves in the central and peripheral nervous systems and is generally caused by malnutrition stemming from habitual alcohol abuse. Korsakoff syndrome is characterized by memory impairment and nerve damage. High doses of thiamine can improve muscle coordination and confusion, but rarely improves memory loss.

Cataracts: Preliminary evidence suggests that thiamine—along with other nutrients—may lower risk of developing cataracts. People with plenty of protein and vitamins A, B1, B2, and B3 (niacin) in their diet are less likely to develop cataracts. Getting enough vitamins C, E, and B complex (particularly B1, B2, B9 [folic acid], and B12 [cobalamin]) may further protect the lens of your eyes from developing cataracts. More research is needed.

Alzheimer's disease: Because lack of thiamine can cause dementia in Wernicke-Korsakoff syndrome, it has been proposed that thiamine might help reduce severity of Alzheimer's disease. Scientific studies have not always shown any benefit from thiamine, however. More research is needed before thiamine can be proposed as an effective treatment for Alzheimer's disease.

Heart failure: Thiamine may be related to heart failure in two ways. First, low levels of thiamine can lead to "wet beriberi," a condition where fluid builds up around the heart. However, it isn't clear that taking thiamin will help people with heart failure not related to beriberi.

Many people with heart failure take diuretics (water pills), which help rid the body of excess fluid. But diuretics may also cause the body to get rid of too much thiamine. A few small studies suggest that taking thiamine supplements may help. A multivitamin, taken regularly, should provide enough thiamine.

Dietary Sources

Most foods contain small amounts of thiamine. Large amounts can be found in pork and organ meats. Other good dietary sources of thiamine include whole-grain or enriched cereals and rice, legumes, wheat germ, bran, brewers yeast, and blackstrap molasses. However, the vitamin is easily destroyed when exposed to heat.

Available Forms

Vitamin B1 can be found in multivitamins (including children's chewable and liquid drops), B complex vitamins, or it can be sold individually. It is available in a variety of forms, including tablets, softgels, and lozenges. It may also be labeled as thiamine hydrochloride or thiamine mononitrate.

How to Take It

As with all medications and supplements, check with a health care provider before giving vitamin B1 supplements to a child.

Daily recommendations for dietary vitamin B1 are listed here.

Pediatric

- Newborns–6 months: 0.2 mg (adequate intake)
- Infants 7 months–1 year: 0.3 mg (adequate intake)
- Children 1–3 years: 0.5 mg (RDA)
- Children 4–8 years: 0.6 mg (RDA)

- Children 9–13 years: 0.9 mg (RDA)
- Males 14–18 years: 1.2 mg (RDA)
- Females 14–18 years: 1 mg (RDA)

Adult

- Males 19 years and older: 1.2 mg (RDA)
- Females 19 years and older: 1.1 mg (RDA)
- Pregnant females: 1.4 mg (RDA)
- Breastfeeding females: 1.5 mg (RDA)

Doses for conditions like beriberi and Wernicke-Korsakoff syndrome are determined by a doctor. For Wernicke-Korsakoff syndrome, thiamine is given intravenously.

A daily dose of 50–100 mg is often taken as a supplement. Thiamine appears safe even at high doses; however, you should talk to your doctor before taking a large amount.

Precautions

Because of the potential for side effects and interactions with medications, you should take dietary supplements only under the supervision of a knowledgeable health care provider.

Thiamine is generally nontoxic. Very high doses may cause stomach upset.

Taking any one of the B vitamins for a long period of time can result in an imbalance of other important B vitamins. For this reason, you may want to take a B complex vitamin, which includes all the B vitamins.

Possible Interactions

If you are currently being treated with any of the following medications, you should not use vitamin B1 without first talking to your health care provider.

Digoxin: Laboratory studies suggest that digoxin (a medication used to treat heart conditions) may reduce the ability of heart cells to absorb and use vitamin B1; this may be particularly true when digoxin is combined with furosemide (Lasix, a loop diuretic).

Diuretics: Diuretics (particularly furosemide, which belongs to a class called loop diuretics) may reduce levels of vitamin B1 in the body. It's possible that other diuretics may have the same effect. If you take a diuretic, ask your doctor if you need a thiamine supplement.

Phenytoin (Dilantin): Some evidence suggests that some people taking phenytoin have lower levels of thiamine in their blood, and that may contribute to the side effects of the drug. However, that is not true of all people who take phenytoin. If you take phenytoin, ask your doctor if you need a thiamine supplement.

Riboflavin

"Facts about Riboflavin," by R. Elaine Turner, PhD, RD, Food Science and Human Nutrition Department, Cooperative Extension Service, Institute of Food and Agriculture Sciences, University of Florida. © 2006, The University of Florida. Reprinted with permission.

Why do we need riboflavin?

Riboflavin is one of the B vitamins. It also is known as vitamin B2. We need riboflavin to use the carbohydrates, fats, and proteins in the foods we eat. Riboflavin helps us use these nutrients for energy in our bodies. Riboflavin also is needed to properly use the vitamins niacin, folate, and vitamin B6.

What happens if we don't get enough riboflavin?

Because riboflavin is found in a variety of foods, most people get plenty in their diets. A deficiency of riboflavin occurs only when the diet is very poor, and lacks many nutrients.

A lack of riboflavin causes sores in the mouth and inflammation of the tongue. Lack of riboflavin also can affect the body's use of other vitamins.

How much riboflavin do we need?

Table 16.3 lists recommended daily intakes of riboflavin.

Table 16.3. Daily Intakes of Riboflavin

Life Stage	Riboflavin (mg/day)
Men, ages 19+	1.3
Women, ages 19+	1.1
Pregnancy	1.4
Breastfeeding	1.6

mg=milligrams

How can we get enough riboflavin?

Milk and milk products are good sources of riboflavin. Riboflavin also is found in whole grains.

Riboflavin is one of four vitamins added to enriched grain products such as enriched flour. The other vitamins added to enriched grains are thiamin, niacin, and folic acid.

Enriched breads and cereals contain riboflavin. Look for the word "riboflavin" in the ingredient list on the label to see if it has been added.

INGREDIENTS: Enriched semolina (iron, thiamin mononitrate, folic acid, **riboflavin,** niacin), tomato, beet and spinach powders, ...

Other good sources of riboflavin are: meat, eggs, and mushrooms. Table 16.4 lists some foods and the amount of riboflavin they contain.

Table 16.4. Riboflavin Content of Foods

Food	Riboflavin (mg per serving)
Yogurt, 8 oz [ounces]	0.5
Milk, 1 cup	0.4
Ready-to-eat cereal, 1 cup	0.4
Egg, cooked, 1 large	0.3
Pork chop, cooked, 3 oz	0.3
Mushrooms, cooked, 1/2 cup	0.2
Cottage cheese, 1/2 cup	0.2

mg=milligrams

How should foods be prepared to retain riboflavin?

Riboflavin is easily destroyed when exposed to light. Milk stored in glass and exposed to light loses much of its riboflavin content. Opaque plastic jugs and paper cartons protect the riboflavin in milk. Only small amounts of riboflavin are lost in cooking.

What about supplements?

Most people get plenty of riboflavin in their diet, so supplements usually are not needed. Most multivitamin supplements contain riboflavin.

Research has not yet found problems from consuming too much riboflavin from food or supplements. However, there is no need to take a supplement with more than 100% to 150% of the Daily Value for riboflavin.

Where can I get more information?

The Family and Consumer Sciences (FCS) agent at your county Extension office may have more written information and nutrition classes for you to attend. Also, a registered dietitian (RD) can provide reliable information to you.

Vitamin B3 (Niacin)

"Vitamin B3 (Niacin)," © 2011 A.D.A.M., Inc. Reprinted with permission.

Vitamin B3 is one of eight B vitamins. It is also known as niacin (nicotinic acid) and has two other forms, niacinamide (nicotinamide) and inositol hexanicotinate, which have different effects from niacin.

All B vitamins help the body to convert food (carbohydrates) into fuel (glucose), which is "burned" to produce energy. These B vitamins, often referred to as B complex vitamins, also help the body metabolize fats and protein. B complex vitamins are necessary for healthy skin, hair, eyes, and liver. They also help the nervous system function properly.

Niacin also helps the body make various sex and stress-related hormones in the adrenal glands and other parts of the body. Niacin is effective in improving circulation and reducing cholesterol levels in the blood.

All the B vitamins are water-soluble, meaning that the body does not store them.

You can meet all of your body's needs for B3 through diet; it is rare for anyone in the developed world to have a B3 deficiency. In the United States, alcoholism is the prime cause of vitamin B3 deficiency.

Symptoms of mild deficiency include indigestion, fatigue, canker sores, vomiting, and depression. Severe deficiency can cause a condition known as pellagra. Pellagra is characterized by cracked, scaly skin, dementia, and diarrhea. It is generally treated with a nutritionally balanced diet and niacin supplements. Niacin deficiency also results in burning in the mouth and a swollen, bright red tongue.

Very high doses of B3 (available by prescription) have been shown to prevent or improve symptoms of the following conditions. However, taken at high doses niacin can be toxic, so you should take doses higher than the Recommended Daily Allowance only under your doctor's supervision. Researchers are trying to determine if inositol hexanicotinate has similar benefits without serious side effects, but so far results are preliminary.

High cholesterol: Niacin (but not niacinamide) has been used since the 1950s to lower elevated LDL [low-density lipoprotein] ("bad") cholesterol and triglyceride (fat) levels in the blood and is more effective in increasing HDL [high-density lipoprotein] ("good") cholesterol levels than other cholesterol-lowering medications. However, side effects can be unpleasant and even dangerous. High doses of niacin cause flushing of the skin (which can be reduced by taking aspirin 30 minutes before the niacin), stomach upset (which usually subsides within a few weeks), headache, dizziness, and blurred vision. There is an increased risk of liver damage. A time-release form of niacin reduces flushing, but its long-term use is associated with liver damage. In addition, niacin can interact with other cholesterol-lowering drugs (see "Possible Interactions"). You should not take niacin at high doses without your doctor's supervision.

Atherosclerosis: Because niacin lowers LDL and triglycerides in the blood, it may help prevent atherosclerosis (hardening of the arteries) and is sometimes prescribed along with other medications. However, niacin also increases homocysteine levels in the blood, which is associated with an increased risk of heart disease. This is another reason you should not take high doses of niacin without your doctor's supervision.

Diabetes: Some evidence suggests that niacinamide (but not niacin) might help delay the onset of insulin dependence (in other words, delay the time that you would need to take insulin) in type 1 diabetes. In type 1 diabetes, the body's immune system mistakenly attacks the cells in the pancreas that make insulin, eventually destroying them. Niacinamide may help protect those cells for a time, but more research is needed to tell for sure.

The effect of niacin on type 2 diabetes is more complicated. People with type 2 diabetes often have high levels of fats and cholesterol in the blood, and niacin, often in conjunction with other drugs, can lower those levels. However, niacin can also raise blood sugar levels, resulting in hyperglycemia, which is particularly dangerous for someone with diabetes. For that reason, anyone with diabetes should take niacin only when directed to do so by their doctor, and should be carefully monitored for hyperglycemia.

Osteoarthritis: One preliminary study suggested that niacinamide may improve arthritis symptoms, including increasing joint mobility and reducing the amount of nonsteroidal anti-inflammatory drugs (NSAIDs) needed. More research is needed to determine whether there is any real benefit.

Alzheimer's disease: Population studies show that people who get higher levels of niacin in their diet have a lower risk of Alzheimer's disease. No studies have evaluated niacin supplements, however.

Skin conditions: Researchers are studying topical forms of niacin as treatments for acne, aging, and prevention of skin cancer, although it's too early to know whether it is effective.

Dietary Sources

The best dietary sources of vitamin B3 are found in beets, brewer's yeast, beef liver, beef kidney, fish, salmon, swordfish, tuna, sunflower seeds, and peanuts. Bread and cereals are usually fortified with niacin. In addition, foods that contain tryptophan, an amino acid the body coverts into niacin, include poultry, red meat, eggs, and dairy products.

Available Forms

Vitamin B3 is available in several different supplement forms: niacinamide, niacin, and inositol hexaniacinate. Niacin is available as a tablet or capsule in both regular and timed-release forms. The timed-release tablets and capsules may have fewer side effects than regular niacin; however, the timed-release versions are more likely to cause liver damage. Regardless of which form of niacin you're using, doctors recommend periodic liver function tests when using high doses (above 100 mg per day) of niacin.

How to Take It

Daily recommendations for niacin in the diet of healthy individuals are listed in the following list.

Generally, high doses of niacin are used to control specific diseases, such as high cholesterol. Such high doses are considered "pharmacologic" and must be prescribed by a doctor, who will have you increase the amount of niacin slowly, over the course of four to six weeks, and take the medicine with meals to avoid stomach irritation.

Pediatric

- Infants birth–6 months: 2 mg (adequate intake)
- Infants 7 months–1 year: 4 mg (adequate intake)
- Children 1–3 years: 6 mg (RDA)
- Children 4–8 years: 8 mg (RDA)

- Children 9–13 years: 12 mg (RDA)
- Males 14–18 years: 16 mg (RDA)
- Females 14–18 years: 14 mg (RDA)

Adult

- Males 19 years and older: 16 mg (RDA)
- Females 19 years and older: 14 mg (RDA)
- Pregnant females: 18 mg (RDA)
- Breastfeeding females: 17 mg (RDA)

Precautions

Because of the potential for side effects and interactions with medications, you should take dietary supplements only under the supervision of a knowledgeable health care provider.

High doses (50 mg or more) of niacin can cause side effects. The most common side effect is called "niacin flush," which is a burning, tingling sensation in the face and chest, and red or "flushed" skin. Taking an aspirin 30 minutes prior to the niacin may help reduce this symptom.

At the very high doses used to lower cholesterol and treat other conditions, liver damage and stomach ulcers can occur. Your health care provider will periodically check your liver function through a blood test.

People with a history of liver disease or stomach ulcers should not take niacin supplements. Those with diabetes or gallbladder disease should do so only under the close supervision of their doctor.

Niacin should not be used if you have gout.

Taking any one of the B complex vitamins for a long period of time can result in an imbalance of other important B vitamins. For this reason, it is generally important to take a B complex vitamin with any single B vitamin.

Possible Interactions

If you are currently taking any of the following medications, you should not use niacin without first talking to your health care provider.

Antibiotics, tetracycline: Niacin should not be taken at the same time as the antibiotic tetracycline because it interferes with the absorption and effectiveness of this medication. (All vitamin B complex supplements act in this way and should therefore be taken at different times from tetracycline.)

Aspirin: Taking aspirin before taking niacin may reduce flushing associated with this vitamin, but should only be done under your doctor's supervision.

Anticoagulants (blood thinners): Niacin may make the effects of these medications stronger, increasing the risk of bleeding.

Blood pressure medications, alpha-blockers: Niacin can make the effects of medications taken to lower blood pressure stronger, leading to the risk of low blood pressure.

Cholesterol-lowering medications: Niacin binds bile-acid sequestrants (cholesterol-lowering medications such as colestipol, colesevelam, and cholestyramine) and may decrease their effectiveness. For this reason, niacin and these medications should be taken at different times of the day.

Recent scientific evidence suggests that taking niacin with simvastatin (a drug that belongs to a class of cholesterol-lowering medications known as HMG-CoA reductase inhibitors, or statins) appears to slow down the progression of heart disease. However, the combination may also increase the likelihood for serious side effects, such as muscle inflammation or liver damage.

Diabetes medications: Niacin may increase blood glucose (sugar) levels. People taking insulin, metformin, glyburide, glipizide, or other medications used to treat high blood sugar levels should monitor their blood sugar levels closely when taking niacin supplements.

Isoniazid (INH): INH, a medication used to treat tuberculosis, may lower levels of niacin in the body and cause a deficiency.

Nicotine patches: Using nicotine patches with niacin may worsen or increase the risk of flushing associated with niacin.

Vitamin B5 (Pantothenic Acid)

"Vitamin B5 (Pantothenic Acid)," © 2011 A.D.A.M., Inc. Reprinted with permission.

Vitamin B5, also called pantothenic acid, is one of eight B vitamins. All B vitamins help the body convert food (carbohydrates) into fuel (glucose), which is "burned" to produce energy. These B vitamins, often referred to as B complex vitamins, also help the body metabolize fats and protein. B complex vitamins are necessary for healthy skin, hair, eyes, and liver. They also help the nervous system function properly.

All B vitamins are water-soluble, meaning that the body does not store them.

In addition to playing a role in the breakdown of fats and carbohydrates for energy, vitamin B5 is critical to the manufacture of red blood cells, as well as sex and stress-related hormones produced in the adrenal glands (small glands that sit atop the kidneys). Vitamin B5 is also important in maintaining a healthy digestive tract, and it helps the body use other vitamins (particularly B2 or riboflavin). It is sometimes referred to as the "anti-stress" vitamin because of its effect on the adrenal glands, but there is no real evidence as to whether it helps the body withstand stressful conditions.

Pantothenic acid is also needed for the body to synthesize cholesterol, and a derivative of pantothenic acid called pantethine is being studied to see if it may help lower cholesterol levels in the body.

It is rare for anyone to be deficient in vitamin B5—a proper diet will give healthy people all they need. Symptoms of a vitamin B5 deficiency may include fatigue, insomnia, depression, irritability, vomiting, stomach pains, burning feet, and upper respiratory infections.

High cholesterol/high triglycerides: Several small, double-blind studies suggest that pantethine may help reduce triglycerides (fats) in the blood in people who have high cholesterol. In some of these studies, pantethine has also helped lower LDL (bad) cholesterol and raise HDL (good) cholesterol. In some open studies, pantethine appears to lower levels of cholesterol and triglycerides in people with diabetes. But not all studies have found any benefit. Larger studies are needed to determine whether pantethine has any real benefit.

Wound healing: Studies, primarily in test tubes and animals but a few on people, suggest that vitamin B5 supplements may speed wound healing, especially following surgery. This may be particularly true if vitamin B5 is combined with vitamin C.

Rheumatoid arthritis: Preliminary evidence suggests that pantothenic acid might help with symptoms of rheumatoid arthritis (RA), but the evidence is weak. One study found that people with RA may have lower levels of B5 in their blood than healthy people, and the lowest levels were associated with the most severe symptoms. A small study conducted in 1980 concluded that 2,000 mg/day of calcium pantothenate improved symptoms of RA, including morning stiffness and pain. More studies are needed to confirm these findings.

Dietary Sources

Pantothenic acid gets its name from the Greek root pantos, meaning "everywhere," because it is available in a wide variety of foods. A lot of vitamin B5 is lost when you food is processed, however. Fresh meats, vegetables, and whole unprocessed grains have more vitamin B5 than refined, canned, and frozen food. The best sources are brewer's yeast, corn, cauliflower, kale, broccoli, tomatoes, avocado, legumes, lentils, egg yolks, beef (especially organ meats such as liver and kidney), turkey, duck, chicken, milk, split peas, peanuts, soybeans, sweet potatoes, sunflower seeds, whole-grain breads and cereals, lobster, wheat germ, and salmon.

Available Forms

Vitamin B5 can be found in multivitamins and B complex vitamins, or sold individually under the names pantothenic acid and calcium pantothenate. It is available in a variety of forms including tablets, softgels, and capsules.

How to Take It

Recommended daily intakes of dietary vitamin B5 are listed in the following:

Pediatric

- Infants birth–6 months: 1.7 mg
- Infants 6 months–1 year: 1.8 mg
- Children 1–3 years: 2 mg
- Children 4–8 years: 3 mg
- Children 9–13 years: 4 mg
- Adolescents 14–18 years: 5 mg

Adult

- 19 years and older: 5 mg
- Pregnant females: 6 mg
- Breastfeeding women: 7 mg

Higher doses may be recommended by a health care provider for the treatment of specific conditions.

- Rheumatoid arthritis: 2,000 mg/day
- High cholesterol/triglycerides: 300 mg pantethine, three times daily (900 mg/day)

Precautions

Because of the potential for side effects and interactions with medications, you should take dietary supplements only under the supervision of a knowledgeable health care provider.

Vitamin B5 is considered safe at doses equivalent to the daily intake, and at moderately higher doses. Very high doses may cause diarrhea and may potentially increase the risk of bleeding.

Pregnant and breastfeeding women should not exceed the daily adequate intake unless directed by their physician.

Vitamin B5 should be taken with water, preferably after eating.

Taking any one of the B vitamins for a long period of time can result in an imbalance of other important B vitamins. For this reason, you may want to take a B complex vitamin, which includes all the B vitamins.

Possible Interactions

If you are being treated with any of the following medications, you should not use vitamin B5 supplements without first talking to your health care provider.

Antibiotics, tetracycline: Vitamin B5 interferes with the absorption and effectiveness of the antibiotic tetracycline. You should take B vitamins at different times from tetracycline. (All vitamin B complex supplements act in this way and should therefore be taken at different times from tetracycline.)

Drugs to treat Alzheimer's disease: Vitamin B5 may increase the effects of a group of drugs called cholinesterase inhibitors, which are used to treat Alzheimer's, potentially leading to severe side effects. These drugs should not be taken with B5 unless under a doctor's supervision. Cholinesterase inhibitors include:

- donepezil (Aricept);
- memantine hydrochloride (Ebixa);
- galantamine (Reminyl);
- rivastigmine (Exelon).

Vitamin B6

"Vitamin B6," August 24, 2007, Office of Dietary Supplements (ods.od .nih.gov).

Vitamin B6 is a water-soluble vitamin that exists in three major chemical forms: pyridoxine, pyridoxal, and pyridoxamine. It performs a wide variety of functions in your body and is essential for your good health. For example, vitamin B6 is needed for more than 100 enzymes involved in protein metabolism. It is also essential for red blood cell metabolism. The nervous and immune systems need vitamin B6 to function efficiently, and it is also needed for the conversion of tryptophan (an amino acid) to niacin (a vitamin).

Hemoglobin within red blood cells carries oxygen to tissues. Your body needs vitamin B6 to make hemoglobin. Vitamin B6 also helps increase the amount of oxygen carried by hemoglobin. A vitamin B6 deficiency can result in a form of anemia that is similar to iron deficiency anemia.

An immune response is a broad term that describes a variety of biochemical changes that occur in an effort to fight off infections. Calories, protein, vitamins, and minerals are important to your immune defenses because they promote the growth of white blood cells that directly fight infections. Vitamin B6, through its involvement in protein metabolism and cellular growth, is important to the immune system. It helps maintain the health of lymphoid organs (thymus, spleen, and lymph nodes) that make your white blood cells. Animal studies show that a vitamin B6 deficiency can decrease your antibody production and suppress your immune response.

Vitamin B6 also helps maintain your blood glucose (sugar) within a normal range. When caloric intake is low your body needs vitamin B6 to help convert stored carbohydrate or other nutrients to glucose to maintain normal blood sugar levels. While a shortage of vitamin B6 will limit these functions, supplements of this vitamin do not enhance them in well-nourished individuals.

What foods provide vitamin B6?

Vitamin B6 is found in a wide variety of foods including fortified cereals, beans, meat, poultry, fish, and some fruits and vegetables.

What is the Recommended Dietary Allowance for vitamin B6 for adults?

The RDA is the average daily dietary intake level that is sufficient to meet the nutrient requirements of nearly all (97% to 98%) healthy individuals in each life-stage and gender group.

Table 16.5. 1998 RDAs for Vitamin B6 for Adults, in Milligrams

Life Stage	Men	Women	Pregnancy	Lactation
Ages 19–50	1.3 mg	1.3 mg		
Ages 51+	1.7 mg	1.5 mg		
All Ages			1.9 mg	2.0 mg

Results of two national surveys, the NHANES III (1988–1994) and the Continuing Survey of Food Intakes by Individuals (1994–1996 CSFII), indicated that diets of most Americans meet current intake recommendations for vitamin B6.

When can a vitamin B6 deficiency occur?

Clinical signs of vitamin B6 deficiency are rarely seen in the United States. Many older Americans, however, have low blood levels of vitamin B6, which may suggest a marginal or suboptimal vitamin B6 nutritional status. Vitamin B6 deficiency can occur in individuals with poor-quality diets that are deficient in many nutrients. Symptoms occur during later stages of deficiency, when intake has been very low for an extended time. Signs of vitamin B6 deficiency include dermatitis (skin inflammation), glossitis (a sore tongue), depression, confusion, and convulsions. Vitamin B6 deficiency also can cause anemia. Some of these symptoms can also result from a variety of medical conditions other than vitamin B6 deficiency. It is important to have a physician evaluate these symptoms so that appropriate medical care can be given.

Who may need extra vitamin B6 to prevent a deficiency?

Individuals with a poor-quality diet or an inadequate B6 intake for an extended period may benefit from taking a vitamin B6 supplement if they are unable to increase their dietary intake of vitamin B6. Alcoholics and older adults are more likely to have inadequate vitamin B6 intakes than other segments of the population because they may have limited variety in their diet. Alcohol also promotes the destruction and loss of vitamin B6 from the body.

Asthmatic children treated with the medicine theophylline may need to take a vitamin B6 supplement. Theophylline decreases body stores of vitamin B6, and theophylline-induced seizures have been linked to low body stores of the vitamin. A physician should be consulted about the need for a vitamin B6 supplement when theophylline is prescribed.

What is the health risk of too much vitamin B6?

Too much vitamin B6 can result in nerve damage to the arms and legs. This neuropathy is usually related to high intake of vitamin B6 from supplements and is reversible when supplementation is stopped. The Food and Nutrition Board of the Institute of Medicine has established an upper tolerable intake level for vitamin B6 of 100 mg per day for all adults.

Folate

"Folate," April 15, 2009, Office of Dietary Supplements (ods.od.nih.gov).

Folate is a water-soluble B vitamin that occurs naturally in food. Folic acid is the synthetic form of folate that is found in supplements and added to fortified foods.

Folate gets its name from the Latin word *folium*, for leaf. A key observation of researcher Lucy Wills nearly 70 years ago led to the identification of folate as the nutrient needed to prevent the anemia of pregnancy. Dr. Wills demonstrated that the anemia could be corrected by a yeast extract. Folate was identified as the corrective substance in yeast extract in the late 1930s and was extracted from spinach leaves in 1941.

Folate helps produce and maintain new cells. This is especially important during periods of rapid cell division and growth such as infancy and pregnancy. Folate is needed to make DNA and RNA, the building blocks of cells. It also helps prevent changes to DNA that may lead to cancer. Both adults and children need folate to make normal red blood cells and prevent anemia. Folate is also essential for the metabolism of homocysteine and helps maintain normal levels of this amino acid.

What foods provide folate?

Leafy green vegetables (like spinach and turnip greens), fruits (like citrus fruits and juices), and dried beans and peas are all natural sources of folate.

In 1996, the Food and Drug Administration (FDA) published regulations requiring the addition of folic acid to enriched breads, cereals, flours, corn meals, pastas, rice, and other grain products. Since cereals and grains are widely consumed in the U.S., these products have become a very important contributor of folic acid to the American diet.

When can folate deficiency occur?

A deficiency of folate can occur when an increased need for folate is not matched by an increased intake, when dietary folate intake does not meet recommended needs, and when folate loss increases. Medications that interfere with the metabolism of folate may also increase the need for this vitamin and risk of deficiency.

Medical conditions that increase the need for folate or result in increased loss of folate include the following:

- Pregnancy and lactation (breast-feeding)
- Alcohol abuse
- Malabsorption
- Kidney dialysis
- Liver disease
- Certain anemias

Medications that interfere with folate utilization include the following:

- Anticonvulsant medications (such as Dilantin, phenytoin, and primidone)
- Metformin (sometimes prescribed to control blood sugar in type 2 diabetes)
- Sulfasalazine (used to control inflammation associated with Crohn disease and ulcerative colitis)
- Triamterene (a diuretic)
- Methotrexate (used for cancer and other diseases such as rheumatoid arthritis)
- Barbiturates (used as sedatives)

What are some common signs and symptoms of folate deficiency?

- Folate-deficient women who become pregnant are at greater risk of giving birth to low-birth-weight or premature infants and/or infants with neural tube defects.

- In infants and children, folate deficiency can slow overall growth rate.

- In adults, a particular type of anemia can result from long-term folate deficiency.

- Other signs of folate deficiency are often subtle. Digestive disorders such as diarrhea, loss of appetite, and weight loss can occur, as can weakness, sore tongue, headaches, heart palpitations,

147

irritability, forgetfulness, and behavioral disorders. An elevated level of homocysteine in the blood, a risk factor for cardiovascular disease, also can result from folate deficiency.

Many of these subtle symptoms are general and can also result from a variety of medical conditions other than folate deficiency. It is important to have a physician evaluate these symptoms so that appropriate medical care can be given.

Do women of childbearing age and pregnant women have a special need for folate?

Folic acid is very important for all women who may become pregnant. Adequate folate intake during the periconceptual period, the time just before and just after a woman becomes pregnant, protects against neural tube defects. Neural tube defects result in malformations of the spine (spina bifida), skull, and brain (anencephaly). The risk of neural tube defects is significantly reduced when supplemental folic acid is consumed in addition to a healthful diet prior to and during the first month following conception. Since January 1, 1998, when the folate food fortification program took effect, data suggest that there has been a significant reduction in neural tube birth defects. Women who could become pregnant are advised to eat foods fortified with folic acid or take a folic acid supplement in addition to eating folate-rich foods to reduce the risk of some serious birth defects. For this population, researchers recommend a daily intake of 400 mcg of synthetic folic acid per day from fortified foods and/or dietary supplements.

Who else may need extra folic acid to prevent a deficiency?

People who abuse alcohol, those taking medications that may interfere with the action of folate, individuals diagnosed with anemia from folate deficiency, and those with malabsorption, liver disease, or who are receiving kidney dialysis treatment may benefit from a folic acid supplement.

Folate deficiency has been observed in alcoholics. A 1997 review of the nutritional status of chronic alcoholics found low folate status in more than 50% of those surveyed. Alcohol interferes with the absorption of folate and increases the amount of folate the kidney gets rid of. In addition, many people who abuse alcohol have poor quality diets that do not provide the recommended intake of folate. Increasing folate intake through diet, or folic acid intake through fortified foods or supplements, may be beneficial to the health of alcoholics.

Anticonvulsant medications such as Dilantin increase the need for folate. Anyone taking anticonvulsants and other medications that interfere with the body's ability to use folate should consult with a medical doctor about the need to take a folic acid supplement.

Anemia is a condition that occurs when there is insufficient hemoglobin in red blood cells to carry enough oxygen to cells and tissues. It can result from a wide variety of medical problems, including folate deficiency. With folate deficiency, your body may make large red blood cells that do not contain adequate hemoglobin, the substance in red blood cells that carries oxygen to your body's cells. Your physician can determine whether an anemia is associated with folate deficiency and whether supplemental folic acid is indicated.

Several medical conditions increase the risk of folic acid deficiency. Liver disease and kidney dialysis increase the loss of folic acid. Malabsorption can prevent your body from using folate in food. Medical doctors treating individuals with these disorders will evaluate the need for a folic acid supplement.

Are there cautions about using folic acid supplements?

Beware of the interaction between vitamin B12 and folic acid. Intake of supplemental folic acid should not exceed 1,000 mcg per day to prevent folic acid from triggering symptoms of vitamin B12 deficiency. Folic acid supplements can correct the anemia associated with vitamin B12 deficiency. Unfortunately, folic acid will not correct changes in the nervous system that result from vitamin B12 deficiency. Permanent nerve damage can occur if vitamin B12 deficiency is not treated.

It is very important for older adults to be aware of the relationship between folic acid and vitamin B12 because they are at greater risk of having a vitamin B12 deficiency. If you are 50 years of age or older, ask your physician to check your B12 status before you take a supplement that contains folic acid. If you are taking a supplement containing folic acid, read the label to make sure it also contains B12 or speak with a physician about the need for a B12 supplement.

What is the health risk of too much folic acid?

Folate intake from food is not associated with any health risk. The risk of toxicity from folic acid intake from supplements and/or fortified foods is also low. It is a water-soluble vitamin, so any excess intake is usually lost in the urine. There is some evidence that high levels of folic acid can provoke seizures in patients taking anticonvulsant medications. Anyone taking such medications should consult with a medical doctor before taking a folic acid supplement.

The Institute of Medicine has established a tolerable upper intake level for folate from fortified foods or supplements (i.e., folic acid) for ages one and above. Intakes above this level increase the risk of adverse health effects. In adults, supplemental folic acid should not exceed the UL to prevent folic acid from triggering symptoms of vitamin B12 deficiency. It is important to recognize that the UL refers to the amount of synthetic folate (i.e., folic acid) being consumed per day from fortified foods and/or supplements. There is no health risk, and no UL, for natural sources of folate found in food. Table 16.6 lists the UL for folate, in micrograms, for children and adults.

Table 16.6. Tolerable Upper Intake Levels for Folate for Children and Adults

Age (years)	Males and Females (mcg/day)	Pregnancy (mcg/day)	Lactation (mcg/day)
1–3	300	N/A	N/A
4–8	400	N/A	N/A
9–13	600	N/A	N/A
14–18	800	800	800
19+	1,000	1,000	1,000

Vitamin B12

"Vitamin B12: QuickFacts," July 8, 2010, Office of Dietary Supplements (ods.od.nih.gov).

What is vitamin B12 and what does it do?

Vitamin B12 is a nutrient that helps keep the body's nerve and blood cells healthy. It also helps prevent a type of anemia that makes people tired and weak.

How much vitamin B12 do I need?

It depends on your age. Here are the amounts people of different ages should get on average each day in micrograms:

- Birth to 6 months: 0.4 mcg

- Infants 7–12 months: 0.5 mcg

- Children 1–3 years: 0.9 mcg

- Children 4–8 years: 1.2 mcg

- Children 9–13 years: 1.8 mcg

- Teens 14–18 years: 2.4 mcg

- Adults: 2.4 mcg

- Pregnant teens and women: 2.6 mcg

- Breast-feeding teens and women: 2.8 mcg

What foods provide vitamin B12?

Foods from animals, but not plants, naturally have vitamin B12. You can get enough vitamin B12 by eating a variety of foods including beef liver, clams, fish, meat, poultry, eggs, milk, and other dairy products. Vitamin B12 is added to some breakfast cereals and other food products (check the product labels).

What kinds of vitamin B12 dietary supplements are available?

Almost all multivitamins have vitamin B12. Some dietary supplements have vitamin B12 only. Others have vitamin B12 with folic acid, vitamin B6, and other nutrients. You can also get vitamin B12 from a shot or a nasal gel with a doctor's prescription. These forms are usually used to treat vitamin B12 deficiency.

Am I getting enough vitamin B12?

Most people get enough vitamin B12 from the foods they eat. But some people have trouble absorbing vitamin B12 and might have a deficiency, even if they get enough vitamin B12. Many older adults, for example, have trouble absorbing the vitamin B12 found naturally in food. However, most older adults can absorb the vitamin B12 that is added to fortified foods, such as some breakfast cereals, and dietary supplements. People over age 50 should get most of their vitamin B12 from these sources. People with pernicious anemia have trouble absorbing vitamin B12 from all foods and dietary supplements. Others who might have trouble getting enough vitamin B12 include people who eat little or no animal foods such as strict vegetarians and vegans; people who have had weight loss surgery; and people with digestive disorders, such as celiac disease or Crohn disease. Your doctor can test your vitamin B12 level to see if you have a deficiency.

What happens if I don't get enough vitamin B12?

People who don't get enough vitamin B12 can have many symptoms. Some of these are tiredness, weakness, memory loss, constipation, loss of appetite, weight loss, and anemia. Nerve problems such as numbness and tingling in the hands and feet can also occur.

What are some effects of vitamin B12 on health?

Scientists are studying vitamin B12 to see how it affects health. Here are a few examples of what this research has shown:

Heart disease: Research on vitamin B12, usually combined with folic acid and vitamin B6, shows that taking vitamin B12 does not reduce the risk of having a heart attack or stroke.

Dementia: As they get older, some people develop dementia or confusion. Scientists don't know yet whether vitamin B12 helps prevent or treat dementia.

Energy and athletic performance: Vitamin B12 supplements do not appear to improve energy or athletic performance, except in people with a vitamin B12 deficiency.

Can vitamin B12 be harmful?

Vitamin B12 has not been shown to cause any harm.

Are there any interactions with vitamin B12 that I should know about?

Yes. For example, metformin for diabetes as well as some medicines that people take for acid reflux and peptic ulcer disease can affect how well the body absorbs vitamin B12.

Bottom line: Tell your doctor, pharmacist, and other health care providers about any dietary supplements and medicines you take. They can tell you if those dietary supplements might interact or interfere with your prescription or over-the-counter medicines or if the medicines might affect how your body uses vitamin B12.

Section 16.3

Vitamin C

"Vitamin C: QuickFacts," Office of Dietary Supplements
(ods.od.nih.gov), July 8, 2010.

What is vitamin C and what does it do?

Vitamin C is a nutrient in food that people need to stay healthy. It helps heal wounds and protects the body from infections, viruses, and damage that naturally occurs when the body turns food into energy.

How much vitamin C do I need?

It depends on your age. Here are the amounts people of different ages should get, on average, each day in milligrams (mg):

- Birth to 6 months: 40 mg
- Infants 7–12 months: 50 mg
- Children 1–3 years: 15 mg
- Children 4–8 years: 25 mg
- Children 9–13 years: 45 mg
- Teens 14–18 years (boys): 75 mg
- Teens 14–18 years (girls): 65 mg
- Adults (men): 90 mg
- Adults (women): 75 mg
- Pregnant teens: 80 mg
- Pregnant women: 85 mg
- Breast-feeding teens: 115 mg
- Breast-feeding women: 120 mg

If you smoke, add 35 mg to the numbers listed here to get the amount you need each day.

What foods provide vitamin C?

Fruits and vegetables are the best sources of vitamin C. You can get enough vitamin C by eating a variety of foods including citrus fruits (such as oranges and grapefruit) and their juices, as well as red and green pepper, kiwifruit, broccoli, strawberries, baked potatoes, and tomatoes. Vitamin C is added to some foods and beverages (check the product labels).

What kinds of vitamin C dietary supplements are available?

Most multivitamins have vitamin C. Vitamin C is also available alone as a dietary supplement or combined with other nutrients.

Am I getting enough vitamin C?

Most people get enough vitamin C. However, people who don't eat a variety of foods might not get as much vitamin C as they need. People who smoke might also have trouble getting enough vitamin C because they need higher amounts. Some people with cancer and people with kidney disease on dialysis might also not get enough vitamin C.

What happens if I don't get enough vitamin C?

Vitamin C deficiency is rare in the United States and Canada. People who get very little vitamin C for many weeks can get a disease called scurvy. Scurvy causes tiredness, swollen gums, small red or purple spots on the skin, joint pain, poor wound healing, and corkscrew hairs. Scurvy can also cause depression, bleeding gums, loose teeth, and anemia. People can die from scurvy if it is not treated.

What are some effects of vitamin C on health?

Scientists are studying vitamin C to see how it affects health. Here are a few examples of what this research has shown.

Cancer: People who get a lot of vitamin C from eating fruits and vegetables might have a lower risk of getting some types of cancer. However, taking vitamin C dietary supplements doesn't seem to help prevent cancer.

It is not clear whether taking high doses of vitamin C helps treat cancer. Vitamin C dietary supplements might interact with chemotherapy and radiation therapy. If you are being treated for cancer, talk with your health care provider before taking vitamin C or other dietary supplements, especially in high doses.

Heart disease: Eating lots of fruits and vegetables might lower your risk of getting heart disease. However, scientists aren't sure whether vitamin C, either from food or supplements, helps protect people from heart disease. It is also not clear whether vitamin C helps keep heart disease from getting worse in people who already have it.

Age-related macular degeneration (AMD) and cataracts: Over time, people with AMD lose the ability to see. In people who have early-stage AMD, a specific supplement with vitamin C and other ingredients might slow down the loss of vision.

Cataracts also cause vision loss. However, it is not clear whether vitamin C, either from food or dietary supplements, affects the risk of getting cataracts.

The common cold: When taken regularly before getting a cold, vitamin C supplements might slightly shorten the length of a cold and reduce symptoms somewhat. However, for most people, taking vitamin C supplements does not seem to lessen the chance of getting colds. Taking vitamin C supplements also doesn't appear to be helpful after someone actually comes down with a cold.

Can vitamin C be harmful?

Too much vitamin C might cause diarrhea, nausea, and stomach cramps. The safe upper limits for vitamin C are listed here:

- Birth to 12 months: Not established
- Children 1–3 years: 400 mg
- Children 4–8 years: 650 mg
- Children 9–13 years: 1,200 mg
- Teens 14–18 years: 1,800 mg
- Adults: 2,000 mg

Are there any interactions with vitamin C that I should know about?

Yes. For example, taking vitamin C supplements might affect how well some medicines work, such as niacin and statins for high cholesterol. Vitamin C supplements might also interact with chemotherapy or radiation therapy for cancer.

Tell your doctor, pharmacist, and other health care providers about any dietary supplements and medicines you take. They can tell you if those dietary supplements might interact or interfere with your prescription or over-the-counter medicines or if the medicines might affect how your body uses vitamin C.

Section 16.4

Vitamin D

This section excerpted from "Vitamin D: QuickFacts,"
Office of Dietary Supplements (ods.od.nih.gov), February 4, 2011.

What is vitamin D and what does it do?

Vitamin D is a nutrient found in some foods that is needed for health and to maintain strong bones. It does so by helping the body absorb calcium (one of bone's main building blocks) from food and supplements.

How much vitamin D do I need?

The amount of vitamin D you need each day depends on your age. Average daily recommended amounts from the Food and Nutrition Board (a national group of experts) for different ages are listed here in International Units (IU):

- Birth to 12 months: 400 IU
- Children 1–13 years: 600 IU
- Teens 14–18 years: 600 IU
- Adults 19–70 years: 600 IU
- Adults 71 years and older: 800 IU
- Pregnant and breast-feeding women: 600 IU

What foods provide vitamin D?

Very few foods naturally have vitamin D. Fortified foods provide most of the vitamin D in American diets.

- Fatty fish such as salmon, tuna, and mackerel are among the best sources.
- Beef liver, cheese, and egg yolks provide small amounts.
- Mushrooms provide some vitamin D.

- Almost all of the U.S. milk supply is fortified with 400 IU of vitamin D per quart. But foods made from milk, like cheese and ice cream, are usually not fortified.

- Vitamin D is added to many breakfast cereals and to some brands of orange juice, yogurt, margarine, and soy beverages; check the labels.

Can I get vitamin D from the sun?

The body makes vitamin D when skin is directly exposed to the sun, and most people meet at least some of their vitamin D needs this way. Skin exposed to sunshine indoors through a window will not produce vitamin D. Cloudy days, shade, and having dark-colored skin also cut down on the amount of vitamin D the skin makes.

However, despite the importance of the sun to vitamin D synthesis, it is prudent to limit exposure of skin to sunlight in order to lower the risk for skin cancer.

Am I getting enough vitamin D?

Some Americans are vitamin D deficient and almost no one has levels that are too high. In general, young people have higher blood levels of vitamin D than older people and males have higher levels than females. By race, non-Hispanic blacks tend to have the lowest levels and non-Hispanic whites the highest.

Certain other groups may not get enough vitamin D:

- Breast-fed infants (breastfed infants should be given a supplement of 400 IU of vitamin D each day)

- Older adults

- People with dark skin

- People with disorders such as Crohn disease or celiac disease

- Obese people

What happens if I don't get enough vitamin D?

People can become deficient in vitamin D because they don't consume enough or absorb enough from food, their exposure to sunlight is limited, or their kidneys cannot convert vitamin D to its active form in the body. In children, vitamin D deficiency causes rickets, where the bones become soft and bend. It's a rare disease but still occurs, especially among African American infants and children. In adults, vitamin D deficiency leads to osteomalacia, causing bone pain and muscle weakness.

What are some effects of vitamin D on health?

Vitamin D is being studied for its possible connections to several diseases and medical problems, including diabetes, hypertension, bone disorders, cancer, and autoimmune conditions such as multiple sclerosis.

Can vitamin D be harmful?

Yes, when amounts in the blood become too high. Signs of toxicity include nausea, vomiting, poor appetite, constipation, weakness, and weight loss. And by raising blood levels of calcium, too much vitamin D can cause confusion, disorientation, and problems with heart rhythm. Excess vitamin D can also damage the kidneys.

Vitamin D toxicity almost always occurs from overuse of supplements. Excessive sun exposure doesn't cause vitamin D poisoning because the body limits the amount of this vitamin it produces.

Are there any interactions with vitamin D that I should know about?

Like most dietary supplements, vitamin D may interact or interfere with other medicines or supplements you might be taking. Tell your doctor, pharmacist, and other health care providers about any dietary supplements and medicines you take.

Section 16.5

Vitamin E

"Vitamin E: QuickFacts," Office of Dietary Supplements
(ods.od.nih.gov), July 19, 2010.

What is vitamin E and what does it do?

Vitamin E is a nutrient in food that people need to stay healthy. The body uses vitamin E, for example, to protect itself from infections and to keep blood flowing through the blood vessels.

How much vitamin E do I need?

It depends on your age. Here are the amounts people should get on average each day, in milligrams and International Units:

- Birth to 6 months: 4 mg (6 IU)

- Infants 7–12 months: 5 mg (7.5 IU)

- Children 1–3 years: 6 mg (9 IU)

- Children 4–8 years: 7 mg (10.4 IU)

- Children 9–13 years: 11 mg (16.4 IU)

- Teens 14–18 years: 15 mg (22.4 IU)

- Adults: 15 mg (22.4 IU)

- Pregnant teens and women: 15 mg (22.4 IU)

- Breast-feeding teens and women: 19 mg (28.4 IU)

What foods provide vitamin E?

You can get enough vitamin E by eating a variety of foods, including vegetable oils (such as wheat germ, sunflower, and safflower oils), nuts (such as almonds), seeds (such as sunflower seeds), and green vegetables (such as spinach and broccoli).

Vitamin E is added to some breakfast cereals, fruit juices, margarines and spreads, and other foods (check the product labels).

What kinds of vitamin E dietary supplements are available?

Most multivitamin-mineral supplements have vitamin E. It is also available alone as a dietary supplement or combined with other nutrients. The doses of vitamin E in these products are often much higher than the recommended amounts.

A chemical name for vitamin E is alpha-tocopherol. Vitamin E from natural (food) sources is listed on food and supplement labels as d-alpha-tocopherol. Synthetic (laboratory-made) vitamin E is listed on labels as dl-alpha-tocopherol. The natural form is stronger. For example, 100 IU of natural vitamin E is equal to about 150 IU of the synthetic form.

Other kinds of vitamin E supplements are named gamma-tocopherol, tocotrienols, and mixed tocopherols. These supplements are often more expensive than alpha-tocopherol. For most people, alpha-tocopherol (natural or synthetic) is fine.

Am I getting enough vitamin E?

Many people do not get recommended amounts of vitamin E from food. But only people with certain diseases become deficient. These include people who have trouble digesting or absorbing fat, such as those with Crohn disease, cystic fibrosis, and certain rare inherited conditions.

What happens if I don't get enough vitamin E?

Usually, nothing obvious happens in the short run if you don't get enough vitamin E. But over time, not getting enough vitamin E can cause nerve and muscle damage and make your body less able to fight off infections.

What are some effects of vitamin E on health?

Scientists are studying vitamin E to see how it affects health. Here are a few examples of what this research has shown.

Heart disease: Vitamin E does not seem to help prevent heart disease in middle-aged or older people or affect the risk of death from this disease. We do not know whether high intakes of vitamin E protect heart health in young, healthy people.

Cancer: Its not clear whether vitamin E prevents cancer. Vitamin E supplements might interact with chemotherapy and radiation therapy. If you are undergoing cancer treatment, talk with your health care provider before taking vitamin E or other dietary supplements, especially in high doses.

Eye disorders: AMD (the loss of straight-ahead vision) and cataracts (clouding of the surface of the eye) cause vision loss in older people. It is not clear whether taking extra vitamin E might help prevent these conditions. In people who have early-stage AMD, a supplement containing vitamin E and other ingredients might help slow vision loss.

Mental function: Vitamin E supplements probably do not help healthy older people stay mentally active and alert. Vitamin E supplements cannot prevent or slow the decline in mental function, or prevent or treat Alzheimer disease.

Can vitamin E be harmful?

In healthy adults, up to 1,500 IU/day of natural vitamin E supplements or up to 1,100 IU/day of the synthetic form is safe. Higher doses can increase the time it takes blood to clot from a cut or injury. Very high doses can increase the risk of serious bleeding in the brain (stroke).

Are there any interactions with vitamin E that I should know about?

Vitamin E can increase the risk of bleeding in people taking anticlotting drugs, such as warfarin (Coumadin®). It might also interact with chemotherapy or radiation therapy. Also, vitamin E might lessen the effectiveness of medicines to lower cholesterol.

Tell your doctor, pharmacist, and other health care providers about any dietary supplements and medicines you take. They can tell you if those supplements might interact or interfere with your prescription or over-the-counter medicines or if the medicines might affect how your body uses vitamin E.

Chapter 17

Important Minerals

Chapter Contents

Section 17.1

Calcium

This section excerpted from "Calcium,"
Office of Dietary Supplements (ods.od.nih.gov),
November 30, 2010.

What is calcium and what does it do?

Calcium is a mineral found in many foods. The body needs calcium to maintain strong bones and to carry out many important functions. Almost all calcium is stored in bones and teeth, where it supports their structure and hardness.

The body also needs calcium for muscles to move and for nerves to carry messages between the brain and every body part. In addition, calcium is used to help blood vessels move blood throughout the body and to help release hormones and enzymes that affect almost every function in the human body.

How much calcium do I need?

The amount of calcium you need each day depends on your age. Average daily recommended amounts are listed here in milligrams (mg):

- Birth to 6 months: 210 mg
- Infants 7–12 months: 270 mg
- Children 1–3 years: 500 mg
- Children 4-8 years: 800 mg
- Children 9–13 years: 1,300 mg
- Teens 14–18 years: 1,300 mg
- Adults 19–50 years: 1,000 mg
- Adults 51 years and older: 1,200 mg
- Pregnant and breast-feeding teens: 1,300 mg
- Pregnant and breast-feeding adults: 1,000 mg

What foods provide calcium?

Calcium is found in many foods. You can get recommended amounts of calcium by eating a variety of foods, including the following:

- Milk, yogurt, and cheese are the main food sources of calcium for the majority of people in the United States.

- Kale, broccoli, and Chinese cabbage are fine vegetable sources of calcium.

- Fish with soft bones that you eat, such as canned sardines and salmon, are fine animal sources of calcium.

- Most grains (such as breads, pastas, and unfortified cereals), while not rich in calcium, add significant amounts of calcium to the diet because people eat them often or in large amounts.

- Calcium is added to some breakfast cereals, fruit juices, soy and rice beverages, and tofu (check the product labels).

What kinds of calcium dietary supplements are available?

Calcium is found in many multivitamin-mineral supplements, though the amount varies by product. Dietary supplements that contain only calcium or calcium with other nutrients such as vitamin D are also available. Check the Supplement Facts label to determine the amount of calcium provided.

The two main forms of calcium dietary supplements are carbonate and citrate. Calcium carbonate is inexpensive but is absorbed best when taken with food. Some over-the-counter antacid products, such as Tums® and Rolaids®, contain calcium carbonate. Each pill or chew provides 200–400 mg of calcium. Calcium citrate, a more expensive form of the supplement, is absorbed well on an empty or a full stomach. In addition, people with low levels of stomach acid (a condition more common in people older than 50) absorb calcium citrate more easily than calcium carbonate. Other forms of calcium in supplements and fortified foods include gluconate, lactate, and phosphate.

Calcium absorption is best when a person consumes no more than 500 mg at one time. So a person who takes 1,000 mg/day of calcium from supplements, for example, should split the dose rather than take it all at once.

Calcium supplements may cause gas, bloating, and constipation in some people. If any of these symptoms occur, try spreading out the calcium dose throughout the day, taking the supplement with meals, or changing the supplement brand or calcium form you take.

Am I getting enough calcium?

Many people don't get recommended amounts of calcium from the foods they eat. This includes women and teenage girls as well as men 60 years of age and older.

Certain groups of people are more likely than others to have trouble getting enough calcium:

- **Postmenopausal women** experience greater bone loss and do not absorb calcium as well. Sufficient calcium intake from food, and supplements if needed, can slow the rate of bone loss.

- **Women of childbearing age whose menstrual periods stop (amenorrhea)** because they exercise heavily, eat too little, or both. They need sufficient calcium to cope with the resulting decreased calcium absorption, increased calcium losses in the urine, and slowdown in the formation of new bone.

- **People with lactose intolerance** cannot digest this natural sugar found in milk and experience symptoms like bloating, gas, and diarrhea when they drink more than small amounts at a time. They usually can eat other calcium-rich dairy products that are low in lactose, such as yogurt and many cheeses, and drink lactose-reduced or lactose-free milk.

- **Vegans (vegetarians who eat no animal products)** avoid the dairy products that are a major source of calcium in other people's diets.

Many factors can affect the amount of calcium absorbed from the digestive tract:

- **Age:** Efficiency of calcium absorption decreases as people age. This explains the higher recommended calcium intakes for people aged 50 and older.

- **Vitamin D intake:** This vitamin, present in some foods and produced in the body when skin is exposed to sunlight, increases calcium absorption.

- **Other components in food:** Both oxalic acid (in some vegetables and beans) and phytic acid (in whole grains) can reduce calcium absorption. People who eat a variety of foods don't have to consider these factors. They are accounted for in the calcium recommended intakes, which take absorption into account.

Many factors can also affect how much calcium the body eliminates in urine, feces, and sweat. These include consumption of alcohol- and caffeine-containing beverages as well as intake of other nutrients (protein, sodium, potassium, and phosphorus). In most people, these factors have little effect on calcium status.

What happens if I don't get enough calcium?

Insufficient intakes of calcium do not produce obvious symptoms in the short term because the body maintains calcium levels in the blood by taking it from bone. Over the long term, intakes of calcium below recommended levels have health consequences, such as low bone mass (osteopenia) and increased risk of osteoporosis and bone fractures.

Symptoms of serious calcium deficiency include numbness and tingling in the fingers, convulsions, and abnormal heart rhythms that can lead to death if not corrected. These symptoms occur almost always in people with serious health problems or who are undergoing certain medical treatments.

What are some effects of calcium on health?

Scientists are studying calcium to understand how it affects health. Here are several examples of what this research has shown:

Bone health and osteoporosis: Bones need plenty of calcium and vitamin D throughout childhood and adolescence to reach their peak strength and calcium content by about age 30. After that, bones slowly lose calcium, but people can help reduce these losses by getting recommended amounts of calcium throughout adulthood and by having healthy, active lifestyles that include weight-bearing physical activity.

Osteoporosis is a disease of the bones in older adults (especially women) in which the bones become porous, fragile, and more prone to fracture. Osteoporosis is a serious public health problem for more than 10 million adults in the United States. Adequate calcium and vitamin D intakes as well as regular exercise are essential to keep bones healthy throughout life.

High blood pressure: Some studies have found that getting recommended intakes of calcium can reduce the risk of developing high blood pressure (hypertension). One large study in particular found that eating a diet high in low-fat and fat-free dairy products, vegetables, and fruits lowered blood pressure.

Cancer: Studies have examined whether calcium supplements or diets high in calcium might lower the risk of developing cancer of the colon or rectum or (in men) increase the risk of prostate cancer. The research to date provides no clear answers. Given that cancer develops over many years, longer term studies are needed.

Kidney stones: Most kidney stones are rich in calcium oxalate. Some studies have found that higher intakes of calcium are linked to a greater risk of kidney stones, but others have found that higher intakes are associated with a lower risk. For most people, other factors (such as not drinking enough fluids) have a larger effect on the risk of kidney stones than calcium intake.

Weight loss: Several studies have shown that getting more calcium helps lower body weight or reduce weight gain over time. However, the best studies have found that calcium—from foods or dietary supplements—has little if any effect on body weight and amounts of body fat.

Can calcium be harmful?

Up to 2,500 mg/day of calcium from foods and dietary supplements is considered to be safe for both children and adults.

When the amount of calcium in the blood is too high, it can damage the kidneys and reduce the absorption of other essential minerals such as iron, zinc, magnesium, and phosphorus. Such high levels of calcium are rarely caused by getting too much calcium from foods or dietary supplements but, rather, by advanced cases of cancer, very excessive intakes of vitamin D from supplements, or hyperparathyroidism.

Are there any interactions with calcium that I should know about?

Calcium dietary supplements can interact or interfere with certain medicines that you take, and some medicines can lower or raise calcium levels in the body. Here are some examples:

- Calcium can reduce the absorption of these drugs when taken together:
  - Bisphosphonates (to treat osteoporosis)
  - Antibiotics of the fluoroquinolone and tetracycline families
  - Levothyroxine (to treat low thyroid activity)
  - Phenytoin (an anticonvulsant)
  - Tiludronate disodium (to treat Paget disease).

- Diuretics differ in their effects. Thiazide-type diuretics (such as Diuril® and Lozol®) reduce calcium excretion by the kidneys, which in turn can raise blood calcium levels too high. But loop diuretics (such as Lasix® and Bumex®) increase calcium excretion and thereby lower blood calcium levels.

- Antacids containing aluminum or magnesium increase calcium loss in the urine.

- Mineral oil and stimulant laxatives reduce calcium absorption.

- Glucocorticoids (such as prednisone) can cause calcium depletion and eventually osteoporosis when people use them for months at a time.

Tell your doctor, pharmacist, and other health care providers about any dietary supplements and medicines you take. They can tell you if those dietary supplements might interact or interfere with your prescription or over-the-counter medicines or if the medicines might interfere with how your body absorbs, uses, or breaks down nutrients.

Section 17.2

Iron

This section excerpted from "Iron," Office of Dietary Supplements (ods.od.nih.gov), August 24, 2007.

Iron, one of the most abundant metals on Earth, is essential to most life forms and to normal human physiology. Iron is an integral part of many proteins and enzymes that maintain good health. In humans, iron is an essential component of proteins involved in oxygen transport. It is also essential for the regulation of cell growth and differentiation. A deficiency of iron limits oxygen delivery to cells, resulting in fatigue, poor work performance, and decreased immunity. On the other hand, excess amounts of iron can result in toxicity and even death.

Almost two-thirds of iron in the body is found in hemoglobin, the protein in red blood cells that carries oxygen to tissues. Smaller amounts of iron are found in myoglobin, a protein that helps supply oxygen to muscle, and in enzymes that assist biochemical reactions.

Iron is also found in proteins that store iron for future needs and that transport iron in blood. Iron stores are regulated by intestinal iron absorption.

What foods provide iron?

There are two forms of dietary iron: heme and nonheme. Heme iron is derived from hemoglobin, the protein in red blood cells that delivers oxygen to cells. Heme iron is found in animal foods that originally contained hemoglobin, such as red meats, fish, and poultry. Iron in plant foods such as lentils, beans, and spinach is arranged in a chemical structure called nonheme iron. This is the form of iron added to iron-enriched and iron-fortified foods. Heme iron is absorbed better than nonheme iron, but most dietary iron is nonheme iron.

According to the 2005 Dietary Guidelines for Americans, "Nutrient needs should be met primarily through consuming foods. Foods provide an array of nutrients and other compounds that may have beneficial effects on health. In certain cases, fortified foods and dietary supplements may be useful sources of one or more nutrients that otherwise might be consumed in less than recommended amounts. However, dietary supplements, while recommended in some cases, cannot replace a healthful diet." It is important for anyone who is considering taking an iron supplement to first consider whether their needs are being met by natural dietary sources of heme and nonheme iron and foods fortified with iron and to discuss their potential need for iron supplements with their physician.

What affects iron absorption?

Iron absorption refers to the amount of dietary iron that the body obtains and uses from food. Healthy adults absorb about 10% to 15% of dietary iron, but individual absorption is influenced by several factors.

Storage levels of iron have the greatest influence on iron absorption. Iron absorption increases when body stores are low. When iron stores are high, absorption decreases to help protect against toxic effects of iron overload. Iron absorption is also influenced by the type of dietary iron consumed. Absorption of heme iron from meat proteins is efficient. Absorption of heme iron ranges from 15% to 35% and is not significantly affected by diet. In contrast, 2% to 20% of nonheme iron in plant foods such as rice, maize, black beans, soybeans, and wheat is absorbed. Nonheme iron absorption is significantly influenced by various food components.

Meat proteins and vitamin C will improve the absorption of non-heme iron. Tannins (found in tea), calcium, polyphenols, and phytates (found in legumes and whole grains) can decrease absorption of nonheme iron. Some proteins found in soybeans also inhibit nonheme iron absorption. It is most important to include foods that enhance nonheme iron absorption when daily iron intake is less than recommended, when iron losses are high (which may occur with heavy menstrual losses), when iron requirements are high (as in pregnancy), and when only vegetarian nonheme sources of iron are consumed.

What is the recommended intake for iron?

Recommendations for iron are provided in the Dietary Reference Intakes (DRIs) developed by the Institute of Medicine of the National Academy of Sciences. Dietary Reference Intakes is the general term for a set of reference values used for planning and assessing nutrient intake for healthy people. Three important types of reference values included in the DRIs are Recommended Dietary Allowances (RDA), Adequate Intakes (AI), and Tolerable Upper Intake Levels (UL). The RDA recommends the average daily intake that is sufficient to meet the nutrient requirements of nearly all (97%–98%) healthy individuals in each age and gender group. An AI is set when there is insufficient scientific data available to establish a RDA. AIs meet or exceed the amount needed to maintain a nutritional state of adequacy in nearly all members of a specific age and gender group. The UL, on the other hand, is the maximum daily intake unlikely to result in adverse health effects. Table 17.1 lists the RDAs for iron, in milligrams, for infants, children, and adults.

Table 17.1. Recommended Dietary Allowances for Iron for Infants (7 to 12 months), Children, and Adults

Age	Males (mg/day)	Females (mg/day)	Pregnancy (mg/day)	Lactation (mg/day)
7 to 12 months	11	11	N/A	N/A
1 to 3 years	7	7	N/A	N/A
4 to 8 years	10	10	N/A	N/A
9 to 13 years	8	8	N/A	N/A
14 to 18 years	11	15	27	10
19 to 50 years	8	18	27	9
51+ years	8	8	N/A	N/A

Healthy full-term infants are born with a supply of iron that lasts for 4 to 6 months. There is not enough evidence available to establish an RDA for iron for infants from birth through 6 months of age. The recommended iron intake (0.27 mg/day) for this age group is based on an AI that reflects the average iron intake of healthy infants fed breast milk.

Iron in human breast milk is well absorbed by infants. It is estimated that infants can use greater than 50% of the iron in breast milk as compared to less than 12% of the iron in infant formula. The amount of iron in cow's milk is low, and infants poorly absorb it. Feeding cow's milk to infants also may result in gastrointestinal bleeding. For these reasons, cow's milk should not be fed to infants until they are at least 1 year old. The American Academy of Pediatrics (AAP) recommends that infants be exclusively breast-fed for the first six months of life. Gradual introduction of iron-enriched solid foods should complement breast milk from 7 to 12 months of age. Infants weaned from breast milk before 12 months of age should receive iron-fortified infant formula. Infant formulas that contain from 4 to 12 milligrams of iron per liter are considered iron-fortified.

Data from the National Health and Nutrition Examination Survey (NHANES) describe dietary intake of Americans 2 months of age and older. NHANES (1988–94) data suggest that males of all racial and ethnic groups consume recommended amounts of iron. However, iron intakes are generally low in females of childbearing age and young children.

Researchers also examine specific groups within the NHANES population. For example, researchers have compared dietary intakes of adults who consider themselves to be food insufficient (and therefore have limited access to nutritionally adequate foods) to those who are food sufficient (and have easy access to food). Older adults from food insufficient families had significantly lower intakes of iron than older adults who are food sufficient. In one survey, 20% of adults age 20 to 59 and 13.6% of adults age 60 and older from food-insufficient families consumed less than 50% of the RDA for iron, as compared to 13% of adults age 20 to 50 and 2.5% of adults age 60 and older from food-sufficient families.

Iron intake is negatively influenced by low nutrient density foods, which are high in calories but low in vitamins and minerals. Sugar-sweetened sodas and most desserts are examples of low nutrient density foods, as are snack foods such as potato chips. Among almost 5,000 children and adolescents between the ages of 8 and 18 who were surveyed, low nutrient density foods contributed almost 30% of daily caloric intake, with sweeteners and desserts jointly accounting for almost 25% of caloric intake. Those children and adolescents who consumed fewer low nutrient density foods were more likely to consume recommended amounts of iron.

Data from the Continuing Survey of Food Intakes by Individuals (CSFII1994–96 and 1998) was used to examine the effect of major food and beverage sources of added sugars on micronutrient intake of U.S. children aged 6 to 17 years. Researchers found that consumption of presweetened cereals, which are fortified with iron, increased the likelihood of meeting recommendations for iron intake. On the other hand, as intake of sugar-sweetened beverages, sugars, sweets, and sweetened grains increased, children were less likely to consume recommended amounts of iron.

When can iron deficiency occur?

The World Health Organization considers iron deficiency the number one nutritional disorder in the world. As many as 80% of the world's population may be iron deficient, while 30% may have iron deficiency anemia.

Iron deficiency develops gradually and usually begins with a negative iron balance, when iron intake does not meet the daily need for dietary iron. This negative balance initially depletes the storage form of iron while the blood hemoglobin level, a marker of iron status, remains normal. Iron deficiency anemia is an advanced stage of iron depletion. It occurs when storage sites of iron are deficient and blood levels of iron cannot meet daily needs. Blood hemoglobin levels are below normal with iron deficiency anemia.

Iron deficiency anemia can be associated with low dietary intake of iron, inadequate absorption of iron, or excessive blood loss. Women of childbearing age, pregnant women, preterm and low-birth-weight infants, older infants and toddlers, and teenage girls are at greatest risk of developing iron deficiency anemia because they have the greatest need for iron. Women with heavy menstrual losses can lose a significant amount of iron and are at considerable risk for iron deficiency. Adult men and postmenopausal women lose very little iron and have a low risk of iron deficiency.

Individuals with kidney failure, especially those being treated with dialysis, are at high risk for developing iron deficiency anemia. This is because their kidneys cannot create enough erythropoietin, a hormone needed to make red blood cells. Individuals who receive routine dialysis treatments usually need extra iron and synthetic erythropoietin to prevent iron deficiency.

Vitamin A helps mobilize iron from its storage sites, so a deficiency of vitamin A limits the body's ability to use stored iron. This results in an apparent iron deficiency because hemoglobin levels are low even though the body can maintain normal amounts of stored iron. While uncommon in the United States, this problem is seen in developing countries where vitamin A deficiency often occurs.

Chronic malabsorption can contribute to iron depletion and deficiency by limiting dietary iron absorption or by contributing to intestinal blood loss. Most iron is absorbed in the small intestines. Gastrointestinal disorders that result in inflammation of the small intestine may result in diarrhea, poor absorption of dietary iron, and iron depletion.

Signs of iron deficiency anemia include the following:

• Feeling tired and weak

• Decreased work and school performance

• Slow cognitive and social development during childhood

• Difficulty maintaining body temperature

• Decreased immune function, which increases susceptibility to infection

• Glossitis (an inflamed tongue)

Eating nonnutritive substances such as dirt and clay, often referred to as pica or geophagia, is sometimes seen in persons with iron deficiency. There is disagreement about the cause of this association. Some researchers believe that these eating abnormalities may result in an iron deficiency. Other researchers believe that iron deficiency may somehow increase the likelihood of these eating problems.

People with chronic infectious, inflammatory, or malignant disorders such as arthritis and cancer may become anemic. However, the anemia that occurs with inflammatory disorders differs from iron deficiency anemia and may not respond to iron supplements. Research suggests that inflammation may over-activate a protein involved in iron metabolism. This protein may inhibit iron absorption and reduce the amount of iron circulating in blood, resulting in anemia.

Who may need extra iron to prevent a deficiency?

Three groups of people are most likely to benefit from iron supplements: people with a greater need for iron, individuals who tend to lose more iron, and people who do not absorb iron normally. These individuals include the following:

- Pregnant women

- Preterm and low-birth-weight infants

- Older infants and toddlers

- Teenage girls

- Women of childbearing age, especially those with heavy menstrual losses

- People with renal failure, especially those undergoing routine dialysis

- People with gastrointestinal disorders who do not absorb iron normally

Celiac disease and Crohn syndrome are associated with gastrointestinal malabsorption and may impair iron absorption. Iron supplementation may be needed if these conditions result in iron deficiency anemia.

Women taking oral contraceptives may experience less bleeding during their periods and have a lower risk of developing an iron deficiency. Women who use an intrauterine device (IUD) to prevent pregnancy may experience more bleeding and have a greater risk of developing an iron deficiency. If laboratory tests indicate iron deficiency anemia, iron supplements may be recommended.

Total dietary iron intake in vegetarian diets may meet recommended levels; however, that iron is less available for absorption than in diets that include meat. Vegetarians who exclude all animal products from their diet may need almost twice as much dietary iron each day as nonvegetarians because of the lower intestinal absorption of nonheme iron in plant foods. Vegetarians should consider consuming nonheme iron sources together with a good source of vitamin C, such as citrus fruits, to improve the absorption of nonheme iron.

There are many causes of anemia, including iron deficiency. There are also several potential causes of iron deficiency. After a thorough evaluation, physicians can diagnose the cause of anemia and prescribe the appropriate treatment.

Does pregnancy increase the need for iron?

Nutrient requirements increase during pregnancy to support fetal growth and maternal health. Iron requirements of pregnant women are approximately double that of nonpregnant women because of increased blood volume during pregnancy, increased needs of the fetus, and blood losses that occur during delivery. If iron intake does not meet increased requirements, iron deficiency anemia can occur. Iron deficiency anemia of pregnancy is responsible for significant morbidity, such as premature deliveries and giving birth to infants with low birth weight.

The RDA for iron for pregnant women increases to 27 mg per day. Unfortunately, data from the 1988–94 NHANES survey suggested that the median iron intake among pregnant women was approximately 15 mg per day. When median iron intake is less than the RDA, more than half of the group consumes less iron than is recommended each day.

Several major health organizations recommend iron supplementation during pregnancy to help pregnant women meet their iron requirements. The Centers for Disease Control and Prevention (CDC) recommends routine low-dose iron supplementation (30 mg/day) for all pregnant women, beginning at the first prenatal visit. When a low hemoglobin or hematocrit is confirmed by repeat testing, the CDC recommends larger doses of supplemental iron. Obstetricians often monitor the need for iron supplementation during pregnancy and provide individualized recommendations to pregnant women.

When is iron supplementation recommended?

Iron supplementation is indicated when diet alone cannot restore deficient iron levels to normal within an acceptable time frame. Supplements are especially important when an individual is experiencing clinical symptoms of iron deficiency anemia. The goals of providing oral iron supplements are to supply sufficient iron to restore normal storage levels of iron and to replenish hemoglobin deficits. When hemoglobin levels are below normal, physicians often measure serum ferritin, the storage form of iron. A serum ferritin level less than or equal to 15 micrograms per liter confirms iron deficiency anemia in women and suggests a possible need for iron supplementation.

Supplemental iron is available in two forms: ferrous and ferric. Ferrous iron salts (ferrous fumarate, ferrous sulfate, and ferrous gluconate) are the best absorbed forms of iron supplements. Elemental iron is the amount of iron in a supplement that is available for absorption.

The amount of iron absorbed decreases with increasing doses. For this reason, it is recommended that most people take their prescribed daily iron supplement in two or three equally spaced doses. For adults who are not pregnant, the CDC recommends taking 50 mg to 60 mg of oral elemental iron (the approximate amount of elemental iron in one 300 mg tablet of ferrous sulfate) twice daily for three months for the therapeutic treatment of iron deficiency anemia. However, physicians evaluate each person individually and prescribe according to individual needs.

Therapeutic doses of iron supplements, which are prescribed for iron deficiency anemia, may cause gastrointestinal side effects such as nausea, vomiting, constipation, diarrhea, dark colored stools, and/ or abdominal distress. Starting with half the recommended dose and gradually increasing to the full dose will help minimize these side effects. Taking the supplement in divided doses and with food also may help limit these symptoms. Iron from enteric-coated or delayed-release preparations may have fewer side effects but is not as well absorbed and is not usually recommended.

Who should be cautious about taking iron supplements?

Iron deficiency is uncommon among adult men and postmenopausal women. These individuals should only take iron supplements when prescribed by a physician because of their greater risk of iron overload. Iron overload is a condition in which excess iron is found in the blood and stored in organs such as the liver and heart. Iron overload is associated with several genetic diseases including hemochromatosis, which affects approximately 1 in 250 individuals of northern European descent. Individuals with hemochromatosis absorb iron very efficiently, which can result in a buildup of excess iron and can cause organ damage such as cirrhosis of the liver and heart failure. Hemochromatosis is often not diagnosed until excess iron stores have damaged an organ. Iron supplementation may accelerate the effects of hemochromatosis, an important reason why adult men and postmenopausal women who are not iron deficient should avoid iron supplements. Individuals with blood disorders that require frequent blood transfusions are also at risk of iron overload and are usually advised to avoid iron supplements.

What is the risk of iron toxicity?

There is considerable potential for iron toxicity because very little iron is excreted from the body. Thus, iron can accumulate in body tissues and organs when normal storage sites are full. For example, people with hemochromatosis are at risk of developing iron toxicity because of their high iron stores.

In children, death has occurred from ingesting 200 mg of iron. It is important to keep iron supplements tightly capped and away from children's reach. Any time excessive iron intake is suspected, immediately call your physician or Poison Control Center, or visit your local emergency room. Doses of iron prescribed for iron deficiency anemia in adults are associated with constipation, nausea, vomiting, and diarrhea, especially when the supplements are taken on an empty stomach.

177

In 2001, the Institute of Medicine of the National Academy of Sciences set a tolerable UL for iron for healthy people. There may be times when a physician prescribes an intake higher than the upper limit, such as when individuals with iron deficiency anemia need higher doses to replenish their iron stores. Table 17.2 lists the ULs for healthy adults, children, and infants 7 to 12 months of age.

Table 17.2. Tolerable Upper Intake Levels for Iron for Infants 7 to 12 months, Children, and Adults

Age	Males (mg/day)	Females (mg/day)	Pregnancy (mg/day)	Lactation (mg/day)
7 to 12 months	40	40	N/A	N/A
1 to 13 years	40	40	N/A	N/A
14 to 18 years	45	45	45	45
19 + years	45	45	45	45

Section 17.3

Magnesium

This section excerpted from "Magnesium," Office of Dietary Supplements (ods.od.nih.gov), July 13, 2009.

Magnesium is the fourth most abundant mineral in the body and is essential to good health. Approximately 50% of total body magnesium is found in bone. The other half is found predominantly inside cells of body tissues and organs. Only 1% of magnesium is found in blood, but the body works very hard to keep blood levels of magnesium constant.

Magnesium is needed for more than 300 biochemical reactions in the body. It helps maintain normal muscle and nerve function, keeps heart rhythm steady, supports a healthy immune system, and keeps bones strong. Magnesium also helps regulate blood sugar levels, promotes normal blood pressure, and is known to be involved in energy metabolism and protein synthesis. There is an increased interest in the role of magnesium in preventing and managing disorders such as hypertension, cardiovascular disease, and diabetes.

What foods provide magnesium?

Green vegetables such as spinach are good sources of magnesium because the center of the chlorophyll molecule (which gives green vegetables their color) contains magnesium. Some legumes (beans and peas), nuts and seeds, and whole, unrefined grains are also good sources of magnesium. Refined grains are generally low in magnesium. When white flour is refined and processed, the magnesium-rich germ and bran are removed. Bread made from whole grain wheat flour provides more magnesium than bread made from white refined flour. Tap water can be a source of magnesium, but the amount varies according to the water supply. Water that naturally contains more minerals is described as hard. Hard water contains more magnesium than soft water.

Eating a wide variety of legumes, nuts, whole grains, and vegetables will help you meet your daily dietary need for magnesium.

What are the Dietary Reference Intakes for magnesium?

Recommendations for magnesium are provided in the Dietary Reference Intakes (DRIs) developed by the Institute of Medicine of the National Academy of Sciences. Dietary Reference Intakes is the general term for a set of reference values used for planning and assessing nutrient intake for healthy people. Three important types of reference values included in the DRIs are Recommended Dietary Allowances (RDA), Adequate Intakes (AI), and Tolerable Upper Intake Levels (UL). The RDA recommends the average daily intake that is sufficient to meet the nutrient requirements of nearly all (97%–98%) healthy people. An AI is set when there is insufficient scientific data available to establish a RDA for specific age/gender groups. AIs meet or exceed the amount needed to maintain a nutritional state of adequacy in nearly all members of a specific age and gender group. The UL, on the other hand, is the maximum daily intake unlikely to result in adverse health effects. Table 17.3 lists the RDAs for magnesium, in milligrams, for children and adults.

There is insufficient information on magnesium to establish a RDA for infants. For infants 0 to 12 months, the DRI is in the form of an Adequate Intake (AI), which is the mean intake of magnesium in healthy, breastfed infants. The AIs for infants are 30 milligrams per day for infants age 0 to 6 months and 75 milligrams per day for infants 7 to 12 months.

Data from the 1999–2000 NHANES survey suggest that substantial numbers of adults in the United States fail to get recommended amounts of magnesium in their diets. Among adult men and women, the diets of Caucasians have significantly more magnesium than do those of African Americans. Magnesium intake is lower among older adults in every racial and ethnic group. Among African American men and Caucasian men and women who take dietary supplements, the intake of magnesium is significantly higher than in those who do not.

Table 17.3. Recommended Dietary Allowances for Magnesium for Children and Adults

Age (years)	Male (mg/day)	Female (mg/day)	Pregnancy (mg/day)	Lactation (mg/day)
1–3	80	80	N/A	N/A
4–8	130	130	N/A	N/A
9–13	240	240	N/A	N/A
14–18	410	360	400	360
19–30	400	310	350	310
31+	420	320	360	320

When can magnesium deficiency occur?

Even though dietary surveys suggest that many Americans do not get recommended amounts of magnesium, symptoms of magnesium deficiency are rarely seen in the United States. However, there is concern that many people may not have enough body stores of magnesium because dietary intake may not be high enough. Having enough body stores of magnesium may be protective against disorders such as cardiovascular disease and immune dysfunction.

The health status of the digestive system and the kidneys significantly influence magnesium status. Magnesium is absorbed in the intestines and then transported through the blood to cells and tissues. Approximately one-third to one-half of dietary magnesium is absorbed into the body. Gastrointestinal disorders that impair absorption such as Crohn disease can limit the body's ability to absorb magnesium. These disorders can deplete the body's stores of magnesium and in extreme cases may result in magnesium deficiency. Chronic or excessive vomiting and diarrhea may also result in magnesium depletion.

Healthy kidneys are able to limit urinary excretion of magnesium to make up for low dietary intake. However, excessive loss of magnesium in urine can be a side effect of some medications and can also occur in cases of poorly controlled diabetes and alcohol abuse.

Early signs of magnesium deficiency include loss of appetite, nausea, vomiting, fatigue, and weakness. As magnesium deficiency worsens, numbness, tingling, muscle contractions and cramps, seizures (sudden changes in behaviors caused by excessive electrical activity in the brain), personality changes, abnormal heart rhythms, and coronary spasms can occur. Severe magnesium deficiency can result in low levels of calcium in the blood (hypocalcemia). Magnesium deficiency is also associated with low levels of potassium in the blood (hypokalemia).

Many of these symptoms are general and can result from a variety of medical conditions other than magnesium deficiency. It is important to have a physician evaluate health complaints and problems so that appropriate care can be given.

Who may need extra magnesium?

Magnesium supplementation may be indicated when a specific health problem or condition causes an excessive loss of magnesium or limits magnesium absorption.

- Some medicines may result in magnesium deficiency, including certain diuretics, antibiotics, and medications used to treat cancer (anti-neoplastic medication).

- Individuals with poorly controlled diabetes may benefit from magnesium supplements because of increased magnesium loss in urine associated with hyperglycemia.

- Magnesium supplementation may be indicated for persons with alcoholism. Low blood levels of magnesium occur in 30% to 60% of alcoholics, and in nearly 90% of patients experiencing alcohol withdrawal. Anyone who substitutes alcohol for food will usually have significantly lower magnesium intakes.

- Individuals with chronic malabsorptive problems such as Crohn disease, gluten sensitive enteropathy, regional enteritis, and intestinal surgery may lose magnesium through diarrhea and fat malabsorption. Individuals with these conditions may need supplemental magnesium.

- Individuals with chronically low blood levels of potassium and calcium may have an underlying problem with magnesium deficiency. Magnesium supplements may help correct the potassium and calcium deficiencies.

- Older adults are at increased risk for magnesium deficiency. The 1999–2000 and 1998–94 NHANES data suggest that older adults have lower dietary intakes of magnesium than younger adults. In addition, magnesium absorption decreases and renal excretion of magnesium increases in older adults. Seniors are also more likely to be taking drugs that interact with magnesium. This combination of factors places older adults at risk for magnesium deficiency. It is very important for older adults to get recommended amounts of dietary magnesium.

Doctors can evaluate magnesium status when the aforementioned medical problems occur and determine the need for magnesium supplementation.

What is the best way to get extra magnesium?

Eating a variety of whole grains, legumes, and vegetables (especially dark green, leafy vegetables) every day will help provide recommended intakes of magnesium and maintain normal storage levels of this mineral. Increasing dietary intake of magnesium can often restore mildly depleted magnesium levels. However, increasing dietary intake of magnesium may not be enough to restore very low magnesium levels to normal.

When blood levels of magnesium are very low, intravenous (by IV) magnesium replacement is usually recommended. Magnesium tablets also may be prescribed, although some forms can cause diarrhea. It is important to have the cause, severity, and consequences of low blood levels of magnesium evaluated by a physician, who can recommend the best way to restore magnesium levels to normal. Because people with kidney disease may not be able to excrete excess amounts of magnesium, they should not take magnesium supplements unless prescribed by a physician.

Oral magnesium supplements combine magnesium with another substance such as a salt. Examples of magnesium supplements include magnesium oxide, magnesium sulfate, and magnesium carbonate. Elemental magnesium refers to the amount of magnesium in each compound. The amount of elemental magnesium in a compound and its bioavailability influence the effectiveness of the magnesium supplement. Bioavailability refers to the amount of magnesium in food, medications, and supplements that is absorbed in the intestines and ultimately available for biological activity in your cells and tissues.

What is the health risk of too much magnesium?

Dietary magnesium does not pose a health risk; however, pharmacologic doses of magnesium in supplements can promote adverse effects such as diarrhea and abdominal cramping. Risk of magnesium toxicity increases with kidney failure, when the kidney loses the ability to remove excess magnesium. Very large doses of magnesium-containing laxatives and antacids also have been associated with magnesium toxicity. There-fore, it is important for medical professionals to be aware of the use of any magnesium-containing laxatives or antacids. Signs of excess magnesium can be similar to magnesium deficiency and include changes in men-tal status, nausea, diarrhea, appetite loss, muscle weakness, difficulty breathing, extremely low blood pressure, and irregular heartbeat.

Physicians may prescribe magnesium in higher doses for specific medical problems. There is no UL for dietary intake of magnesium, only for magnesium supplements.

Section 17.4

Zinc

This section excerpted from "Zinc: QuickFacts,"
Office of Dietary Supplements (ods.od.nih.gov), April 18, 2011.

What is zinc and what does it do?

Zinc is a nutrient that people need to stay healthy. Zinc is found in cells throughout the body. It helps the immune system fight off invading bacteria and viruses. The body also needs zinc to make proteins and DNA, the genetic material in all cells. During pregnancy, infancy, and childhood, the body needs zinc to grow and develop properly. Zinc also helps wounds heal and is important for proper senses of taste and smell.

How much zinc do I need?

The amount of zinc you need each day depends on your age. Aver-age daily recommended amounts for different ages are listed here in milligrams (mg):

- Birth to 6 months : 2 mg
- Infants 7–12 months: 3 mg
- Children 1–3 years: 3 mg
- Children 4–8 years: 5 mg
- Children 9–13 years: 8 mg

- Teens 14–18 years (boys): 11 mg
- Teens 14–18 years (girls): 9 mg
- Adults (men): 11 mg
- Adults (women): 8 mg
- Pregnant teens: 12 mg
- Pregnant women: 11 mg
- Breast-feeding teens: 13 mg
- Breast-feeding women: 12 mg

What foods provide zinc?

Zinc is found in a wide variety of foods. You can get recommended amounts of zinc by eating a variety of foods including the following:

- Oysters, which are the best source of zinc
- Red meat, poultry, seafood such as crab and lobsters, and fortified breakfast cereals, which are also good sources of zinc
- Beans, nuts, whole grains, and dairy products, which provide some zinc

Am I getting enough zinc?

Most people in the United States get enough zinc from the foods they eat. However, certain groups of people are more likely than others to have trouble getting enough zinc:

- People who have had gastrointestinal surgery, such as weight loss surgery, or who have digestive disorders, such as ulcerative colitis or Crohn disease
- Vegetarians
- Older infants who are breast-fed (older infants who do not take formula should be given foods that have zinc such as pureed meats; formula-fed infants get enough zinc from infant formula)
- Alcoholics
- People with sickle cell disease

What happens if I don't get enough zinc?

Zinc deficiency is rare in North America. It causes slow growth in infants and children, delayed sexual development in adolescents, and impotence in men. Zinc deficiency also causes hair loss, diarrhea, eye and skin sores, and loss of appetite.

What are some effects of zinc on health?

Scientists are studying zinc to learn about its effects on the immune system (the body's defense system against bacteria, viruses, and other foreign invaders). Scientists are also researching possible connections between zinc and other health problems, including wound healing, diarrhea, the common cold, and age-related macular degeneration.

Can zinc be harmful?

Yes, if you get too much. Signs of too much zinc include nausea, vomiting, loss of appetite, stomach cramps, diarrhea, and headaches. When people take too much zinc for a long time, they sometimes have problems such as low copper levels, lower immunity, and low levels of HDL cholesterol (the "good" cholesterol).

Are there any interactions with zinc that I should know about?

Yes. Zinc dietary supplements can interact or interfere with medicines that you take, and, in some cases, medicines can lower zinc levels in the body. Tell your doctor, pharmacist, and other health care providers about any dietary supplements and medicines you take.

Chapter 18

Phytochemicals, Antioxidants, and Other Functional Foods

Chapter Contents

Section 18.1

Phytochemicals

"Phytochemicals," Navy and Marine Corps Public
Health Center (www-nehc.med.navy.mil), undated.
Reviewed by David A. Cooke, MD, FACP, February 2011.

What are phytochemicals?

Phytochemicals are plant chemicals that contain protective, disease-preventing compounds. Nearly 1,000 of these chemicals have already been identified, and many more continue to be identified today. This is an exciting and promising area of nutrition research, as phytochemicals are associated with the prevention and/or treatment of at least four of the leading causes of death in the United States—heart disease, cancer, diabetes, and hypertension. They have been proven to be involved in many processes, including ones that help prevent cell damage, prevent cancer cell replication, and decrease LDL (low-density lipoprotein) cholesterol levels.

What are some of the most commonly studied phytochemicals and what are examples of their food sources?

- **Flavonoids** are one subgroup of phytochemicals and are included in such foods as apples, cherries, soy beans, soy products, chickpeas, licorice, and tea. These are being studied to evaluate their effectiveness against cancer and heart disease.

  - **Phenolic flavonoids** found in red wine and red grape juice can act as antioxidants, protect against LDL oxidation, and inhibit blood clotting, which provides protection against heart disease.

- **Carotenoids**, which lend carrots, cantaloupe, yams, and apricots their orange color, are promoted as anticancer chemicals.

- **Lycopene** is found in tomatoes, red peppers, and red grapefruit and is also touted as a powerful antioxidant.

- **Ellagic acid** is found in strawberries, raspberries, blackberries, walnuts, and cranberries and is also said to be anticancerous.

- **Sulfides**, found in garlic and onions, are reputed to stimulate enzymes that inhibit the growth of bacteria and may reduce the incidence of stomach cancer, lower blood pressure, and strengthen the immune system.

* This is only a partial list of phytochemicals and foods containing them. There are many, many more!

What is the evidence?

It has long been established that a diet rich in fruits, vegetables, and whole grains is beneficial to health. However, it is only very recently that serious research has started trying to understand the roles phytochemicals play in disease prevention. Many studies have shown that people who eat higher amounts of fruits and vegetables have about one-half the risk of cancer. This protective effect has also been observed in hormone-related cancers, like breast and prostate cancers. In addition to countless studies showing the anti-tumor activity of several of these compounds, some have potent anti-inflammatory properties (which may be an important finding for people with asthma, arthritis, lupus, etc.) and immune-strengthening abilities.

Furthermore, studies show that people who consume about one to two ounces of soy protein for about four weeks can experience a decrease in total and LDL (bad) cholesterol levels of as much as 10% to 20% when initial levels are elevated. This is especially impressive considering that while LDL levels are reduced, good HDL (high-density lipoprotein) levels remain constant. Soy also lowers triglyceride levels, especially in persons with elevated levels.

What about supplements?

Though supplements would seem an easy way to increase phytochemical intake, there is no evidence to support that taking supplements is as beneficial as consuming the whole foods from which they are derived. This is likely because consuming such supplements will only provide certain components in a concentrated form, not the diversity of these compounds that occur naturally in fruits, vegetables, and grains; besides, scientists are still trying to understand the combined effect these compounds have, and optimal levels of phytochemicals have yet to be determined.

How do I work phytochemicals into my diet?

Many Americans eat far below the five servings of fruits and vegetables recommended by the National Cancer Institute. People need to realize just how few servings they eat daily and then look at simple strategies for incorporating fruits and vegetables into their diets. The slogan "eat your colors" is also useful here, as the vivid red, green, yellow, and orange pigments found in these plant foods are often markers for the protective compounds they contain. Some easy suggestions for increasing phytochemical intake are listed here:

- Add chopped fruit to cereal, oatmeal, and yogurt.

- Add fresh greens, carrots, celery, broccoli, beans, and peppers to soups and spaghetti sauce.

- Keep dried fruits like raisins, apricots, and prunes for snacking instead of chips.

- Try replacing sodas and sports drinks with green or black teas.

- Add salsa to eggs, and use it in place of creamy dips for raw vegetables.

- Replaced processed grains for whole grains. (Refining wheat reduces phytochemical content by 200%–300%.)

Are phytochemicals destroyed by cooking?

Most of the chemicals are heat stable and are not significantly lost in cooking water. Interestingly, some chemicals are actually more easily used by the body when they have been cooked; for example, the lycopene in processed tomatoes (such as in pasta sauces and ketchup) is more available than in raw tomatoes.

Finally, although research is ongoing about the benefits of these chemicals and their role against disease, studies do support that the risks of cancer and heart disease are significantly reduced with increased consumption of fruits, vegetables, and whole grains. Furthermore, they are naturally low in fat, calories, and sodium and supply an abundance of flavors and textures.

Section 18.2

Antioxidants

Background

Plant foods, such as fruits, vegetables, and whole grains, contain many components that are beneficial to human health. Research supports that some of these foods, as part of an overall healthful diet, have the potential to delay the onset of many age-related diseases. These observations have led to continuing research aimed at identifying specific bioactive components in foods, such as antioxidants, which may be responsible for improving and maintaining health.

Antioxidants are present in foods as vitamins, minerals, carotenoids, and polyphenols, among others. Many antioxidants are often identified in food by their distinctive colors—the deep red of cherries and of tomatoes; the orange of carrots; the yellow of corn, mangos, and saffron; and the blue-purple of blueberries, blackberries, and grapes. The most well-known components of food with antioxidant activities are vitamins A, C, and E; β-carotene; the mineral selenium; and more recently, the compound lycopene.

Health Effects

The research continues to grow regarding the knowledge of antioxidants as healthful components of food. Oxidation, or the loss of an electron, can sometimes produce reactive substances known as free radicals that can cause oxidative stress or damage to the cells. Antioxidants, by their very nature, are capable of stabilizing free radicals before they can react and cause harm, in much the same way that a buffer stabilizes an acid to maintain a normal pH. Because oxidation is a naturally occurring process within the body, a balance with antioxidants must exist to maintain health.

191

Table 18.1. Examples of Functional Components*

Class/Components	Source*	Potential Benefit
Carotenoids		
Beta-carotene	carrots, various fruits	neutralizes free radicals, which may damage cells; bolsters cellular antioxidant defenses
Lutein, zeaxanthin	kale, collards, spinach, corn, eggs, citrus	may contribute to maintenance of healthy vision
Lycopene	tomatoes and processed tomato products	may contribute to maintenance of prostate health
Flavonoids		
Anthocyanidins	berries, cherries, red grapes	bolster cellular antioxidant defenses; may contribute to maintenance of brain function
Flavanols— catechins, epicatechins, procyanidins	tea, cocoa, chocolate, apples, grapes	may contribute to maintenance of heart health
Flavanones	citrus foods	neutralize free radicals, which may damage cells; bolster cellular antioxidant defenses
Flavonols	onions, apples, tea, broccoli	neutralize free radicals, which may damage cells; bolster cellular antioxidant defenses
Proanthocyanidins	cranberries, cocoa, apples, strawberries, grapes, wine, peanuts, cinnamon	may contribute to maintenance of urinary tract health and heart health
Isothiocyanates		
Sulforaphane	cauliflower, broccoli, Brussels sprouts, cabbage, kale, horseradish	may enhance detoxification of undesirable compounds and bolster cellular antioxidant defenses
Phenols		
Caffeic acid, ferulic acid	apples, pears, citrus fruits, some vegetables	may bolster cellular antioxidant defenses; may contribute to maintenance of healthy vision and heart health
Sulfides/Thiols		
Diallyl sulfide, allyl methyl trisulfide	garlic, onions, leeks, scallions	may enhance detoxification of undesirable compounds; may contribute to maintenance of heart health and healthy immune function
Dithiolethiones	cruciferous vegetables— broccoli, cabbage, bok choy, collards	contribute to maintenance of healthy immune function
Whole Grains		
Whole grains	cereal grains	may reduce risk of coronary heart disease and cancer; may contribute to reduced risk of diabetes

Chart adapted from International Food Information Council Foundation: Media Guide on Food Safety and Nutrition: 2004–2006.

* Not a representation of all sources

For more information on additional beneficial components of food, visit Background on Functional Foods [at http://www.foodinsight.org/Content/6/functionalfoodsbackgrounder.pdf].

Research

While the body has its defenses against oxidative stress, these defenses are thought to become less effective with aging as oxidative stress becomes greater. Research suggests there is involvement of the resulting free radicals in a number of degenerative diseases associated with aging, such as cancer, cardiovascular disease, cognitive impairment, Alzheimer's disease, immune dysfunction, cataracts, and macular degeneration. Certain conditions, such as chronic diseases and aging, can tip the balance in favor of free radical formation, which can contribute to ill effects on health.

Consumption of antioxidants is thought to provide protection against oxidative damage and contribute positive health benefits. For example, the carotenoids lutein and zeaxanthin engage in antioxidant activities that have been shown to increase macular pigment density in the eye. Whether this will prevent or reverse the progression of macular degeneration remains to be determined. An increasing body of evidence suggests beneficial effects of the antioxidants present in grapes, cocoa, blueberries, and teas on cardiovascular health, Alzheimer's disease, and even reduction of the risk of some cancers.

Until recently, it appeared that antioxidants were almost a panacea for continued good health. It is only as more research has probed the mechanisms of antioxidant action that a far more complex story continues to be unraveled. Although recent research has attempted to establish a causal link between indicators of oxidative stress and chronic disease, none has yet been validated. A new area of research, led by the study of the human genome, suggests that the interplay of human genetics and diet may play a role in the development of chronic diseases. This science, while still in its infancy, seeks to provide an understanding of how common dietary nutrients such as antioxidants can affect health through gene-nutrient interactions.

There still remains a lack of direct experimental evidence from randomized trials that antioxidants are beneficial to health, which has led to different recommendations for different populations. For example, the use of supplemental β-carotene has been identified as a contributing factor to increased risk of lung cancer in smokers. However, because the risk has not been indicated in non-smokers, these studies suggest that a precaution regarding the use of supplemental β-carotene is not warranted for non-smokers. If supplementation is desired, the use of a daily multivitamin-mineral supplement containing antioxidants has been recommended for the general public as the best advice at this time.

A recent review of current literature suggests that fruits and vegetables in combination have synergistic effects on antioxidant activities leading to greater reduction in risk of chronic disease, specifically for cancer and heart disease. For some time, health organizations have recognized the beneficial roles fruits and vegetables play in the reduced risk of disease and developed communication programs to encourage consumers to eat more antioxidant-rich fruits and vegetables. The American Heart Association recommends healthy adults "Eat a variety of fruits and vegetables. Choose five or more servings per day." The American Cancer Society recommends to "Eat five or more servings of fruits and vegetables each day." The World Cancer Research Fund and the American Institute for Cancer Research 1997 report *Food, Nutrition, and the Prevention of Cancer: A Global Perspective* states, "Evidence of dietary protection against cancer is strongest and most consistent for diets high in vegetables and fruits." The potential for antioxidant-rich fruits and vegetables to help improve the health of Americans led the National Cancer Institute (NCI) to start the "Five-a-Day for Better Health" campaign to promote consumption of these foods.

Given the high degree of scientific consensus about consumption of a diet that is high in fruits and vegetables—particularly those which contain dietary fiber and vitamins A and C; the Food and Drug Administration (FDA) released a health claim for fruits and vegetables in relation to cancer. Food packages that meet FDA criteria may now carry the claim "Diets low in fat and high in fruits and vegetables may reduce the risk of some cancers." In addition the FDA, in cooperation with NCI, released a dietary guidance message for consumers, "Diets rich in fruits and vegetables may reduce the risk of some types of cancer and other chronic diseases." Most recently the *Dietary Guidelines for Americans* stated, "Increased intakes of fruits, vegetables, whole grains and fat-free or low-fat milk and milk products are likely to have important health benefits for most Americans."

Antioxidant research continues to grow and emerge as new beneficial components of food are discovered. Reinforced by current research, the message remains that antioxidants obtained from food sources, including fruits, vegetables, and whole grains, are potentially active in disease risk reduction and can be beneficial to human health.

The Bottom Line

Most research indicates that there are overall health benefits from antioxidant-rich foods consumed in the diet. The results of clinical trials with antioxidant supplements have yet to provide conclusive indication of health benefits. Current recommendations by the U.S. government and health organizations are to consume a varied diet with at least 5 servings of fruits and vegetables per day and 6–11 servings of grains per day, with at least 3 of those being whole grains.

Table 18.2. Examples of Antioxidant Vitamins and Minerals

Vitamins	Daily Reference Intakes (DRIs)*	Antioxidant Activity	Sources
Vitamin A	300–900 µg/d [microgram/deciliter]	Protects cells from free radicals	Liver, dairy products, fish
Vitamin C	15–90 mg/d	Protects cells from free radicals	Bell peppers, citrus fruits
Vitamin E	6–15 mg/d	Protects cells from free radicals, helps with immune function and DNA repair	Oils, fortified cereals, sunflower seeds, mixed nuts
Selenium	20–55 µg/d	Helps prevent cellular damage from free radicals	Brazil nuts, meats, tuna, plant foods

Chart adapted from Food and Nutrition Board Institute of Medicine DRI reports and National Institutes of Health Office of Dietary Supplements.

* DRIs provided are a range for Americans ages 2–70.

For information on Daily Reference Intakes for specific populations visit http://www.iom.edu.

Section 18.3

Health Benefits and Risks of Soy Foods

"Herbs at a Glance: Soy," National Center for Complementary and
Alternative Medicine (nccam.nih.gov), July 2010.

Soy, a plant in the pea family, has been common in Asian diets for thousands of years. It is found in modern American diets as a food or food additive. Soybeans, the high-protein seeds of the soy plant, contain isoflavones—compounds similar to the female hormone estrogen. The following information highlights what is known about soy when used by adults for health purposes.

What Soy Is Used For

People use soy products to prevent or treat a variety of health conditions, including high cholesterol levels, menopausal symptoms such as hot flashes, osteoporosis, memory problems, high blood pressure, breast cancer, and prostate cancer.

How Soy Is Used

- Soy is available in dietary supplements, in forms such as tablets and capsules. Soy supplements may contain isoflavones or soy protein or both.

- Soybeans can be cooked and eaten or used to make tofu, soy milk, and other foods. Also, soy is sometimes used as an additive in various processed foods, including baked goods, cheese, and pasta.

What the Science Says

- Research suggests that daily intake of soy protein may slightly lower levels of LDL (bad) cholesterol.

- Some studies suggest that soy isoflavone supplements may reduce hot flashes in women after menopause. However, the results have been inconsistent.

- There is not enough scientific evidence to determine whether soy supplements are effective for any other health uses.

- National Center for Complimentary and Alternative Medicine (NCCAM) supports studies on soy, including its effects in cardio-vascular disease and breast cancer and on menopause-related symptoms and bone loss.

Side Effects and Cautions

- Soy is considered safe for most people when used as a food or when taken for short periods as a dietary supplement (a product that contains vitamins, minerals, herbs or other botanicals, amino acids, enzymes, and/or other ingredients intended to supplement the diet). The FDA has special labeling requirements for dietary supplements and treats them as foods, not drugs.

- Minor stomach and bowel problems such as nausea, bloating, and constipation are possible.

- Allergic reactions such as breathing problems and rash can occur in rare cases.

- The safety of long-term use of soy isoflavones has not been established. Evidence is mixed on whether using isoflavone supplements over time can increase the risk of endometrial hyperplasia (a thickening of the lining of the uterus that can lead to cancer). Studies show no effect of dietary soy on risk for endometrial hyperplasia.

- Soy's possible role in breast cancer risk is uncertain. Until more is known about soy's effect on estrogen levels, women who have or who are at increased risk of developing breast cancer or other hormone-sensitive conditions (such as ovarian or uterine cancer) should be particularly careful about using soy and should discuss it with their health care providers.

- Tell all your health care providers about any complementary and alternative practices you use. Give them a full picture of what you do to manage your health. This will help ensure coordinated and safe care.

Sources

Balk E, Chung M, Chew P, et al. *Effects of Soy on Health Outcomes.* Evidence Report/Technology Assessment no. 126. Rockville, MD: Agency for Health-care Research and Quality; 2005. AHRQ publication no. 05-E024-1.

Low Dog T. Menopause: a review of botanical dietary supplements. *American Journal of Medicine*. 2005;118(suppl 12B):98S–108S.

Sacks FM, Lichtenstein A, Van Horn L, et al. Soy protein, isoflavones, and cardiovascular health: an American Heart Association Science Advisory for professionals from the Nutrition Committee. *Circulation*. 2006;113(7):1034–1044.

Soy. Natural Medicines Comprehensive Database Website. Accessed at www.naturaldatabase.com on July 23, 2009.

Soy (Glycine max [L.] Merr.). Natural Standard Database Website. Accessed at www.naturalstandard.com on July 23, 2009.

Part Three

Nutrition Through
the Life Span

Chapter 19

Feeding Infants and Toddlers

Chapter Contents

Section 19.1

Infants: Breastfeeding and Bottle Feeding

A Personal Decision

Choosing whether to breastfeed or formula feed your baby is one of the first decisions expectant parents will make. The American Academy of Pediatrics (AAP) joins other organizations such as the American Medical Association (AMA), the American Dietetic Association (ADA), and the World Health Organization (WHO) in recommending breastfeeding as the best for babies. Breastfeeding helps defend against infections, prevent allergies, and protect against a number of chronic conditions.

The AAP says babies should be breastfed exclusively for the first 6 months. Beyond that, the AAP encourages breastfeeding until at least 12 months, and longer if both the mother and baby are willing.

Although experts believe breast milk is the best nutritional choice for infants, breastfeeding may not be possible for all women. For many women, the decision to breastfeed or formula feed is based on their comfort level, lifestyle, and specific medical considerations that they might have.

For mothers who are unable to breastfeed or who decide not to, infant formula is a good alternative. Some women feel guilty if they don't breastfeed. But if you feed your baby with a commercially prepared formula, be assured that your baby's nutritional needs will be met. And you'll still bond with your baby just fine. After all, whether with breast milk or formula, feeding is an important time of connection between mother and baby.

The decision to breastfeed or formula feed your baby is a very personal one. But here are some points you may want to consider as you decide which is best for you and your new addition.

Breastfeeding: The Advantages

Nursing can be a wonderful experience for both mother and baby. It provides ideal nourishment and a special bonding experience that many nursing mothers cherish.

Here are some of the many benefits of breastfeeding:

Infection-fighting: Antibodies passed from a nursing mother to her baby can help lower the occurrence of many conditions, including:

- ear infections;
- diarrhea;
- respiratory infections;
- meningitis.

Other factors help to protect a breastfed baby from infection by contributing to the infant's immune system by increasing the barriers to infection and decreasing the growth of organisms like bacteria and viruses.

Breastfeeding is particularly beneficial for premature babies and also may protect children against:

- allergies;
- asthma;
- diabetes;
- obesity;
- sudden infant death syndrome (SIDS).

As a group, breastfed babies have fewer infections and hospitalizations than formula-fed infants.

Nutrition and ease of digestion: Often called the "perfect food" for a human baby's digestive system, breast milk's components—lactose, protein (whey and casein), and fat—are easily digested by a newborn's immature system.

As a group, breastfed infants have less difficulty with digestion than do formula-fed infants. Breast milk tends to be more easily digested so that breastfed babies have fewer incidences of diarrhea or constipation.

Breast milk also naturally contains many of the vitamins and minerals that a newborn requires. A healthy mother does not need any additional vitamins or nutritional supplements, with the exception of vitamin D. Breast milk does contain some vitamin D, and vitamin D is produced by the body when the skin is exposed to sunlight. However, sun exposure increases the risk of skin damage, so parents are advised to minimize exposure. As a result, the AAP recommends that all breastfed babies begin receiving vitamin D supplements during the first two months and continuing until the infant consumes enough vitamin D–fortified formula or milk (after one year of age).

The U.S. Food and Drug Administration (FDA) regulates formula companies to ensure that they provide all the known necessary nutrients (including vitamin D) in their formulas. Commercial formulas do a pretty good job of trying to duplicate the ingredients in breast milk—and are coming closer—but haven't matched their exact combination and composition. Why? Because some of breast milk's more complex substances are too difficult to manufacture and some have not yet been identified.

Free: Breast milk doesn't cost a cent, while the cost of formula quickly adds up. And because of the immunities and antibodies passed onto them through their mothers' breast milk, breastfed infants are sick less often than infants who receive formula. For example, researchers have determined that infants who are breastfed exclusively have fewer episodes of ear infections. That may mean they make fewer trips to the doctor's office, which equates to fewer co-pays and less money doled out for prescriptions and over-the-counter medications.

Likewise, women who breastfeed are less likely to have to take time off from work to care for their sick babies.

Different tastes: A nursing mother will usually need 500 extra calories per day, which means that she should eat a wide variety of well-balanced foods. This introduces breastfed babies to different tastes through their mothers' breast milk, which has different flavors depending on what their mothers have eaten.

Convenience: With no last-minute runs to the store for more formula, breast milk is always fresh and available. And when women breastfeed, there's no need to warm up bottles in the middle of the night. It's also easy for breastfeeding mothers to be active—and go out and about—with their babies and know that they'll have food available for whenever their little one is hungry.

Obesity prevention: Some studies have found that breastfeeding may help prevent obesity.

Smarter babies: Some studies suggest that children who were exclusively breastfed have slightly higher IQs than children who were formula fed.

"Skin-to-skin" contact: Many nursing mothers really enjoy the experience of bonding so closely with their babies. And the skin-to-skin contact can enhance the emotional connection between mother and infant.

Beneficial for mom, too: The ability to nourish a baby totally can also help a new mother feel confident in her ability to care for her baby. Breastfeeding also burns calories and helps shrink the uterus, so nursing moms may be able to return to their pre-pregnancy shape and weight quicker. In addition, studies show that breastfeeding helps lower the risk of breast cancer, high blood pressure, diabetes, and cardiovascular disease, and also may help decrease the risk of uterine and ovarian cancer. In one long-term study of the National Institutes of Health Women's Health Initiative, women who breastfed for at least 7 to 12 months after giving birth had a lower risk of cardiovascular disease.

Breastfeeding: The Challenges

Although it is the best nutritional source for babies, breastfeeding does come with some concerns that many new mothers share. Whereas it's easy from the get-go for some, it can be challenging. Sometimes, both mother and baby need plenty of patience and persistence to get used to the routine of breastfeeding. But all the effort is often worth it in the long run—for both the mother and her baby.

Common concerns of new moms, especially during the first few weeks and months, may include:

Personal comfort: Initially, as with any new skill, many moms feel uncomfortable with breastfeeding. But with adequate education, support, and practice, most moms overcome this. The bottom line is that breastfeeding shouldn't hurt.

Latch-on pain is normal for the first week to 10 days and should last less than a minute with each feeding. But if breastfeeding hurts throughout feedings, or if the nipples and/or breasts are sore, it's a good idea for breastfeeding mothers to seek the help of a lactation consultant or their doctor. Many times, it's just a matter of using the proper technique, but sometimes pain can mean that something else is going on, like an infection.

Time and frequency of feedings: There's no question that breastfeeding does require a substantial time commitment from mothers. Then again, many things in parenting do. Some women may be concerned that nursing will make it hard for them to work, run errands, or travel because of a breastfeeding schedule or a need to pump breast milk during the day.

And breastfed babies do need to eat more often than babies who are fed formula, because breast milk digests faster than formula. This means Mom may find herself in demand every two or three hours (maybe more, maybe less) in the first few weeks.

This can be tiring, but once breastfeeding has been established (usually in about a month), other family members may be able to help out by giving the baby pumped breast milk if Mom needs a break or is going back to work outside the home. And it's not long before babies feed less frequently and sleep through the night (usually around three months). Also, with a little organization and time management, it becomes easier to work out a schedule to breastfeed and/or pump.

Diet: Women who are breastfeeding need to be careful about what they eat and drink, since things can be passed to the baby through the breast milk. Just like during pregnancy, breastfeeding women should avoid fish that are high in mercury and limit lower mercury fish intake. If a woman has alcohol, a small amount can be passed to the baby through breast milk. She should wait to breastfeed at least two hours after a single alcoholic drink in order to avoid passing any alcohol to the baby. Caffeine intake should be kept to no more than 300 milligrams (about one to three cups of regular coffee) per day for breastfeeding women because it may cause problems such as restlessness and irritability in some babies. Some infants are sensitive enough to caffeine to have problems even with smaller amounts of caffeine.

Maternal medical conditions, medicines, and breast surgery: Medical conditions such as HIV or AIDS or those that involve chemotherapy or treatment with certain medications may make breastfeeding unsafe. A woman should check with her doctor or a lactation consultant if she's unsure if she should breastfeed with a specific condition. Women should always check with the doctor about the safety of taking medications while breastfeeding, including over-the-counter and herbal medicines.

Mothers who've had breast surgery, such as a reduction, may have difficulty with supply if their milk ducts have been severed. In this situation, a woman should to talk to her doctor about her concerns and work with a lactation specialist.

Formula Feeding: The Advantages

Breastfeeding is considered the best nutritional option for babies by the major medical organizations, but it's not right for every mother. Commercially prepared infant formulas are a nutritious alternative to breast milk and even contain some vitamins and nutrients that breastfed babies need to get from supplements.

Manufactured under sterile conditions, commercial formulas attempt to duplicate mother's milk using a complex combination of proteins, sugars, fats, and vitamins that would be virtually impossible to create at home. So, if you don't breastfeed your baby, it's important that you use only a commercially prepared formula and that you do not try to create your own.

In addition to medical concerns that may prevent breastfeeding, for some women, breastfeeding may be too difficult or stressful.

Here are a few other reasons women may choose to formula feed:

Convenience: Either parent (or another caregiver) can feed the baby a bottle at any time (although this is also true for women who pump their breast milk). This allows the mother to share the feeding duties and helps her partner to feel more involved in the crucial feeding process and the bonding that often comes with it.

Flexibility: Once the bottles are made, a formula-feeding mother can leave her baby with a partner or caregiver and know that her little one's feedings are taken care of. There's no need to pump or to schedule work or other obligations and activities around the baby's feeding schedule. And formula-feeding moms don't need to find a private place to nurse in public. However, if Mom is out and about with baby, she will need to bring supplies for making bottles.

Time and frequency of feedings: Because formula digests slower than breast milk, formula-fed babies usually need to eat less often than do breastfed babies.

Diet: Women who opt to formula feed don't have to worry about the things they eat or drink that could affect their babies.

Formula Feeding: The Challenges

As with breastfeeding, there are some challenges to consider when deciding whether to formula feed.

Organization and preparation: Enough formula must be on hand at all times and bottles must be prepared. The powdered and condensed formulas must be prepared with sterile water (which needs to be boiled until the baby is at least six months old). Ready-to-feed formulas that can be poured directly into a bottle without any mixing or water tend to be expensive.

Bottles and nipples need to be sterilized before the first use and then washed after every use after that (this is also true for breastfeeding women who give their babies bottles of pumped breast milk). Bottles and nipples can transmit bacteria if they aren't cleaned properly, as can formula if it isn't stored in sterile containers.

Bottles left out of the refrigerator longer than one hour and any formula that a baby doesn't finish must be thrown out. And prepared bottles of formula should be stored in the refrigerator for no longer than 24 to 48 hours (check the formula's label for complete information).

Some parents warm bottles up before feeding the baby, although this often isn't necessary. The microwave should never be used to warm a baby's bottle because it can create dangerous "hot spots."

Instead, run refrigerated bottles under warm water for a few minutes if the baby prefers a warm bottle to a cold one. Or the baby's bottles can be put in a pan of hot water (away from the heat of the stove) with the temperature tested by squirting a drop or two of formula on the inside of the wrist.

Lack of antibodies: None of the important antibodies found in breast milk are found in manufactured formula, which means that formula doesn't provide the baby with the added protection against infection and illness that breast milk does.

Expense: Formula can be costly. Powdered formula is the least expensive, followed by concentrated, with ready-to-feed being the most expensive. And specialty formulas (i.e., soy and hypoallergenic) cost more—sometimes far more—than the basic formulas. During the first year of life, the cost of basic formula can run about $1,500.

Possibility of producing gas and constipation: Formula-fed babies may have more gas and firmer bowel movements than breast-fed babies.

Can't match the complexity of breast milk: Manufactured formulas have yet to duplicate the complexity of breast milk, which changes as the baby's needs change.

Whatever nutritional option you choose, be sure to talk to your doctor about the choices available to help you make the decision that's best for both you and your baby.

Section 19.2

Introducing Solids and Table Foods

Feeding Your 4- to 7-Month-Old

This is the age when most babies are introduced to solid foods. The AAP currently recommends gradually introducing solid foods when a baby is about six months old. Your doctor, however, may recommend starting as early as four months depending on your baby's readiness and nutritional needs. Be sure to check with your doctor before starting any solid foods.

Is My Baby Ready to Eat Solids?

How can you tell if your baby is ready for solids? Here are a few hints:

• Is your baby's tongue-thrust reflex gone or diminished? This reflex, which prevents infants from choking on foreign objects, also causes them to push food out of their mouths.

• Can your baby support his or her own head? To eat solid food, an infant needs good head and neck control and should be able to sit up.

• Is your baby interested in food? A six-month-old baby who stares and grabs at your food at dinnertime is clearly ready for some variety in the food department.

If your doctor gives the go-ahead but your baby seems frustrated or uninterested as you're introducing solid foods, try waiting a few days or even weeks before trying again. Since solids are only a supplement at this point, breast milk and formula will still fill your baby's basic nutritional needs.

How to Start Feeding Solids

When your baby is ready and the doctor has given you the okay to try solid foods, pick a time of day when your baby is not tired or cranky. You want your baby to be a little hungry, but not all-out starving; you might want to let your baby breastfeed a while, or provide part of the usual bottle.

Have your baby sit supported in your lap or in an upright infant seat. Infants who sit well, usually around six months, can be placed in a high chair with a safety strap.

Most babies' first food is a little iron-fortified infant rice cereal mixed with breast milk or formula. The first feeding may be nothing more than a little cereal mixed in a whole lot of liquid. Place the spoon near your baby's lips, and let the baby smell and taste. Don't be surprised if this first spoonful is rejected. Wait a minute and try again. Most food offered to your baby at this age will end up on the baby's chin, bib, or high-chair tray. Again, this is just an introduction.

Do not add cereal to your baby's bottle unless your doctor instructs you to do so, as this can cause babies to become overweight and doesn't help the baby learn how to eat solid foods.

Once your little one gets the hang of eating cereal off a spoon, it may be time to introduce a fruit or vegetable. When introducing new foods, go slow. Introduce one food at a time and wait several days before trying something else new. This will allow you to identify foods that your baby may be allergic to.

Your baby may take a little while to "learn" how to eat solids. During these months you'll still be providing the usual feedings of breast milk or formula, so don't be concerned if your baby refuses certain foods at first or doesn't seem interested. It may just take some time.

Foods to Avoid for Now

Some foods are generally withheld until later. Do not give eggs, cow's milk, citrus fruits and juices, and honey until after a baby's first birthday.

Eggs (especially the whites) may cause an allergic reaction, especially if given too early. Citrus is highly acidic and can cause painful diaper rashes for a baby. Honey may contain certain spores that, while harmless to adults, can cause botulism in babies. Regular cow's milk does not have the nutrition that infants need.

Fish and seafood, peanuts and peanut butter, and tree nuts are also considered allergenic for infants, and shouldn't be given until after the child is two or three years old, depending on whether the child is at higher risk for developing food allergies. A child is at higher risk for food allergies if one or more close family members have allergies or allergy-related conditions, like food allergies, eczema, or asthma.

Some possible signs of food allergy or allergic reactions include:

- rash;

- bloating or an increase in intestinal gas;

- diarrhea;

- fussiness after eating.

For more severe allergic reactions, like hives or breathing difficulty, get medical attention right away. If your child has any type of reaction to a food, don't offer that food until you talk with your doctor.

Tips for Introducing Solids

With the hectic pace of family life, most parents opt for commercially prepared baby foods at first. They come in small, convenient containers, and manufacturers must meet strict safety and nutrition guidelines. Avoid brands with added fillers and sugars.

If you do plan to prepare your own baby foods at home, pureeing them with a food processor or blender, here are some things to keep in mind:

- Protect your baby and the rest of your family from foodborne illness by following the rules for food safety (including frequent hand washing).

- Try to preserve the nutrients in your baby's food by using cooking methods that retain the most vitamins and minerals. Try steaming or baking fruits and vegetables instead of boiling, which washes away the nutrients.

- Freeze portions that you aren't going to use right away rather than canning them.

- Avoid home-prepared beets, collard greens, spinach, and turnips. They can contain high levels of nitrates, which can cause anemia in infants. Serve jarred varieties of those vegetables.

Whether you buy the baby food or make it yourself, remember that texture and consistency are important. At first, babies should have finely pureed single foods. (Just applesauce, for example, not apples and pears mixed together.) After you've successfully tried individual foods, it's okay to offer a pureed mix of two foods. When your child is about nine months old, coarser, chunkier textures are going to be tolerated as he or she begins transitioning to a diet that includes more table foods.

If you are using commercially prepared baby food in jars, spoon some of the food into a bowl to feed your baby. Do not feed your baby directly from the jar, because bacteria from the baby's mouth can contaminate the remaining food. It's also smart to throw away opened jars of baby food within a day or two.

Juice can be given after six months of age, which is also a good age to introduce your baby to a cup. Buy one with large handles and a lid (a "sippy cup"), and teach your baby how to maneuver and drink from it. You might need to try a few different cups to find one that works for your child. Use water at first to avoid messy clean-ups.

Serve only 100% fruit juice, not juice drinks or powdered drink mixes. Do not give juice in a bottle and remember to limit the amount of juice your baby drinks to less than four total ounces (120 ml) a day. Too much juice adds extra calories without the nutrition of breast milk or formula. Drinking too much juice can contribute to overweight and can cause diarrhea.

Infants usually like fruits and sweeter vegetables, such as carrots and sweet potatoes, but don't neglect other vegetables. Your goal over the next few months is to introduce a wide variety of foods. If your baby doesn't seem to like a particular food, reintroduce it at later meals. It can take quite a few tries before kids warm up to certain foods.

Feeding Your 8- to 12-Month-Old

By about eight months old, most babies are pros at handling the iron-fortified infant cereals and pureed vegetables and fruits that have been introduced as part of their diet along with breast milk or formula.

Over the next few months, they start to explore table foods.

Changing Eating Habits

As you expand your baby's palate, continue to give new foods a trial run (a few days to a week) to look for any allergic reactions. Do not feed your little one eggs, citrus fruits, fish and seafood, nuts (including peanuts and peanut butter), or honey.

During this transition, you may want to introduce meats and offer your child new, coarser textures that require a little more chewing.

You can buy baby foods that offer new tastes and textures or you can fork-mash, cut up, or grind whatever foods the rest of the family eats. You should cook it a little longer, until it's very soft, and cut it into small pieces that your baby can handle to decrease the risk of choking.

By the time babies are around nine months old, they usually have the dexterity and coordination to take food between forefinger and thumb so that they can try feeding themselves with their fingers. (You may want to provide a safe baby spoon as well.)

If you haven't already, have your baby join the rest of the family at meals. At this age, they enjoy being at the table.

By the first birthday, babies usually are ready to go from formula to cow's milk. If you're breastfeeding, you can continue or you may decide to stop now.

You've probably already introduced your baby to a sippy cup, so let him or her keep working on it. (Juice should always be given in a cup, not a bottle.) After 12 months, you can serve whole milk in a cup, which will help with the transition from the bottle.

Feeding Safety

Never leave your baby unattended while eating in case he or she chokes. Avoid foods that could present a choking hazard such as whole grapes, raw vegetables, hard fruits, raisins, white bread, pieces of hard cheese, hot dogs, popcorn, and hard candies.

If you're unsure about whether a finger food is safe, ask yourself:

- Does it melt in the mouth? Some dry cereals will melt in the mouth, and so will light and flaky crackers.

- Is it cooked enough so that it mashes easily? Well-cooked vegetables and fruits will mash easily. So will canned fruits and vegetables. (Make sure to choose canned foods that don't have added sugar or salt.)

- Is it naturally soft? Cottage cheese, shredded cheese, and small pieces of tofu are soft.

- Can it be gummed? Pieces of ripe banana and well-cooked pasta can be gummed.

Making Meals Work

Keep your baby's temperament in mind when introducing new foods. If your baby balks at new textures, serve them in small portions and mix them with food you know your child likes. A child who likes a lot of stimulation may enjoy it when you "play airplane" with the spoon to get the food into his or her mouth. A more sensitive tot, however, may need the focus kept on eating with minimum distractions.

How Much Should My Baby Eat?

Infant formula and breast milk continue to provide important nutrients for growing infants, but babies will start to drink less as they approach the first birthday. They're getting more nutrients now from the variety of foods they've learned to eat and enjoy.

You may be concerned that you're feeding your child too much or not enough. Pay attention to your child's cues of hunger and fullness. A child who is full may suck with less enthusiasm, stop, or turn away from the breast or the bottle. With solid foods, your baby may turn away, refuse to open his or her mouth, or spit the food out.

Let your baby finger feed or hold a spoon while you do the actual feeding. This is good preparation for the toddler years when kids take charge of self-feeding. And if you haven't already, consider establishing more regular mealtimes.

Section 19.3

Healthy Nutrition for Toddlers

"Nutrition Guide for Toddlers," October 2008, reprinted with permission from www.kidshealth.org. Copyright © 2008 The Nemours Foundation. This information was provided by KidsHealth, one of the largest resources online for medically reviewed health information written for parents, kids, and teens. For more articles like this one, visit www.KidsHealth.org, or www.TeensHealth.org.

Nutrition through Variety

Babies grow at a lightning pace—three inches or so every three months. A toddler, in contrast, grows at a much slower rate—only three to five inches in an entire year.

While growth slows somewhat, nutrition remains a top priority. It's also a time for parents to shift gears, leaving bottles behind and moving into a new era where kids will eat and drink more independently.

The toddler years are a time of transition, especially between 12–24 months, when they're learning to eat table food and accepting new tastes and textures. Breast milk and formula provided adequate nutrition for your child as an infant, but now it's time for toddlers to start getting what they need through a variety of foods.

Lower-fat toddlers: Fat intake shouldn't be restricted in an infant's diet. But by age two, a toddler should only get 30%–35% of daily calories from fat.

How Much Food Do They Need?

Depending on their age, size, and activity level, toddlers need about 1,000–1,400 calories a day. Refer to the following chart to get an idea of how much your child should be eating and what kinds of foods would satisfy the requirements.

Use Table 19.1 as a guide, but trust your own judgment and a toddler's cues to tell if he or she is satisfied and getting adequate nutrition. Nutrition is all about averages so don't panic if you don't hit every mark every day—just strive to provide a wide variety of nutrients in your child's diet.

The amounts provided are based on the Food Guide Pyramid [My-Pyramid was replaced by MyPlate (www.choosemyplate.gov) on June 2, 2011] for the average two- and three-year-old. For kids between 12 and 24 months, the two-year-old recommendations can serve as a guide, but during this year toddler diets are still in transition.

Talk with your doctor about specifics for your child. And younger toddlers may not be eating this much—at least at first. When a range of amounts is given, the higher amount applies to kids who are older, bigger, or more active and need more calories.

Table 19.1. Daily Nutrition Needs for Toddlers

Food Group	Daily Amount for Two-Year-Olds	Daily Amount for Three-Year-Olds	Help with Servings
Grains	3 ounces, half from whole-grain sources	4–5 ounces, half from whole-grain sources	One ounce equals: 1 slice of bread, 1 cup of ready-to-eat cereal, or 1/2 cup of cooked rice, cooked pasta, or cooked cereal.
Vegetables	1 cup	1 1/2 cups	Use measuring cups to check amounts. Serve veggies that are soft, cut in small pieces, and well cooked to prevent choking.
Fruits	1 cup	1–1 1/2 cups	Use measuring cups to check amounts. An 8- to 9-inch banana equals 1 cup.
Milk	2 cups	2 cups	One cup equals: 1 cup of milk or yogurt, 1 1/2 ounces of natural cheese, or 2 ounces of processed cheese.
Meat and Beans	2 ounces	3–4 ounces	One ounce equals: 1 ounce of meat, poultry, or fish; 1/4 cup cooked dry beans; or 1 egg.

Milk Matters

An important part of a toddler's diet, milk provides calcium and vitamin D to help build strong bones. Toddlers should have 500 milligrams of calcium and 400 IU (international units) vitamin D (which aids in calcium absorption) a day.

The calcium requirement is easily met if your child gets the recommended two servings of dairy foods every day, but this amount provides only half of the vitamin D requirement. The AAP recommends vitamin D supplementation of 400 IU per day if a child is drinking less than one liter (about four cups) of milk a day.

In general, kids ages 12 to 24 months should drink whole milk to help provide the dietary fats they need for normal growth and brain development. Reduced fat (2%) milk may be given if overweight or obesity is a concern, or if there is a family history of obesity, high cholesterol, or heart disease. After age two, most kids can switch to low-fat (1%) or non-fat milk. Your doctor will help you decide which kind of milk to serve your toddler.

Some kids initially reject cow's milk because it doesn't taste like the familiar breast milk or formula. If your child is at least 12 months and having this difficulty, mix whole milk with some formula or breast milk. Gradually adjust the mixture over time so it becomes 100% cow's milk.

Some kids don't like milk or are unable to drink or eat dairy products. Explore other calcium sources, such as fortified cereals, calcium-fortified soy beverages, broccoli, and calcium-fortified orange juice.

Meeting Iron Requirements

Toddlers should have seven milligrams of iron each day. After 12 months of age, they're at risk for iron deficiency because they no longer drink iron-fortified formula and may not be eating iron-fortified infant cereal or enough other iron-containing foods to make up the difference.

Cow's milk is low in iron. Drinking a lot of cow's milk also can put a child at risk of developing iron deficiency. Toddlers who drink a lot of cow's milk may be less hungry and less likely to eat iron-rich foods. Milk decreases the absorption of iron and can also irritate the lining of the intestine, causing small amounts of bleeding and the gradual loss of iron in the stool.

Iron deficiency can affect growth and may lead to learning and behavioral problems. And it can progress to anemia (a decreased number of red blood cells in the body). Iron is needed to make red blood cells, which carry oxygen throughout the body. Without enough iron and red blood cells, the body's tissues and organs get less oxygen and don't function as well.

To help prevent iron deficiency:

- Limit your child's milk intake to about 16–24 ounces a day.

- Serve more iron-rich foods (meat, poultry, fish, enriched grains, beans, tofu).

- When serving iron-rich meals, include foods that contain vitamin C (tomatoes, broccoli, oranges, and strawberries), which improve the body's iron absorption.

- Continue serving iron-fortified cereal until your child is 18–24 months of age.

Talk to your doctor if you're concerned that your child isn't eating a balanced diet. Many toddlers are checked for iron-deficiency anemia, but never give your child a vitamin or mineral supplement without first discussing it with your doctor.

Chapter 20

Children and Food

Chapter Contents

Section 20.1

Healthy Nutrition for Children

This section excerpted from "Helping Your Child: Tips for Parents,"
Weight-Control Information Network, National Institute of Diabetes and
Digestive and Kidney Diseases (win.niddk.nih.gov), January 2007.

Eating well and being physically active are key to your child's well-being. Eating too much and exercising too little can lead to overweight and related health problems that can follow children into their adult years. You can take an active role in helping your child—and your whole family—learn healthy eating and physical activity habits.

How Will Healthy Eating and Physical Activity Help My Child?

All children benefit from healthy eating and physical activity. A balanced diet and being physically active help children do the following:

- Grow
- Learn
- Build strong bones and muscles
- Have energy
- Maintain a healthy weight
- Avoid obesity-related diseases like type 2 diabetes
- Get plenty of nutrients
- Feel good about themselves

How Are My Child's Eating and Activity Habits Formed?

Parents play a big role in shaping children's eating habits. When parents eat a variety of foods that are low in fat and sugar and high in fiber, children learn to like these foods as well. It may take 10 or more tries before a child accepts a new food, so do not give up if your child does not like a new food right away.

Parents have an effect on children's physical activity habits as well. You can set a good example by going for a walk or bike ride after dinner instead of watching TV. Playing ball or jumping rope with your children shows them that being active is fun.

With many parents working outside the home, child care providers also help shape children's eating and activity habits. Make sure your child care provider offers well-balanced meals and snacks, as well as plenty of active play time.

If your child is in school, find out more about the school's breakfast and lunch programs and ask to have input into menu choices, or help your child pack a lunch that includes a variety of foods. Get involved in the parent-teacher association (PTA) to support physical education and after-school sports.

Your child's friends and the media can also affect his or her eating and activity choices. Children may go to fast food places or play video games with their friends instead of playing tag, basketball, or other active games. TV commercials try to persuade kids to choose high-fat snacks and high-sugar drinks and cereals. When parents help their children be aware of peer and media pressures, youngsters are more likely to make healthy choices outside the home.

What Should My Child Eat?

Just like adults, children need to eat a wide variety of foods for good health. The *Dietary Guidelines for Americans* encourage Americans over two years of age to eat a variety of nutrient-dense foods. Recommended items include fruits, vegetables, fat-free or low-fat milk and milk products, lean meats, poultry, fish, beans, eggs, nuts, and whole grains. The guidelines also recommend a diet low in saturated fats, trans fats, cholesterol, salt (sodium), and added sugars.

Sources of Calcium

Calcium helps build strong bones and teeth. Milk and milk products are great sources of calcium. If your child cannot digest milk or if you choose not to serve milk products, there are other ways to make sure he or she gets enough calcium.

- Serve calcium-rich vegetables like broccoli, mustard greens, kale, collard greens, and Brussels sprouts.

- Include high-calcium beans like great northern beans, black turtle beans, navy beans, and baked beans in casseroles and salads.

221

- Try calcium-enriched soy- and rice-based drinks. Serve chilled, use in place of cow's milk in your favorite recipes, or add to hot or cold cereals.

- Serve lactose-reduced or lactose-free dairy products like low-fat or fat-free milk, yogurt, and ice cream. (Lactose is the sugar in milk and foods made with milk. People who cannot digest lactose often have stomach pain and bloating when they drink milk.)

- Try low-fat yogurt or cheese in small amounts—they may be easier to digest than milk.

How Can I Help My Child Eat Better?

- Give your child a snack or two in addition to his or her three daily meals.

- Offer your child a wide variety of foods, such as grains, vegetables and fruits, low-fat dairy products, and lean meat or beans.

- Serve snacks like dried fruit, low-fat yogurt, and air-popped popcorn.

- Let your child decide whether and how much to eat. Keep serving new foods even if your child does not eat them at first.

- Cook with less fat—bake, roast, or poach foods instead of frying.

- Limit the amount of added sugar in your child's diet. Choose cereals with low or no added sugar. Serve water or low-fat milk more often than sugar-sweetened sodas and fruit-flavored drinks.

- Choose and prepare foods with less salt. Keep the salt shaker off the table. Have fruits and vegetables on hand for snacks instead of salty snack foods.

- Involve your child in planning and preparing meals. Children may be more willing to eat the dishes they help fix.

- Have family meals together and serve everyone the same thing.

- Do not be too strict. In small amounts, sweets or food from fast-food restaurants can still have a place in a healthy diet.

- Make sure your child eats breakfast. Breakfast provides children with the energy they need to listen and learn in school.

Simple Snack Ideas*

- Dried fruit and nut mix

- Fresh, frozen, or canned vegetables or fruit served plain or with low-fat yogurt

- Rice cakes, whole-grain crackers, or whole-grain bread served with low-fat cheese, fruit spread, peanut butter, almond butter, or soy nut butter

- Pretzels or air-popped popcorn sprinkled with salt-free seasoning mix

- Homemade fruit smoothie made with low-fat milk or yogurt and frozen or fresh fruit

- Dry cereals served plain or with low-fat or fat-free milk

* Children of preschool age and younger can easily choke on foods that are hard to chew, small and round, or sticky, such as hard vegetables, whole grapes, hard chunks of cheese, raisins, nuts and seeds, and popcorn. Carefully select snacks for children in this age group.

What about Physical Activity?

Like adults, children should be physically active most, if not all, days of the week. Experts suggest at least 60 minutes of moderate physical activity daily for most children. Walking fast, bicycling, jumping rope, dancing fast, and playing basketball are all good ways for your child to be active.

As children spend more time watching TV and playing computer and video games, they spend less time being active. Parents play a big role in helping kids get up and get moving.

What If My Child Is Overweight?

Children who are overweight are more likely to become overweight adults. They may develop type 2 diabetes, high blood pressure, heart disease, and other illnesses that can follow them into adulthood. Overweight in children can also lead to stress, sadness, and low self-esteem.

Because children grow at different rates at different times, it is not always easy to tell if a child is overweight. For example, it is normal for boys to have a growth spurt in weight and catch up in height later. Your health care provider can measure your child's height and weight and tell you if your child is in a healthy range for his or her gender and age. If your provider finds that your child is overweight, you can help.

How Can I Help My Overweight Child?

- Do not put your child on a weight-loss diet unless your health care provider tells you to. Limiting what children eat may interfere with their growth.

- Involve the whole family in building healthy eating and physical activity habits. It benefits everyone and does not single out the child who is overweight.

- Accept and love your child at any weight. It will boost his or her self-esteem.

- Help your child find ways other than food to handle setbacks or successes.

- Talk with your health care provider if you are concerned about your child's eating habits or weight.

Remember, you play the biggest role in your child's life. You can help your children learn healthy eating and physical activity habits that they can follow for the rest of their lives.

Section 20.2

Food Allergies in Children on the Rise

"CDC Study Finds Three Million U.S. Children Have Food
or Digestive Allergies," Centers for Disease Control and
Prevention (www.cdc.gov), October 22, 2008.

The number of young people who had a food or digestive allergy increased 18% between 1997 and 2007, according to a new report by the Centers for Disease Control and Prevention (CDC). In 2007, approximately 3 million U.S. children and teenagers under age 18—or nearly 4% of that age group—were reported to have a food or digestive allergy in the previous 12 months, compared to just over 2.3 million (3.3%) in 1997.

The findings are published in a new data brief, "Food Allergy among U.S. Children: Trends in Prevalence and Hospitalizations." The data are from the National Health Interview Survey and the National Hospital Discharge Survey, both conducted by CDC's National Center for Health Statistics.

The report found that eight types of food account for 90% of all food allergies: milk, eggs, peanuts, tree nuts, fish, shellfish, soy, and wheat. Reactions to these foods by an allergic person can range from a tingling sensation around the mouth and lips, to hives and even death, depending on the severity of the reaction.

Children with food allergy are two to four times more likely to have other related conditions such as asthma and other allergies, compared to children without food allergies, the report said.

Other highlights include the following:

- Boys and girls had similar rates of food allergy—3.8% for boys and 4.1% for girls.

- Approximately 4.7% of children younger than 5 years had a reported food allergy compared to 3.7% of children and teens aged 5 to 17 years.

- Hispanic children had lower rates of reported food allergy (3.1%) than non-Hispanic white (4.1%) or non-Hispanic black children (4%).

225

- In 2007, 29% of children with food allergy also had reported asthma compared to 12% of children without food allergy.

- Approximately 27% of children with food allergy had reported eczema or skin allergy, compared to 8% of children without food allergy.

- Over 30% of children with food allergy also had reported respiratory allergy, compared with 9% of children with no food allergy.

- From 2004 to 2006, there were approximately 9,537 hospital discharges per year with a diagnosis related to food allergy among children from birth to 17 years. Hospital discharges with a diagnosis related to food allergy increased significantly over time between 1998–2000 through 2004–2006.

The mechanisms by which a person develops an allergy to specific foods are largely unknown. Food allergy is more prevalent in children than adults. Most affected children will outgrow food allergies, although food allergy can be a lifelong concern.

The full report is available at www.cdc.gov/nchs.

Section 20.3

School Lunches

Buying lunch at school may be the first time kids get to call the shots on which foods they'll eat. Luckily, school lunches have improved over the years, both in taste and nutrition, with many serving healthier dishes, such as grilled chicken sandwiches and salads.

But some still exceed recommendations for fat. In the typical school cafeteria, kids can still choose an unhealthy mix of foods, especially the less nutritious fare often available a la carte or in the vending machine. For instance, a kid might decide to buy a hot dog, day after day.

Lunchtime Opportunities

Use school lunches as a chance to steer your kids toward good choices. Especially with younger kids, explain how a nutritious lunch will give them energy to finish the rest of the schoolday and enjoy after-school activities.

Here are some other tips:

- Look over the cafeteria menu together. Ask what a typical lunch includes and which meals your kids particularly like. Recommend items that are healthier, but be willing to allow them to buy favorite lunch items occasionally, even if that includes a hot dog.

- Ask about foods like chips, soda, and ice cream. Find out if and when these foods are available at school.

- Encourage kids to take a packed lunch, at least occasionally. This can put you back in the driver's seat and help ensure that kids get a nutritious midday meal.

Healthier Alternatives

Encourage kids to choose cafeteria meals that include fruits, vegetables, lean meats, and whole grains, such as whole wheat bread instead of white. Also, they should avoid fried foods when possible and choose low-fat milk or water as a drink.

If you're helping pack a lunch, start by brainstorming foods and snacks that your kids would like to eat. In addition to old standbys, such as peanut butter and jelly, try pitas or wrap sandwiches stuffed with grilled chicken or veggies. Try soups and salads, and don't forget last night's leftovers as an easy lunchbox filler.

You also can perform a lunch makeover. These small changes do make a nutritional difference.

Table 20.1. Healthy Lunch Substitutes

Instead of	Consider
Higher-fat lunch meats	Lower-fat deli meats, such as turkey
White bread	Whole-grain breads (wheat, oat, multi-grain)
Mayonnaise	Light mayonnaise or mustard
Fried chips and snacks	Baked chips, air-popped popcorn, trail mix, veggies and dip
Fruit in syrup	Fruit in natural juices or fresh fruit
Cookies and snack cakes	Trail mix, yogurt, or homemade baked goods such as oatmeal cookies or fruit muffins
Fruit drinks and soda	Low-fat milk, water, or 100% fruit juice

Nutritional Upgrades

Table 20.2 shows how two lunches stack up after a typical lunch received a nutritional upgrade.

Healthy Packed Lunches

Prepackaged lunches for kids are popular and convenient, but they're also expensive and often less than nutritious. Instead, create your own packable lunch using healthier ingredients. Consider these components and pack them in plastic containers, resealable plastic bags, or colorful plastic wrap:

- Cold-cut roll ups (lean, low-fat turkey, ham, or roast beef with low-fat cheese on whole wheat tortillas)

- Cold pizza (shredded mozzarella cheese with pizza sauce on a flour tortilla, whole wheat pita, English muffin, or mini pizza shell)

- Cracker sandwiches (whole-grain crackers filled with low-fat cream cheese or peanut butter and jelly)

- Peanut butter and celery sticks

- Veggie sticks with low-fat dip or dressing

- 100% fruit juice box or bottle of water

- Optional dessert (choose one): flavored gelatin, low-fat pudding, oatmeal raisin cookie, graham crackers, fresh fruit

Be sure to check with the school to make sure that there aren't any restrictions on what kids can pack in their lunches. And don't forget to involve your kids in the process so that healthier lunches can become a goal they strive for, too.

Table 20.2. Nutritional Upgrades

Typical Lunch	Nutritional Upgrade	Why It's Better
Beef bologna on white	Lean turkey on whole wheat	Less fat and more fiber
Mayonnaise	Lettuce and mustard	Less fat and fewer calories
Potato chips	Carrots and celery with light dressing	Less fat and a serving of vegetables
Fruit cup in light syrup	Fresh grapes	Less sugar and fewer calories
Chocolate sandwich cookies	Homemade trail mix	Less fat and more fiber
Fruit punch drink	Skim milk	Fewer calories, less sugar, plus calcium
980 calories	725 calories	255 fewer calories
48 g fat	13.5 g fat	34.5 fewer grams of fat
13.5 g saturated fat	2.5 g saturated fat	11 fewer grams of saturated fat
125 g carbohydrates	120 g carbohydrates	5 fewer grams of carbohydrates
59 g sugar	52 g sugar	7 fewer grams of sugar
3 g fiber	13 g fiber	10 more grams of fiber

Safe Packing

A packed lunch carries the added responsibility of keeping the food safe to eat. That means keeping hot foods hot and cold foods cold. One study found that fewer than a third of parents included a cold pack when packing yogurt, deli-meat sandwiches, and other foods that need refrigeration.

Here are some suggestions to keep lunch foods safe:

• Wash your hands first.

• Use a thermos for hot foods.

• Use cold packs or freeze some foods and drinks overnight. They'll thaw in the lunchbox.

• Wash out lunchboxes every day or use brown paper bags that can be discarded or recycled.

• Toss in some moist towelettes to remind kids to wash their hands before eating and to clean up after.

Chapter 21

Nutrition Information for Teens and Young Adults

Chapter Contents

Section 21.1

Teens and Healthy Eating

This section excerpted from "Take Charge of Your Health," Weight-Control Information Network, National Institute of Diabetes and Digestive and Kidney Diseases (win.niddk.nih.gov), August 2009.

Does Your Life Move at a Hectic Pace?

You may feel stressed from school, after-school activities, peer pressure, and family relationships. Your busy schedule may lead you to skip breakfast, buy lunch from vending machines, and grab whatever is in the refrigerator for dinner when you get home. Yet healthy behaviors, like nutritious eating and regular physical activity, may help you meet the challenges of your life. In fact, healthy eating and regular exercise may help you feel energized, learn better, and stay alert in class. These healthy habits may also lower your risk for diseases such as diabetes, asthma, heart disease, and some forms of cancer.

From 2003 to 2004, approximately 17.4% of U.S. teens between the ages of 12 and 19 were overweight. Overweight children and teens are at high risk for developing serious diseases. Type 2 diabetes and heart disease were considered adult diseases, but they are now being reported in children and teens.

Dieting is not the answer. The best way to lose weight is to eat healthfully and be physically active. It is a good idea to talk with your health care provider if you want to lose weight. Many teens turn to unhealthy dieting methods to lose weight, including eating very little, cutting out whole groups of foods (like grain products), skipping meals, and fasting. These methods can leave out important foods you need to grow. Other weight-loss tactics such as smoking, self-induced vomiting, or using diet pills or laxatives can lead to health problems. In fact, unhealthy dieting can actually cause you to gain more weight because it often leads to a cycle of eating very little, then overeating or binge eating. Also, unhealthy dieting can put you at greater risk for growth and emotional problems.

Healthy Eating

Eating healthfully means getting the right balance of nutrients your body needs to perform every day. You can find out more about your nutritional needs by checking out the *Dietary Guidelines for Americans*. This U.S. government publication explains how much of each type of food you should eat, along with great information on nutrition and physical activity. The guidelines suggest the number of calories you should eat daily based on your gender, age, and activity level.

According to the guidelines, a healthy eating plan includes the following:

- Fruits and vegetables

- Fat-free or low-fat milk and milk products

- Lean meats, poultry, fish, beans, eggs, and nuts

- Whole grains

In addition, a healthy diet is low in saturated and trans fats, cholesterol, salt, and added sugars. When it comes to food portions, the *Dietary Guidelines* use the word "servings" to describe a standard amount of food. Serving sizes are measured as ounce- or cup-equivalents. The tips in this chapter are based on the guidelines and can help you develop healthy eating habits for a lifetime.

Eat Fruits and Vegetables Every Day

When consumed as part of a well-balanced and nutritious eating plan, fruits and vegetables can help keep you healthy. You may get your servings from fresh, frozen, dried, and canned fruits and vegetables. Teenagers who are consuming 2,000 calories per day should aim for 2 cups of fruit and 2 1/2 cups of vegetables every day. You may need fewer or more servings depending on your individual calorie needs, which your health care provider can help you determine.

Count Your Calcium

Calcium helps strengthen bones and teeth. This nutrient is very important, since getting enough calcium now can reduce the risk for broken bones later in life. Yet most teens get less than the recommended 1,200 mg of calcium per day. Aim for at least 3 cup-equivalents of low-fat or fat-free calcium-rich foods and beverages each day.

Power up with Protein

Protein builds and repairs body tissue like muscles and organs. Eating enough protein can help you grow strong and sustain your energy levels. Teens need 5 1/2 ounce-equivalents of protein-rich foods each day.

Go Whole Grain

Grain foods help give you energy. Whole-grain foods like whole-wheat bread, brown rice, and oatmeal usually have more nutrients than refined grain products. They give you a feeling of fullness and add bulk to your diet. Try to get 6 ounce-equivalents of grains every day, with at least 3 ounce-equivalents coming from whole-grain sources.

Know Your Fats

Fat is also an important nutrient. It helps your body grow and develop, and it is a source of energy as well—it even keeps your skin and hair healthy. But be aware that some fats are better for you than others. Limit your fat intake to 25% to 35% of your total calories each day.

Unsaturated fat can be part of a healthy diet—as long as you do not eat too much since it is still high in calories. Good sources include the following:

- Olive, canola, safflower, sunflower, corn, and soybean oils
- Fish like salmon, trout, tuna, and whitefish
- Nuts like walnuts, almonds, peanuts, and cashews

Limit saturated fat, which can clog your arteries and raise your risk for heart disease. Saturated fat is found primarily in animal products and in a few plant oils, such as the following:

- Butter
- Full-fat cheese
- Whole milk
- Fatty meats
- Coconut, palm, and palm kernel oils

Limit trans fat, which is also bad for your heart. Trans fat is often found in these foods:

- Baked goods like cookies, muffins, and doughnuts
- Snack foods like crackers and chips
- Vegetable shortening
- Stick margarine
- Fried foods

Look for words like "shortening," "partially hydrogenated vegetable oil," or "hydrogenated vegetable oil" in the list of ingredients. These ingredients tell you that the food contains trans fat. Packaged food products are required to list trans fat on their Nutrition Facts.

Replenish Your Body with Iron

Teen boys need iron to support their rapid growth—most boys double their lean body mass between the ages of 10 and 17. Teen girls also need iron to support growth and replace blood lost during menstruation.

To get the iron you need, try eating these foods:

- Fish and shellfish
- Lean beef
- Iron-fortified cereals
- Enriched and whole-grain breads
- Cooked dried beans and peas like black beans, kidney beans, black-eyed peas, and chickpeas/garbanzo beans
- Spinach

Control Your Food Portions

The portion sizes that you get away from home at a restaurant, grocery store, or school event may contain more food than you need to eat in one sitting. Research shows that when people are served more food, they eat more food. So, how can you control your food portions? Try these tips:

- When eating out, share your meal, order a half-portion, or order an appetizer as a main meal. Be aware that some appetizers are larger than others and can have as many calories as an entree.
- Take at least half of your meal home.

- When eating at home, take one serving out of a package (read the Nutrition Facts to find out how big a serving is) and eat it off a plate instead of eating straight out of a box or bag.

- Avoid eating in front of the TV or while you are busy with other activities. It is easy to lose track of how much you are eating if you eat while doing other things.

- Eat slowly so your brain can get the message that your stomach is full.

- Do not skip meals. Skipping meals may lead you to eat more high-calorie, high-fat foods at your next meal or snack. Eat breakfast every day.

Read Food Labels.

When you read a food label, pay special attention to these elements:

- **Serving Size:** Check the amount of food in a serving. Do you eat more or less? The "servings per container" line tells you the number of servings in the food package.

- **Calories and other nutrients:** Remember, the number of calories and other listed nutrients are for one serving only. Food packages often contain more than one serving.

- **Percent Daily Value:** Look at how much of the recommended daily amount of a nutrient (%DV) is in one serving of food—5% DV or less is low and 20% DV or more is high. For example, if your breakfast cereal has 25% DV for iron, it is high in iron.

Plan Meals and Snacks

You and your family have busy schedules, which can make eating healthfully a challenge. Planning ahead can help. Think about the meals and snacks you would like for the week—including bag lunches to take to school—and help your family make a shopping list. You may even want to go grocery shopping and cook together.

Jumpstart Your Day with Breakfast

Did you know that eating breakfast can help you do better in school? By eating breakfast you can increase your attention span and memory, have more energy, and feel less irritable and restless. A breakfast that is part of a healthy diet can also help you maintain an appropriate weight now and in the future.

Pack Your Lunch

Whether you eat lunch from school or pack your own, this meal should provide you with one-third of the day's nutritional needs. A lunch of chips, cookies, candy, or soda just gives you lots of calories, but not many nutrients. Instead of buying snacks from vending machines at school, bring food from home. Try packing your lunch with a lean turkey sandwich on whole-grain bread and healthy foods like fruits, vegetables, low-fat yogurt, and nuts.

Snack Smart

A healthy snack can contribute to a healthy eating plan and give you the energy boost you need to get through the day. Try these snack ideas, but keep in mind that most of these foods should be eaten in small amounts:

- Fruit—any kind—fresh, canned, dried, or frozen
- Peanut butter on rice cakes or whole-wheat crackers
- Baked potato chips or tortilla chips with salsa
- Veggies with low-fat dip
- String cheese, low-fat cottage cheese, or low-fat yogurt
- Frozen fruit bars, fruit sorbet, or low-fat frozen yogurt
- Vanilla wafers, graham crackers, animal crackers, or fig bars
- Popcorn (air popped or low-fat microwave)

Eat Dinner with Your Family

For many teens, dinner consists of eating on the run, snacking in front of the TV, or nonstop munching from after school to bedtime. Try to eat dinner as a family instead. Believe it or not, when you eat with your family you are more likely to get more fruits, vegetables, and other foods with the vitamins and minerals your body needs. Family meals also help you reconnect after a busy day. Talk to your family about fitting in at least a few meals together throughout the week.

Limit Fast Food and Choose Wisely

Like many teens, you may eat at fast food restaurants often. If so, you are probably taking in a lot of extra calories from added sugar and fat. Just one value-sized fast food meal of a sandwich, fries, and sweetened soda can have more calories, fat, and added sugar than anyone needs.

The best approach is to limit the amount of fast food you eat. If you do order fast food, try these tips:

- Skip "value-sized" or "super-sized" meals.

- Choose a grilled chicken sandwich or a plain, small burger.

- Use mustard instead of mayonnaise.

- Limit fried foods or remove breading from fried chicken, which can cut half the fat.

- Order garden or grilled chicken salads with light or reduced-calorie dressings.

- Choose water or fat-free or low-fat milk instead of sweetened soda.

Rethink Your Drinks

Soda and other sugary drinks have replaced milk and water as the drinks of choice for teens and adults alike. Yet these drinks are actually more like desserts because they are high in added sugar and calories. In fact, soda and sugar-laden drinks may contribute to weight problems in kids and teens. Try sticking to water, low-fat milk, or fat-free milk.

Making It Work

Look for chances to move more and eat better at home, at school, and in the community. It is not easy to maintain a healthy weight in today's environment. Fast food restaurants on every corner, vending machines at schools, and not enough safe places for physical activity can make it difficult to eat healthfully and be active. Busy schedules may also keep families from fixing and eating dinners together.

What You Can Do at Home

Talk to your family about making changes that encourage healthy eating and regular physical activity. Dance to music, run around the park, or play basketball together. Help your family plan weekly menus and shopping lists. Get involved with shopping and cooking, too.

1. Is the kitchen stocked with fruits, vegetables, low-fat or fat-free milk and milk products, whole-grain items, and other foods you need to eat healthy?

2. Can you get water and low-fat or fat-free milk instead of soda, sweetened tea, and sugary fruit drinks?

3. Do you pack healthy lunches to take to school?

4. Does your family eat dinner together a few times per week?

What You Can Do at School

Form a group of students and ask the principal for healthier food choices in the cafeteria or in vending machines. You can also ask for more P.E. classes or school-sponsored physical activities.

1. Does the cafeteria offer healthy foods such as salads and fruit?

2. Are there vending machines in school where you can buy snacks and drinks like baked chips, fig bars, and bottled water?

Section 21.2

The Importance of Calcium for Tweens and Teens

This section excerpted from "Tweens and Teens Need Calcium Now More Than Ever!" National Institute of Child Health and Human Development (www.nichd.nih.gov), 2005. Reviewed by David A. Cooke, MD, FACP, January 2011.

Tweens (kids ages 9–12) and teens need calcium now more than ever! All they need is three cups of low-fat or fat-free milk every day, plus other calcium-rich foods.

What's the Problem?

Ages 11–15 are a time when fast-growing bones need calcium. Unfortunately, most boys and girls are not getting the calcium they need.

Why Are the Tween and Teen Years So Critical?

It takes calcium to build strong bones. So calcium is especially important during the tween and teen years, when bones are growing their fastest.

Boys and girls in these age groups have calcium needs that they can't make up for later in life. In fact, by the time teens finish their growth spurts around age 17, 90% of their adult bone mass is established.

Unfortunately, fewer than 1 in 10 girls and only 1 in 4 boys ages 9 to 13 are at or above their adequate intake of calcium. This lack of calcium has a big impact on bones and teeth.

Calcium Is Critical for Lifelong Bone Health

Having a calcium-rich diet when you're young makes a big difference in health, now and later. By getting the calcium they need now, tweens and teens will accomplish the following:

Strengthen bones now: Some researchers suspect that the rise in forearm fractures in children is due to decreased bone mass, which may result because children are drinking less milk and more soda and are getting less physical activity. Making sure young people get the calcium they need will help strengthen their bones against the bumps and thumps of being an active teen.

Help prevent osteoporosis later in life: Osteoporosis is a condition that makes bones weak so they break more easily. Bones rely on calcium they store to stay strong throughout life. But the "bone bank" for storing calcium is only open for a short time. Tweens and teens can help prevent osteoporosis by filling their bone banks with calcium when they are young, so that their bones can use it throughout life.

Calcium Is Critical for Teeth

Even before they come in, baby teeth and adult teeth need calcium to develop fully. And after the teeth are in, calcium may also help protect them against decay. Calcium makes jawbones strong and healthy too!

Besides making sure your children get enough calcium, there are other things you can do to keep their teeth healthy:

- Make sure your children brush with fluoride toothpaste. Fluoride protects teeth from decay and helps heal early decay.

- Ask your child's dental care provider or health care provider if there is fluoride in your town or city's drinking water. If there is not, ask about fluoride tablets or drops for your child.

- Ask your child's dental care provider about proper brushing and flossing techniques and other ways your tween and teen can make sure teeth stay healthy.

How Much Calcium Do Kids Need?

Tweens and teens can get most of their daily calcium from three cups of low-fat or fat-free milk (900 mg of calcium) and additional servings of calcium-rich foods (400 mg of calcium) to get the 1,300 mg of calcium necessary to build strong bones for life.

Starting around age nine, young people need almost twice as much calcium as younger kids.

What Are Good Sources of Calcium?

There are lots of different calcium-rich foods to choose from, making it easy for tweens and teens to get the calcium they need every day.

Calcium from Milk

Low-fat or fat-free milk is a great source of calcium for a number of reasons:

- Milk contains a lot of calcium in a form that the body can easily absorb.

- Milk has other important nutrients that are good for bones and teeth. One especially important nutrient is vitamin D, which helps the body absorb more calcium.

- Milk is widely available and is already a part of many people's diets.

Today, tweens and teens have more milk choices than ever before. Most types of milk have approximately 300 mg of calcium per eight fluid ounces (one cup)—about 25% of the calcium that children and teenagers need every day.

The best choices are low-fat or fat-free milk and milk products. Because these items contain little or no fat, it's easy to get enough calcium without adding extra fat to the diet.

Calcium from Other Foods

Milk isn't the only way for tweens and teens to get the calcium they need every day. Experts report that the best way to get calcium is by eating calcium-rich foods. But for people who have lactose intolerance or who don't eat dairy products, foods with calcium added are also an option.

Check the ingredient list for added calcium in these foods:

- Tofu (with added calcium sulfate)

- Calcium-fortified orange juice

- Soy beverages with added calcium

- Calcium-fortified cereals or breads

Calcium supplements are also an alternative way to get calcium for children and adults who don't or can't have milk or milk products.

Food labels can tell you how much calcium is in one serving of food. Look at the % Daily Value (%DV) next to the calcium number on the food label. For more information on food labels, go to www.fda.gov/Food/LabelingNutrition/ConsumerInformation/ucm078889.htm.

What Small Changes Make a Big Difference?

The tween and teen years are an important time for young people to learn smart eating habits that will last a lifetime. Making low-fat and fat-free milk and other calcium-rich foods a part of the diet now teaches tweens and teens to make healthy choices. And, learning to make healthy food choices at home will carry over into school and adulthood.

Make Calcium Easy to Get at Home

Just a few simple and easy changes can bring great calcium benefits. Try one or all of the following ideas for making it easy to get calcium at home.

If you enjoy milk, chances are your children will, too. Tweens and teens look up to their parents and want to be like them. Young people make many food choices by watching their parents, so if you want your children to enjoy the bone-building benefits of calcium, show it. Drink milk yourself, and offer calcium-rich meals and snacks.

Put calcium on the menu at every meal. One way to make it easier for tweens and teens to get enough calcium is to serve low-fat or fat-free milk and other calcium-rich foods throughout the day. When low-fat or fat-free milk is the main beverage for meals, tweens and teens will choose it more often.

Ideas for calcium-rich meals and snacks.

Breakfast
- Pour low-fat or fat-free milk over your breakfast cereal.
- Have a cup of low-fat or fat-free yogurt.
- Drink a glass of orange juice with added calcium.
- Add low-fat or fat-free milk instead of water to oatmeal and hot cereal.

Lunch
- Add low-fat or fat-free cheese to a sandwich.
- Have a glass of low-fat or fat-free milk instead of soda.
- Have pizza or macaroni and cheese.
- Add low-fat or fat-free milk instead of water to tomato soup.

Snack

- Make a smoothie with fruit, ice, and low-fat or fat-free milk.
- Try flavored low-fat or fat-free milk such as chocolate or strawberry.
- Have a low-fat or fat-free frozen yogurt.
- Try some pudding made with low-fat or fat-free milk.
- Dip fruits and vegetables into yogurt.
- Have some low-fat or fat-free string cheese.

Dinner

- Make a salad with dark green, leafy vegetables.
- Serve broccoli or cooked, dry beans as a side dish.
- Top salads, soups, and stews with low-fat shredded cheese.
- Toss tofu with added calcium into stir fry and other dishes.

Grab-n-Go Calcium

Busy tweens and teens may skip meals or grab what is on hand for a quick meal or snack. But, with some guidance, they can still keep calcium in mind for meals and snacks on the go. Introduce kids to foods containing calcium that they can eat on the run. Keep portable, calcium-rich foods on hand for easy on-the-go snacks:

- Low-fat or fat-free string cheese
- Low-fat or fat-free pudding
- A handful of almonds
- A cereal bar with calcium added

Even gas stations and convenience stores carry calcium-rich options.

What If Milk Is a Problem for My Kids?

For some tweens and teens, getting 1,300 mg of calcium a day isn't easy. Some people have lactose intolerance, which limits how much milk and milk products they can have. Others dislike the taste of milk or avoid it because they think it is fattening. But even kids with these concerns can still get the calcium they need each day to build strong bones for life.

244

Concerns about Lactose Intolerance

Someone with lactose intolerance has trouble digesting lactose, the natural sugar found in dairy foods. Symptoms of lactose intolerance include stomach pain, diarrhea, bloating, and gas.

The best way for someone with lactose intolerance to get the health benefits of milk is to choose lactose-free milk and milk products. There are also a variety of pills and drops, which are available without a prescription, that help people digest lactose.

Even if your child has problems digesting lactose, he or she can probably still eat or drink these options:

- Eight fluid ounces (one cup) of low-fat or fat-free milk taken with meals

- Low-fat or fat-free yogurt or cheese

- Low-fat or fat-free milk poured on hot or cold cereal

People with lactose intolerance can also get some of their needed calcium from dark green, leafy vegetables, such as spinach, broccoli, and bok choy. Calcium supplements also provide an alternative way of getting calcium.

Foods with calcium added are also an option. Check the ingredient list for added calcium in tofu, orange juice, soy beverages, and breakfast cereals or breads.

My Child Doesn't Like the Taste of Milk

Even if your tweens or teens don't like the taste of plain milk, there are still plenty of ways to get calcium in the diet:

- Try a flavored low-fat or fat-free milk, such as chocolate, vanilla, or strawberry. Flavored milk has just as much calcium as plain.

- Serve foods that go with milk, such as fruit bars and fig bars.

- Drink low-fat or fat-free milk or yogurt smoothies for breakfast or a snack. You can make these at home or try one of the ready-made versions now available at many grocery stores.

- Keep portable, calcium-rich foods on hand for snacks on the run, such as low-fat or fat-free string cheese or individual pudding cups with calcium added.

- In moderation, low-fat or fat-free ice cream and frozen yogurt are calcium-rich treats.

- Serve non-milk sources of calcium, such as calcium-fortified soy beverages or orange juice with added calcium.

- Try a spinach salad or have fresh or cooked broccoli.

Concerns about Weight Control

Some tweens and teens avoid milk because they think it is fattening. Low-fat and fat-free milk and milk products are healthy food choices that are not high in fat or calories. They can be included in a healthy diet without adding to overall fat.

Section 21.3

Healthy Eating for College Students

"Beating the Freshman 15," July 2010, reprinted with permission from www.kidshealth.org. Copyright © 2010 The Nemours Foundation. This information was provided by KidsHealth, one of the largest resources online for medically reviewed health information written for parents, kids, and teens. For more articles like this one, visit www.KidsHealth.org, or www .TeensHealth.org.

What's Behind First-Year Weight Gain?

Everyone's heard warnings about the "freshman 15." But is it true that many college students pack on 15 pounds during their first year at school?

Recent studies find that some first-year students are indeed likely to gain weight—but it might not be the full freshman 15 and it may not all happen during freshman year. That might sound like good news, but it's not. Doctors are concerned that students who gradually put on pounds are establishing a pattern of weight gain that could spell trouble if it continues.

Studies show that students on average gain 3 to 10 pounds during their first two years of college. Most of this weight gain occurs during the first semester of freshman year.

College offers many temptations. You're on your own and free to eat what you want, when you want it. You can pile on the portions in the dining hall, eat dinners of french fries and ice cream, and indulge in sugary and salty snacks to fuel late-night study sessions. In addition, you may not get as much exercise as you did in high school.

College is also a time of change, and the stress of acclimating to school can trigger overeating. People sometimes eat in response to anxiety, homesickness, sadness, or stress, and all of these can be part of adapting to being away at school.

Should I Worry about the Weight?

Some weight gain is normal as an adolescent body grows and metabolism shifts. But pronounced or rapid weight gain may become a problem.

Weight gain that pushes you above the body's normal range carries health risks. People who are overweight are more likely to have high blood pressure, high cholesterol, breathlessness, and joint problems. People who are overweight when they're younger have a greater likelihood of being overweight as adults. Poor diet and exercise habits in college can start you on a path that could later lead to heart disease, type 2 diabetes, or obesity and may increase your risk for developing certain cancers.

Even without weight gain, unhealthy food choices also won't give you the balance of nutrients you need to keep up with the demands of college. You may notice that your energy lags and your concentration and memory suffer. Studies have found that most students get fewer than the recommended five servings of fruits and vegetables each day.

Balanced Lifestyle, Healthy Bones

College-age adults are still building bone mass. Eating calcium-rich foods (like dairy products) and doing weight-bearing exercises (like running) can help build bone mass. But some college habits, like smoking and drinking alcohol, can interfere with bone health. And cola, often a staple of late-night studying, interferes with the absorption of calcium.

What If I Gain Weight?

If you do gain weight, don't freak out. Take a look at your eating and exercise habits and make adjustments. In a study in which freshmen gained four pounds in 12 weeks, the students were only eating an average of 174 extra calories each day. So cutting out one can of soda or a midnight snack every day and being more active will help you get back on track.

It may be tempting to go for the easy fix, like skipping meals or trying the latest fad diet. But these approaches don't work to keep weight off in the long run. It's best to make small adjustments to your diet that you know you can stick with.

How Can I Avoid Gaining Weight?

The best way to beat weight gain is to prevent it altogether. Good habits like a balanced diet, regular exercise, and getting enough sleep can do more than keep the pounds off—they can also help you stay healthy and avoid problems down the line. Adopting some simple practices can have a big impact today and years from now.

Take a sound approach to eating. Here are some easy ways to adopt a healthy food attitude:

- Avoid eating when stressed, while studying, or while watching TV.
- Eat slowly.
- Eat at regular times and try not to skip meals.
- Keep between-meal and late-night snacking to a minimum.
- Choose a mix of nutritious foods.
- Pick lower-fat options when you can, such as low-fat milk instead of whole milk or light salad dressing instead of full-fat dressing.
- Watch the size of your portions.
- Resist going back for additional servings.
- Steer clear of vending machines and fast food.
- Keep healthy snacks like fruit and vegetables on hand in your room.
- Replace empty-calorie soft drinks with water or skim milk.

Be aware of your attitude toward food. If you find yourself fixating on food or your weight, or feeling guilty about what you eat, talk to your doctor or ask someone at the student health center for advice.

Learn about nutrition. Many schools have nutrition counselors. If yours does not, talk to someone on the student health services staff about nutrition and how to make good choices in the dining hall.

Lifestyle Changes to Manage Weight

Making some lifestyle changes can help people to manage their weight. Here are some things you can do:

Keep an eye on your alcohol consumption. Not only can excess drinking lead to health problems, but beer and alcohol are high in calories and can cause weight gain. (Why do you think it's called a beer belly?)

Smoking is another culprit. Although cigarettes may suppress the appetite, smoking can make exercise and even normal activity such as walking across campus or climbing stairs more difficult—not to mention causing heart and lung problems and increasing your risk of cancer.

Many smokers who quit find they have more energy, so battle the extra pounds by exercising. You can avoid gaining weight and increase your chances of quitting if you do. If you want to stop smoking, you don't have to go it alone. Someone at your student health center can direct you to smoking-cessation programs and give you the tips and support you need to quit.

Get enough exercise. Researchers found that students who exercised at least three days a week were more likely to report better physical health, as well as greater happiness, than those who did not exercise. They were also more likely to report using their time productively.

Reaping the benefits of exercise does not have to be as difficult as it might seem. Try to work 30 minutes of moderate exercise into your schedule each day (like walking, jogging, swimming, or working out at the gym) and you'll feel and see the results. For other options, check out biking or hiking trails or sign up for a martial arts class. Attending a class on a regular schedule can motivate some people to stick with their fitness goals.

If you don't like organized forms of exercise, you can also work at least 30 minutes of exercise into your daily schedule by walking briskly across campus instead of taking the bus, taking the stairs instead of the elevator, or cycling to class. And take time—even just a few minutes here and there—to move around and stretch when you've been sitting for a long time, such as during study sessions.

Get enough sleep. Recent studies have linked getting enough sleep to maintaining a healthy weight. Sleep is also a great way to manage the stress that can prompt overeating. So make sleep a priority, and try to work in a regular seven or eight hours each night.

Here are some ways to make the most of your sleep:

• Keep a regular sleeping schedule by getting up and going to bed at about the same time every day.

• Don't nap too much.

• Avoid caffeine in the evening.

• Avoid exercising, watching TV, or listening to loud music before bed.

Late night eating fuels more than the brain. In one 2005 study, food eaten between 8 p.m. and 4 a.m. was a leading contributor to weight gain. Fuel late-night study sessions with fruit, veggies, or sugar-free drinks.

Gaining weight during the first year of college is not inevitable. You may have your ups and downs, but a few simple changes to your daily routine can help you fend off excess weight while keeping you physically and mentally healthy.

Chapter 22

Nutrition Needs for Women

Chapter Contents

251

Section 22.1

Nutrition for Pregnancy and Breastfeeding

This section excerpted from "Healthy Pregnancy: Staying Healthy and Safe," September 27, 2010, and "Nutrition and Fitness," August 1, 2010, Department of Health and Human Services Office of Women's Health (www.womenshealth.gov).

Eating for Two

Eating healthy foods is more important now than ever! You need more protein, iron, calcium, and folic acid than you did before pregnancy. You also need more calories. But "eating for two" doesn't mean eating twice as much. Rather, it means that the foods you eat are the main source of nutrients for your baby. Sensible, balanced meals combined with regular physical fitness is still the best recipe for good health during your pregnancy.

Weight Gain

The amount of weight you should gain during pregnancy depends on your body mass index (BMI) before you became pregnant. The Institute of Medicine provides these guidelines:

- If you were at a normal weight before pregnancy, you should gain about 25 to 30 pounds.

- If you were underweight before pregnancy, you should gain between 28 and 40 pounds.

- If you were overweight before pregnancy, you should gain between 15 and 25 pounds.

- If you were obese before pregnancy, you should gain between 11 and 20 pounds.

Check with your doctor to find out how much weight gain during pregnancy is healthy for you. You should gain weight gradually during your pregnancy, with most of the weight gained in the last trimester. Generally, doctors suggest women gain weight at the following rate:

- Two to four pounds *total* during the first trimester
- Three to four pounds per month for the second and third trimesters

Where does the added weight go?

- **Baby:** Six to eight pounds
- **Placenta:** One and one-half pounds
- **Amniotic fluid:** Two pounds
- **Uterus growth:** Two pounds
- **Breast growth:** Two pounds
- **Your blood and body fluids:** Eight pounds
- **Your body's protein and fat:** Seven pounds

Recent research shows that women who gain more than the recommended amount during pregnancy and who fail to lose this weight within six months after giving birth are at much higher risk of being obese nearly 10 years later. Findings from another large study suggest that gaining more weight than the recommended amount during pregnancy may raise your child's odds of being overweight in the future. If you find that you are gaining weight too quickly, try to cut back on foods with added sugars and solid fats. If you are not gaining enough weight, you can eat a little more from each food group.

Calorie Needs

Your calorie needs will depend on your weight gain goals. Most women need 300 calories a day more during at least the last six months of pregnancy than they do pre-pregnancy. Keep in mind that not all calories are equal. Your baby needs healthy foods that are packed with nutrients—not "empty calories" such as those found in soft drinks, candies, and desserts.

Although you want to be careful not to eat more than you need for a healthy pregnancy, make sure not to restrict your diet during pregnancy either. If you don't get the calories you need, your baby might not get the right amounts of protein, vitamins, and minerals. Low-calorie diets can break down a pregnant woman's stored fat. This can cause your body to make substances called ketones. Ketones can be found in the mother's blood and urine and are a sign of starvation. Constant production of ketones can result in a child with mental deficiencies.

Foods Good for Mom and Baby

A pregnant woman needs more of many important vitamins, minerals, and nutrients than she did before pregnancy. Making healthy food choices every day will help you give your baby what he or she needs to develop. The MyPlate for Pregnant and Breastfeeding Women (www.choosemy plate.gov/mypyramidmoms/index.html) can show you what to eat as well as how much you need to eat from each food group based on your pre-pregnancy BMI and activity level. Use your personal MyPlate plan to guide your daily food choices. Here are some foods to choose often:

- **Grains:** Fortified, cooked, or ready-to-eat cereals; wheat germ

- **Vegetables:** Carrots, sweet potatoes, pumpkin, spinach, cooked greens, winter squash, tomatoes, red pepper

- **Fruits:** Cantaloupe, honeydew melon, mangoes, prunes or prune juice, bananas, apricots, oranges or orange juice, grapefruit, avocado

- **Dairy:** Nonfat or low-fat yogurt; nonfat milk (skim milk); low-fat milk (1% milk)

- **Meat and beans:** Cooked dried beans and peas; nuts and seeds; lean beef, lamb, and pork; shrimp, clams, oysters, and crab; cod, salmon, pollock, and catfish

Talk to your doctor if you have special diet needs for these reasons:

- **Diabetes:** Make sure you review your meal plan and insulin needs with your doctor. High blood glucose levels can be harmful to your baby.

- **Lactose intolerance:** Find out about low-lactose or reduced-lactose products and calcium supplements to ensure you are getting the calcium you need.

- **Vegetarian:** Ensure that you are eating enough protein, iron, vitamin B12, and vitamin D.

- **Phenylketonuria (PKU):** Keep good control of phenylalanine levels in your diet.

Food Safety

Most foods are safe for pregnant women and their babies. But you will need to use caution or avoid eating certain foods. Follow these guidelines:

- Clean, handle, cook, and chill food properly to prevent foodborne illness, including listeria and toxoplasmosis.
- Wash hands with soap after touching soil or raw meat.
- Keep raw meats, poultry, and seafood from touching other foods or surfaces.
- Cook meat completely.
- Wash produce before eating.
- Wash cooking utensils with hot, soapy water.

Do not eat these foods:

- Refrigerated smoked seafood like whitefish, salmon, and mackerel
- Hot dogs or deli meats unless steaming hot
- Refrigerated meat spreads
- Unpasteurized milk or juices
- Store-made salads, such as chicken, egg, or tuna salad
- Unpasteurized soft cheeses, such as unpasteurized feta, Brie, queso blanco, queso fresco, and blue cheeses
- Shark, swordfish, king mackerel, or tile fish (also called golden or white snapper); these fish have high levels of mercury.
- More than six ounces per week of white (albacore) tuna
- Herbs and plants used as medicines without your doctor's okay (the safety of herbal and plant therapies isn't always known; some herbs and plants might be harmful during pregnancy, such as bitter melon [karela], noni juice, and unripe papaya)
- Raw sprouts of any kind (including alfalfa, clover, radish, and mung bean)

Fish Facts

Fish and shellfish can be an important part of a healthy diet. They are a great source of protein and heart-healthy omega-3 fatty acids. What's more, some researchers believe low fish intake may be linked to depression in women during and after pregnancy. Research also suggests that omega-3 fatty acids consumed by pregnant women may aid in babies' brain and eye development.

Women who are or may become pregnant and nursing mothers need 12 ounces of fish per week to reap the health benefits. Unfortunately, some pregnant and nursing women do not eat any fish because they worry about mercury in seafood. Mercury is a metal that at high levels can harm the brain of your unborn baby—even before it is conceived. Mercury mainly gets into our bodies by eating large, predatory fish. Yet many types of seafood have little or no mercury at all. So the risk of mercury exposure depends on the amount and type of seafood you eat.

Women who are nursing, pregnant, or who may become pregnant can safely eat a variety of cooked seafood, but should steer clear of fish with high levels of mercury. Keep in mind that removing all fish from your diet will rob you of important omega-3 fatty acids. To reach 12 ounces while limiting exposure to mercury, follow these tips:

Do not eat: Avoid these fish that are high in mercury.

- Swordfish
- Tilefish
- King mackerel
- Shark

Limit: Eat up to 6 ounces (about one serving) per week.

- Canned albacore or chunk white tuna (also sold as tuna steaks), which has more mercury than canned light tuna

Little or no mercury: Eat up to 12 ounces (about two servings) per week of cooked* fish and shellfish with little or no mercury.

- Shrimp
- Crab
- Clams
- Oysters
- Scallops
- Canned light tuna
- Salmon
- Pollock
- Catfish
- Cod
- Tilapia

* Don't eat uncooked fish or shellfish (such as clams, oysters, scallops), including refrigerated uncooked seafood labeled nova-style, lox, kippered, smoked, or jerky.

- **Check before eating fish caught in local waters.** State health departments have guidelines on fish from local waters. Or get local fish advisories at the U.S. Environmental Protection Agency. If you are unsure about the safety of a fish from local waters, only eat six ounces per week and don't eat any other fish that week.

- **Eat a variety of cooked seafood rather than just a few types.**

Foods supplemented with DHA/EPA [docosahexaenoic acid/eicosapentaenoic acid] (such as "omega-3 eggs") and prenatal vitamins supplemented with DHA are other sources of the type of omega-3 fatty acids found in seafood.

Vitamins and Minerals

In addition to making healthy food choices, ask your doctor about taking a prenatal vitamin and mineral supplement every day to be sure you are getting enough of the nutrients your baby needs. You also can check the label on the foods you buy to see how much of a certain nutrient the product contains. Women who are pregnant need more of these nutrients than women who are not pregnant:

- **Folic acid:** 400 to 800 micrograms (mcg) (0.4 to 0.8 mg) in the early stages of pregnancy, which is why all women who are capable of pregnancy should take a daily multivitamin that contains 400 to 800 mcg of folic acid; pregnant women should continue taking folic acid throughout pregnancy

- **Iron:** 27 milligrams (mg)

- **Calcium:** 1,000 mg; 1,300 mg if 18 or younger

- **Vitamin A:** 770 mcg; 750 mcg if 18 or younger

- **Vitamin B12:** 2.6 mcg

Women who are pregnant also need to be sure to get enough vitamin D. The current recommendation for all adults under 50 (including pregnant women) is 5 micrograms of vitamin D each day. But many health experts don't think this is enough. Ask your doctor how much vitamin D you need each day. Because vitamin D is important to your unborn baby's development, your doctor might want to measure your vitamin D levels to be sure you are getting enough.

Keep in mind that taking too much of a supplement can be harmful. For example, too much of the nutrient vitamin A can cause birth defects. For this reason, only take vitamins and mineral supplements that your doctor recommends.

Don't Forget Fluids

All of your body's systems need water. When you are pregnant, your body needs even more water to stay hydrated and support the life inside you. Water also helps prevent constipation, hemorrhoids, excessive swelling, and urinary tract or bladder infections. Not getting enough water can lead to premature or early labor.

Your body gets the water it needs through the fluids you drink and the foods you eat. How much fluid you need to drink each day depends on many factors, such as your activity level, the weather, and your size. Your body needs more fluids when it is hot and when you are physically active. It also needs more water if you have a fever or if you are vomiting or have diarrhea.

The Institute of Medicine recommends that pregnant women drink about 10 cups of fluids daily. Water, juices, coffee, tea, and soft drinks all count toward your fluid needs. But keep in mind that some beverages are high in sugar and "empty" calories. A good way to tell if your fluid intake is okay is if your urine is pale yellow or colorless and you rarely feel thirsty. Thirst is a sign that your body is on its way to dehydration. Don't wait until you feel thirsty to drink.

Alcohol

There is no known safe amount of alcohol a woman can drink while pregnant. When you are pregnant and you drink beer, wine, hard liquor, or other alcoholic beverages, alcohol gets into your blood. The alcohol in your blood gets into your baby's body through the umbilical cord. Alcohol can slow down the baby's growth, affect the baby's brain, and cause birth defects.

Caffeine

Small amounts of caffeine (about one 12-ounce cup of coffee a day) appear to be safe during pregnancy. Some studies have shown a link between higher amounts of caffeine and miscarriage and preterm birth. But there is no solid proof that caffeine causes these problems.

The effects of too much caffeine are unclear. Ask your doctor whether drinking a limited amount of caffeine is okay for you.

Cravings

Many women have strong desires for specific foods during pregnancy. The desire for "pickles and ice cream" and other cravings might be caused by changes in nutritional needs during pregnancy. The fetus needs nourishment. And a woman's body absorbs and processes nutrients differently while pregnant. These changes help ensure normal development of the baby and fill the demands of breastfeeding once the baby is born.

Some women crave nonfood items such as clay, ice, laundry starch, or cornstarch. A desire to eat nonfood items is called pica. Eating nonfood items can be harmful to your pregnancy. Talk to your doctor if you have these urges.

Breastfeeding: Nutrition and Fitness

Many new mothers wonder if they should be on a special diet while breastfeeding, but the answer is no. You can take in the same number of calories that you did before becoming pregnant, which helps with weight loss after birth. There are no foods you have to avoid. In fact, you can continue to enjoy the foods that are important to your family— the special meals you know and love.

As for how your diet affects your baby, there are no special foods that will help you make more milk. You may find that some foods cause stomach upset in your baby. You can try avoiding those foods to see if your baby feels better and ask your baby's doctor for help.

Keep these important nutrition tips in mind:

- Drink plenty of fluids to stay hydrated (but fluid intake does not affect the amount of breast milk you make). Drink when you are thirsty, and drink more fluids if your urine is dark yellow. A common suggestion is to drink a glass of water or other beverage every time you breastfeed. Limit beverages that contain added sugars, such as soft drinks and fruit drinks.

- Drinking a moderate amount (up to two or three cups a day) of coffee or other caffeinated beverages does not cause a problem for most breastfeeding babies. Too much caffeine can cause the baby to be fussy or not sleep well.

- Vitamin and mineral supplements can not replace a healthy diet. In addition to healthy food choices, some breastfeeding women may need a multivitamin and mineral supplement. Talk with your doctor to find out if you need a supplement.

Is It Safe to Smoke, Drink, or Use Drugs?

If you smoke, it is best for you and your baby to quit as soon as possible. If you can't quit, it is still better to breastfeed because it can help protect your baby from respiratory problems and SIDS (sudden infant death syndrome). Be sure to smoke away from your baby and change your clothes to keep your baby away from the chemicals smoking leaves behind. Ask a health care provider for help quitting smoking!

You should avoid alcohol, especially in large amounts. An occasional small drink is okay, but avoid breastfeeding for two hours after the drink.

It is not safe for you to use or be dependent upon an illicit drug. Drugs such as cocaine and marijuana, heroine, and PCP harm your baby. Some reported side effects in babies include seizures, vomiting, poor feeding, and tremors.

Can a Baby Be Allergic to Breast Milk?

Research shows that a mother's milk is affected only slightly by the foods she eats. Breastfeeding mothers can eat whatever they have eaten during their lifetimes and do not need to avoid certain foods. Babies love the flavors of foods that come through in your milk. Sometimes a baby may be sensitive to something you eat, such as dairy products like milk and cheese. Symptoms in your baby of an allergy or sensitivity to something you eat include some or all of the following:

- Green stools with mucus and/or blood, diarrhea, vomiting
- Rash, eczema, dermatitis, hives, dry skin
- Fussiness during and/or after feedings
- Crying for long periods without being able to feel consoled
- Sudden waking with discomfort
- Wheezing or coughing

Babies who are highly sensitive usually react to the food the mother eats within minutes or within 4 to 24 hours afterwards. These signs do not mean the baby is allergic to your milk itself, only to something you are eating. If you stop eating whatever is bothering your baby or eat less of it, the problem usually goes away on its own. You also can talk with your baby's doctor about any symptoms. If your baby ever has problems breathing, call 911 or go to your nearest emergency room.

Vegan Diets

If you follow a vegan diet or one that does not include any forms of animal protein, you or your baby might not get enough vitamin B12 in your bodies. This can also happen if you eat meat, but not enough. In a baby, this can cause symptoms such as loss of appetite, slow motor development, being very tired, weak muscles, vomiting, and blood problems. You can protect your and your baby's health by taking vitamin B12 supplements while breastfeeding. Talk to your doctor about your B12 needs.

Section 22.2

The Importance of Folic Acid for Women of Childbearing Age

"Folic Acid," Centers for Disease Control and Prevention
(www.cdc.gov), May 7, 2010.

Why can't I wait until I'm pregnant—or planning to get pregnant—to start taking folic acid?

Birth defects of the brain and spine (anencephaly and spina bifida) happen in the first few weeks of pregnancy; often before you find out you're pregnant. By the time you realize you're pregnant, it might be too late to prevent those birth defects. Also, half of all pregnancies in the United States are unplanned.

These are two reasons why it is important for all women who can get pregnant to be sure to get 400 mcg of folic acid every day, even if they aren't planning a pregnancy any time soon.

I'm planning to get pregnant this month. Is it too late to start taking folic acid?

The Centers for Disease Control and Prevention (CDC) recommends women to take 400 mcg of folic acid every day, starting at least one month before getting pregnant. If you are trying to get pregnant this month, or planning to get pregnant soon, start taking 400 mcg of folic acid today!

I already have a child with spina bifida. Should I do anything different to prepare for my next pregnancy?

Women who had one pregnancy affected by a birth defect of the brain or spine might have another. Talk to your doctor about taking 4,000 mcg (4.0 milligrams) of folic acid each day at least one month before getting pregnant and during the first few months of being pregnant. This is 10 times the amount most people take. Your doctor will give you a prescription. You should not take more than one multivitamin each day. Taking more than one each day over time could be harmful to you and your baby.

Can't I get enough folic acid by eating a well-balanced, healthy diet?

It is hard to eat a diet that has all the nutrients you need every day. Even with careful planning, you might not get all the vitamins you need from your diet alone. That's why it's important to take a vitamin with folic acid every day.

A single serving of many breakfast cereals also has the amount of folic acid that a woman needs each day. Check the label! Look for cereals that have 100% Daily Value (DV) of folic acid (400 mcg) in a serving.

Vitamins cost too much. How can I get the folic acid that I need?

Many stores offer a single folic acid supplement for just pennies a day. Another good choice is a store brand multivitamin, which includes more of the vitamins a woman needs each day. Unless your doctor suggests a special type, you do not have to choose among vitamins for women or active people. A basic multivitamin meets the needs of most women.

How can I remember to take a vitamin with folic acid every day?

Make it easy to remember by taking your vitamin at the same time every day. Try taking your vitamin when you do one of your daily tasks.

Seeing the vitamin bottle on the bathroom or kitchen counter can help you remember it, too. If you use a cell phone or PDA, you can program it to give you a daily reminder. If you have children, you can take your vitamin when they take theirs.

Are there other health benefits of taking folic acid?

Folic acid might help prevent some other birth defects, such as cleft lip and palate and some heart defects. There might also be other health benefits of taking folic acid for both women and men. More research is needed to confirm these other health benefits. All adults should take 400 mcg of folic acid every day.

Is it better to take more than 400 mcg of folic acid every day?

When taking supplements, more is not better. Women who can get pregnant (whether planning to or not) need just 400 mcg of folic acid daily, and they can get this amount from vitamins or fortified foods. This is in addition to eating foods rich in folate. But your doctor might ask you to take more for certain reasons.

What is folate and how is it different from folic acid?

Folate is a form of the B vitamin folic acid. Folate is found naturally in some foods, such as leafy, dark green vegetables; citrus fruits and juices; and beans.

The body does not use folate as easily as folic acid. We cannot be sure that eating folate has the same benefits as getting 400 mcg of manmade (synthetic) folic acid. Women who can get pregnant should consume 400 mcg of synthetic folic acid in addition to the natural food folate from a varied diet.

Synthetic folic acid is the simple, manmade form of the B vitamin folate. Folic acid is found in most multivitamins and has been added in U.S. foods labeled as "enriched" such as bread, pasta, rice, and breakfast cereals. The words "folic acid" and "synthetic folic acid" mean the same thing.

Section 22.3

Nutrition for Menopause

"Menopause: Staying Healthy through Good Nutrition," © 2010 The Cleveland Clinic Foundation, 9500 Euclid Avenue, Cleveland, OH 44195, http://my.clevelandclinic.org. Additional information is available from the Cleveland Clinic Health Information Center, 216-444-3771, toll-free 800-223-2273 extension 43771, or at http://my.clevelandclinic.org/health.

Some risk factors associated with aging and menopause cannot be changed. However, healthy eating can prevent or reduce certain conditions that may develop during and after menopause.

What are some basic dietary guidelines?

Eat a variety of foods to get all the nutrients you need. Since women's diets are often low in iron and calcium, follow these guidelines:

- **Get enough calcium.** Eating and drinking two to four servings of dairy products and calcium-rich foods a day will help ensure that you are getting enough calcium in your daily diet. Calcium is found in dairy products, clams, sardines, broccoli, and legumes.

- **Pump up your iron intake.** Eating at least three servings of iron-rich foods a day will help ensure that you are getting enough iron in your daily diet. Iron is found in lean red meat, poultry, fish, eggs, leafy green vegetables, nuts, and enriched grain products.

- **Get enough fiber.** Help yourself to foods high in fiber such as whole-grain breads, cereals, pasta, rice, fresh fruits, and vegetables.

- **Eat fruits and vegetables.** Include at least two to four servings of fruits and three to five servings of vegetables in your daily diet.

- **Read labels.** Use the package label information to help you to make the best selections for a healthy lifestyle.

- **Drink plenty of water.** Drink at least eight 8-ounce glasses of water a day.

- **Maintain a healthy weight.** Lose weight if you are overweight by cutting down on portion sizes and reducing foods high in fat, not by skipping meals. A registered dietitian or your doctor can help you determine your ideal body weight.

- **Reduce foods high in fat.** Fat should provide 30% or less of your total daily calories. Also, limit saturated fat to less than 10% of your total daily calories. Saturated fat raises cholesterol and increases your risk of heart disease. Saturated fat is found in fatty meats, whole milk, ice cream, and cheese. Limit cholesterol intake to 300 mg or less per day.

- **Use sugar and salt in moderation.** Too much sodium in the diet is linked to high blood pressure. Also, go easy on smoked, salt-cured, and charbroiled foods—these foods contain high levels of nitrates, which have been linked to cancer.

- **Limit alcohol intake.** Women should limit their consumption of alcohol to one or fewer drinks per day (three to five drinks per week maximum).

What foods can reduce menopausal symptoms?

Plant-based foods that contain isoflavones (plant estrogens) work in the body like a weak form of estrogen and may help relieve menopausal symptoms in some women. Some may lower cholesterol levels and have been suggested to relieve hot flashes and night sweats. Currently, most research indicates that soy isoflavones are not particularly effective for treating several menopausal symptoms. Aside from soy products, isoflavones can also be found in foods such as whole grains and beans.

Should I avoid certain foods while I am going through menopause?

If you are experiencing hot flashes, you may find that avoiding certain "trigger" foods and beverages—spicy foods, caffeine, and alcohol—may lessen the severity and frequency of hot flashes.

Are there dietary supplements I can take to ease symptoms/prevent disease?

Because there is a direct relationship between the lack of estrogen after menopause and the development of osteoporosis, the following supplements, combined with a healthy diet, may help prevent the onset of this condition.

- **Calcium:** If you think you need to take a supplement to get enough calcium, check with your doctor first. Calcium carbonate and calcium citrate are good forms of calcium supplements. Be careful not to get more than 2,000 mg of calcium a day very often. That amount can increase your chance of developing kidney problems.

- **Vitamin D3 (cholecalciferol):** Your body uses vitamin D to absorb calcium. People aged 51 to 70 should have at least 1,000 IU [International Units] daily. Those over 70 or with a history of vitamin D deficiency who have followed a replacement program should take at least 2,000 IU daily. Vitamin D intake helps with mood disorders, autoimmune problems, and prevention of certain cancers in addition to keeping the bones healthy.

Chapter 23

Nutrition for Older Persons

Chapter Contents

Section 23.1

Healthy Eating after 50

Food for thought: Think healthy eating is all about dieting and sacrifice? Think again. Eating well is a lifestyle that embraces colorful food, creativity in the kitchen, and eating with friends.

For seniors, the benefits of healthy eating include increased mental acuteness, resistance to illness and disease, higher energy levels, a more robust immune system, faster recuperation times, and better management of chronic health problems. As we age, eating well can also be the key to a positive outlook and staying emotionally balanced.

You are the boss when it comes to food choices! Read on for tips on how to supercharge your life with the right food.

Senior Nutrition: Feeding the Body, Mind, and Soul

Remember the old adage, *you are what you eat*? Make it your motto. When you choose a variety of colorful fruits and veggies, whole grains, and lean proteins you'll feel simply marvelous inside and out.

- **Live longer and stronger:** Good nutrition keeps muscles, bones, organs, and other body parts strong for the long haul. Eating vitamin-rich food boosts immunity and fights illness-causing toxins. A proper diet reduces the risk of heart disease, stroke, high blood pressure, type-2 diabetes, bone loss, cancer, and anemia. Also, eating sensibly means consuming fewer calories and more nutrient-dense foods, keeping weight in check.

- **Sharpen the mind:** Scientists know that key nutrients are essential for the brain to do its job. Research shows that people who eat a selection of brightly colored fruit, leafy veggies, certain fish, and nuts packed with omega-3 fatty acids can improve focus and decrease the risk for Alzheimer's disease.

- **Feel better:** Eating well is a feast for your five senses! Wholesome meals give you more energy and help you look better, resulting in a self-esteem boost. It's all connected—when your body feels good you feel happier inside and out.

How Many Calories Do Seniors Need?

There is a right number of calories for your body. Use the following as a guideline.

A woman over 50 who is:

- not physically active needs about 1,600 calories a day;
- somewhat physically active needs about 1,800 calories a day;
- very active needs about 2,000 calories a day.

A man over 50 who is:

- not physically active needs about 2,000 calories a day;
- somewhat physically active needs about 2,200–2,400 calories a day;
- very active needs about 2,400–2,800 calories a day.

Source: National Institute of Aging

Remember that balanced nutrition is more than calorie counting. Read on for more tips on creating a nutritious lifestyle.

Senior Nutrition: What Your Body Needs

Older adults can feel better immediately and stay healthy for the future by choosing healthy foods. A balanced diet and physical activity contribute to a higher quality of life and enhanced independence as you age.

Senior Food Pyramid Guidelines

[Ed. Note: The federal Food Guide Pyramid, MyPyramid, was replaced by MyPlate (www.choosemyplate.gov) on June 2, 2011.]

Fruit: Focus on whole fruits rather than juices for more fiber and vitamins and aim for around 1 1/2 to 2 servings each day. Break the apple and banana rut and go for color-rich pickings like berries or melons.

Veggies: Color is your credo in this category. Choose antioxidant rich dark leafy greens, such as kale, spinach, and broccoli as well as oranges and yellows, such as carrots, squash, and yams. Try for 2 to 2 1/2 cups of veggies every day.

Calcium: Aging bone health depends on adequate calcium intake to prevent osteoporosis and bone fractures. Seniors need 1,200 milligrams of calcium a day through servings of milk, yogurt, or cheese. Non-dairy sources include tofu, broccoli, almonds, and kale.

Grains: Be smart with your carbs and choose whole grains over processed white flour for more nutrients and a higher fiber count. If you're not sure, look for pasta, breads, and cereals that list "whole" in the ingredient list. Seniors need six to seven ounces of grains each day, and one ounce is about one slice of bread.

Protein: Seniors need about .5 grams per pound of bodyweight. Simply divide your bodyweight in half to know how many grams you need. A 130-pound woman will need around 65 grams of protein a day. A serving of tuna, for example, has about 40 grams of protein. Vary your sources with more fish, beans, peas, nuts, eggs, milk, cheese, and seeds.

Important Vitamin and Minerals

Water: Seniors are prone to dehydration because our bodies lose some of its ability to regulate fluid levels and our sense of thirst is dulled. Post a note in your kitchen reminding you to sip water every hour and with meals to avoid urinary tract infections, constipation, and possibly confusion.

Vitamin B: After 50, your stomach produces less gastric acid making it difficult to absorb vitamin B12—needed to help keep blood and nerves vital. Get the recommended daily intake (2.4 micrograms) of B12 from fortified foods or a vitamin.

Vitamin D: We get most of vitamin D—essential to absorbing calcium—through sun exposure and a few foods (fatty fish, egg yolk, and fortified milk). With age, our skin is less efficient at synthesizing vitamin D, so consult your doctor about supplementing with fortified foods or a multivitamin.

Senior Nutrition: Tips for Wholesome Eating

Once you've made friends with nutrient-dense food, your body will feel slow and sluggish if you eat less wholesome fare. Here's how to get in the habit of eating well.

- **Reduce sodium** (salt) to help prevent water retention and high blood pressure. Look for the "low sodium" label and season meals with a few grains of course sea salt instead of cooking with salt.

- **Enjoy good fats.** Reap the rewards of olive oil, avocados, salmon, walnuts, flaxseed, and other monounsaturated fats. Research shows that the fat from these delicious sources protects your body against heart disease by controlling "bad" LDL [low-density lipoprotein] cholesterol levels and raising "good" HDL [high-density lipoprotein] cholesterol levels.

- **Fiber up.** Avoid constipation, lower the risk of chronic diseases, and feel fuller longer by increasing fiber intake. Your go-to fiber-foods are raw fruits and veggies, whole grains, and beans.

- **Look for hidden sugar.** Added sugar can be hidden in foods such as bread, canned soups and vegetables, pasta sauce, instant mashed potatoes, frozen dinners, fast food, and ketchup. Check food labels for alternate terms for sugar such as corn syrup, molasses, brown rice syrup, cane juice, fructose, sucrose, dextrose, or maltose. Opt for fresh or frozen vegetables instead of canned goods, and choose low-carb or sugar-free versions of products such as tortillas, bread, pasta, and ice cream.

- **Cook smart.** The best way to prepare veggies is by steaming or sautéing in olive oil—it preserves nutrients. Forget boiling—it leeches nutrients.

- **Put five colors on your plate.** Take a tip from Japanese food culture and try to include five colors on your plate. Fruits and veggies rich in color correspond to rich nutrients (think: blackberries, melons, yams, spinach, tomato, zucchini).

Senior Nutrition: Changing Dietary Needs

Every season of life brings changes and adjustments to the body. Understanding what is happening will help you take control of your nutrition requirements.

Physical Changes

- **Metabolism.** Every year over the age of 40, our metabolism slows. This means that even if you continue to eat the same amount as when you were younger, you're likely to gain weight because you're burning fewer calories. In addition, you may be less physically active. Consult your doctor to decide if you should cut back on calories.

- **Weakened senses.** Your taste and smell senses diminish with age. Seniors tend to lose sensitivity to salty and bitter tastes first, so you may be inclined to salt your food more heavily than before—even though seniors need less salt than younger people. Use herbs and healthy oils—like olive oil—to season food instead of salt. Similarly, seniors tend to retain the ability to distinguish sweet tastes the longest, leading some to overindulge in sugary foods and snacks. Instead of adding sugar, try increasing sweetness to meals by using naturally sweet food such as fruit, peppers, or yams.

- **Medicines and illnesses.** Prescription medications and illnesses often negatively influence appetite and may also affect taste, again leading seniors to add too much salt or sugar to their food. Ask your doctor about overcoming side effects of medications or specific physical conditions.

- **Digestion.** Due to a slowing digestive system, you generate less saliva and stomach acid as you get older, making it more difficult for your body to process certain vitamins and minerals, such as B12, B6, and folic acid, which are necessary to maintain mental alertness, a keen memory, and good circulation. Up your fiber intake and talk to your doctor about possible supplements.

Lifestyle Changes

- **Loneliness and depression.** Loneliness and depression affect your diet. For some, feeling down leads to not eating, and in others it may trigger overeating. Be aware if emotional problems are affecting your diet, and take action by consulting your doctor or therapist.

- **Death or divorce.** Newly single seniors may not know how to cook or may not feel like cooking for one. People on limited budgets might have trouble affording a balanced, healthy diet. See the resources at helpguide.org/life/senior_nutrition.htm for suggestions on cooking for one and easy, healthy menu selections.

Understanding Malnutrition

Malnutrition is a critical senior health issue caused by eating too little food, too few nutrients, and by digestive problems related to aging.

Malnutrition causes fatigue; depression; weak immune system; anemia; weakness; digestive, lung, and heart problems; and skin concerns.

Tips for Preventing Malnutrition

- Eat nutrient-packed food
- Have flavorful food available
- Snack between meals
- Eat with company as much as possible
- Get help with food prep
- Consult your doctor

Senior Nutrition: Tips for Creating a Well-Balanced Diet

Thinking of trading a tired eating regime for a nutrient-dense menu? Good for you! It's easy and delicious.

Avoid skipping meals: This causes your metabolism to slow down, which leads to feeling sluggish and poorer choices later in the day.

Breakfast: Select high-fiber breads and cereals, colorful fruit, and protein to fill you with energy for the day. Try yogurt with muesli and berries, a veggie-packed omelet, peanut butter on whole grain toast with a citrus salad, or old-fashioned oatmeal made with dried cherries, walnuts, and honey.

Lunch: Keep your body fueled for the afternoon with a variety of whole-grain breads, lean protein, and fiber. Try a veggie quesadilla on a whole-wheat tortilla, veggie stew with whole-wheat noodles, or a quinoa salad with roasted peppers and mozzarella cheese.

Dinner: End the day on a wholesome note. Try warm salads of roasted veggies and a side of crusty brown bread and cheese, grilled salmon with spicy salsa, or whole-wheat pasta with asparagus and shrimp. Opt for sweet potatoes instead of white potatoes and grilled meat instead of fried.

Snacks: It's okay, even recommended, to snack. But make sure you make it count by choosing high-fiber snacks to healthfully tide you over to your next meal. Choose almonds and raisins instead of chips, and fruit instead of sweets. Other smart snacks include yogurt, cottage cheese, apples and peanut butter, and veggies and hummus.

Senior Nutrition: Overcoming Obstacles to Healthy Eating

Let's face it. There's a reason why so many seniors have trouble eating nutritiously every day. It's not always easy! The following tips will help you "speak the language" of good nutrition and help you feel in control.

Say "No" to Eating Alone

Eating with company can be as important as vitamins. Think about it: a social atmosphere stimulates your mind and helps you enjoy meals. When you enjoy mealtimes, you're more likely to eat better. If you live alone, eating with company will take some strategizing, but the effort will pay off.

- **Make a date** to share lunch or dinners with grandchildren, nieces, nephews, friends, and neighbors on a rotating basis.

- **Join in** by taking a class, volunteering, or going on an outing, all of which can lead to new friendships and dining buddies.

- **Adult day care** centers provide both companionship and nutritious meals for seniors who are isolated and lonely, or unable to prepare their own meals. See Helpguide's "Adult Day Care Centers: A Guide to Options and Selecting the Best Center for Your Needs" (at helpguide.org/elder/adult_day_care_centers.htm) for more information.

- **Senior meal programs** are a great way to meet others. Contact your local Senior Center, YMCA, congregation, or high school and ask about senior meal programs.

Loss of Appetite

First, check with your doctor to see if your loss of appetite could be due to medication you're taking, and whether the dosage can be adjusted or changed. Then let the experimenting begin. Try natural flavor enhancers such as olive oil, vinegar, garlic, onions, ginger, and spices.

Difficulty Chewing

Make chewing easier by drinking smoothies made with fresh fruit, yogurt, and protein powder. Eat steamed veggies and soft food such as couscous, rice, and yogurt. Consult your dentist to make sure your dentures are properly fitted.

Dry Mouth

Drink 8–10 glasses of water each day. Period. Take a drink of water after each bite of food, add sauces and salsas to foods to moisten, avoid commercial mouthwash, and ask your doctor about artificial saliva products.

I Don't Like Healthy Food

If you were raised eating lots of meat and white bread, a new way of eating might sound off-putting. Don't beat yourself up. Eating healthfully is a new adventure. Start with small steps:

- First and foremost, commit to keeping an open mind.
- Try including a healthy fruit or veggie at every meal.
- Focus on how you feel after eating well—this will help foster new habits and tastes.

Stuck in a Rut

Rekindle inspiration by perusing produce at a farmers market, reading a cooking magazine, buying a new-to-you spice, or chatting with friends about what they eat. By making variety a priority, you'll soon look forward to getting creative with healthy meals.

If You Can't Shop or Cook for Yourself

There are a number of possibilities, depending on your living situation, finances, and needs:

- **Take advantage of home delivery:** Many grocery stores have internet or phone delivery services.
- **Swap services:** Ask a friend, neighborhood teen, or college student if they would be willing to shop for you.
- **Share your home:** If you live alone in a large home, consider having a housemate / companion who would be willing to do the grocery shopping and cooking.
- **Hire a homemaker:** Try to find someone who can do the shopping and meal preparation for you. For more information, see Helpguide's "Services to Help Seniors Remain at Home" (at helpguide.org/elder/senior_services_living_home.htm).

Meals on Wheels: Meals on Wheels provides nutritious meals to people who are homebound and/or disabled, or would otherwise be unable to maintain their dietary needs. The daily delivery generally consists of two meals: a nutritionally balanced hot meal to eat at lunch time and a dinner, consisting of a cold sandwich and milk along with varying side dishes. Generally, Meals on Wheels is available to those persons who are not able to provide for themselves, for whatever reason. Meals on Wheels: Find a Local Program (at www.mowaa.org/Page.aspx?pid=253) is a searchable database that allows you to find a Meals on Wheels program in your area.

Senior Nutrition: Tips for Staying on Track

Healthy eaters have their personal rules for keeping with the program. Here are some to keep in mind.

- **Ask for help for your health's sake.** Know when you need a hand to make shopping, cooking, and meal planning assistance.

- **Variety, variety, variety!** Try eating and cooking something new as soon as boredom strikes.

- **Make every meal "do-able."** Healthy eating needn't be a big production. Keep it simple and you'll stick with it. Stocking the pantry and fridge with wholesome choices will make "do-able" even easier.

- **Set the mealtime mood.** Set the table, light candles, play music, or eat outside or by a window when possible. Tidying yourself and your space will help you enjoy the moment.

- **Break habits.** If you eat watching TV, try eating while reading. If you eat at the counter, curl up to a movie and a slice of veggie pizza.

Section 23.2

Nutrition Concerns for the Elderly

This section excerpted from "Older Americans Need to Make Every Calorie Count," U.S. Department of Agriculture (www.usda.gov), 2002. Reviewed by David A. Cooke, MD, FACP, January 2011. The federal Food Guide Pyramid, MyPyramid, was replaced with the MyPlate system (www.choosemyplate. gov) on June 2, 2011.

As individuals age, their declining energy needs mean they must eat better while eating less. U.S. Department of Agriculture (USDA) food consumption survey data indicate that most older Americans are having trouble fitting the recommended number of daily food group servings into their decreased "calorie budgets."

While the basic nutrition advice in the *Dietary Guidelines for Americans* and the Food Guide Pyramid applies to healthy adults of all ages, the elderly face some special challenges, particularly declining energy (calorie) needs as metabolism slows down.

Because the amount of food they can eat while maintaining calorie balance is more limited than when they were younger, older individuals must choose wisely, selecting nutrient-dense foods and limiting "extras." A quantitative way of providing food choice guidance would be to compute benchmark food densities for younger and older men and women. A benchmark food density is the number of servings per 1,000 calories an individual consuming a given number of calories would need to consume to meet the Food Guide Pyramid recommendations. For example, a person who consumes 2,200 calories daily should consume 4 servings of vegetables, according to the Food Guide Pyramid. This consumption level would translate into a benchmark density of 1.8 servings of vegetables per 1,000 calories.

Data from USDA's Continuing Survey of Food Intakes by Individuals, 1994–96 (CSFII) were used to examine food intakes of younger men and women, age 19–59, and seniors, age 60 and older.

As expected, younger adults ate considerably more than their older counterparts. Men age 19–59 reported consuming an average of 2,535 calories per day, compared with 1,940 calories consumed by men age 60 and older. Women age 19–59 reported average intakes of 1,676 calories daily, compared with 1,413 calories per day for women age 60 and older.

Benchmark servings for the five food groups are lowest for young men and highest for older women, the group with the lowest calorie intake. These numbers show just how important it is that older individuals, particularly women, make every calorie count.

More Older Men Than Women Meet Food Guide Pyramid Recommendations

Comparisons of average food group intakes of older men and women with intakes of younger men and women indicate that older individuals eat fewer servings of most food groups than their younger counterparts.

On a per-1,000-calories basis, intake of some but not all food groups is higher for older men and women than their younger counterparts, although not as high as our benchmark densities. Older men have higher densities than younger men for grains; vegetables; milk, yogurt, and cheese; and, especially, fruit. Older women's diets have higher food group densities than diets of younger women for all food groups except milk, yogurt, and cheese; however, their diets are not sufficiently more dense to make up for older women's low energy intakes.

As might be expected, on a given day, older individuals are less likely than their younger counterparts to consume recommended numbers of servings of most food groups. The difference was particularly dramatic for the milk, yogurt, and cheese group. Only 6% of older men consumed recommended numbers of servings from this group, compared with 26% of younger men. Even fewer older women—3%— met servings recommendations for the milk, cheese, and yogurt group, compared with 15% of younger women.

Fruit consumption is a notable exception to the general decline in proportion of individuals meeting serving recommendations as they age. As individuals age, they may become more health conscious and actively increase consumption of healthful foods, such as fruit. Also, today's elderly may have grown up when fruit was more heavily consumed and are simply continuing habits developed over a lifetime.

Older Men More Likely Than Younger Men to Take Dietary Supplements

Older adults have been reported to be more likely to take vitamin and/or mineral supplements than younger individuals. The *Dietary*

Guidelines for Americans stress the importance of wise food choices as the basis of good nutrition; therefore, supplement intake would not be considered an alternative to consuming more nutrient-dense foods. Some older adults, however, may benefit from selected supplements, such as vitamins D and B12 or calcium.

As part of the CSFII interview, individuals were asked if they took vitamin or mineral supplements. More older men than younger men reported taking supplements—47% compared with 40%. Fifty-five percent of women reported taking supplements, but there was no difference by age. Most individuals reported taking a multivitamin or a multivitamin-mineral product but provided little or no specific information about the nutrients contained in such products.

Illness and Low Income May Add Further Nutrition Challenges

Many of the elderly also face other nutritional challenges. Many older individuals suffer from chronic health conditions that may complicate nutrition needs and may require dietary modifications. In a previous analysis of CSFII 1994–96 data, we found that almost half of all older Americans reported suffering from high blood pressure. Substantial numbers of the elderly also reported suffering from diabetes, high blood cholesterol, and cardiovascular disease. Despite this high prevalence of nutrition-related chronic conditions, only about one-quarter of the elderly reported following a special diet.

For many elderly, especially the "oldest old," physical limitations may impair the ability to shop for and prepare nutritious meals. Programs that deliver groceries to seniors or bring "mobile markets" to senior housing complexes can ease the difficulties in acquiring foods. Congregate and home-delivered meal programs may help those individuals who also have difficulty with food preparation.

Low-income elderly also may face more difficulty in maintaining a nutritious diet. In a previous study, we found that low-income elderly consumed fewer servings of Food Guide Pyramid food groups than higher income elderly. The low-income segment of the elderly tend to be older, less educated, and more likely to live alone than other elderly—all factors that are also associated with lower diet quality.

Section 23.3

Elderly and Foodborne Illnesses

This section excerpted from "Older Adults at Risk of Complications from Microbial Foodborne Illness," U.S. Department of Agriculture (www.usda .gov), 2002. Reviewed by David A. Cooke, MD, FACP, January 2011.

Although younger individuals usually face far higher rates of infection from foodborne pathogens (bacteria, fungi, parasites, viruses, and their toxins), older adults, along with the very young and the immuno-compromised, are more likely to have some of the more severe complications from these infections. In particular, some research has shown that the elderly are more vulnerable to gastroenteritis-induced deaths.

Data from the Centers for Disease Control and Prevention's (CDC) FoodNet surveillance system show that for some pathogens, older adults have lower culture-confirmed rates of infection than most or all of the other age groups, despite many age-related factors, such as decreased immune functioning and decreased stomach acid production, that predispose older persons to gastrointestinal infections and their more severe complications. These low rates may be partly due to older persons being more careful about food handling and food consumption than younger persons.

Foodborne Illness Can Have Secondary Complications

CDC estimates that each year in the United States, nine microbial pathogens cause an estimated 3.5 million foodborne illnesses, 33,000 associated hospitalizations, and over 1,200 deaths. Data are unavailable on what proportion of these illnesses and deaths afflict older adults.

Most cases of foodborne illnesses are classified as "acute." These cases are usually self-limiting and of short duration, although they can range from mild to severe.

The U.S. Food and Drug Administration estimates that 2%–3% of all acute foodborne illnesses develop secondary long-term illnesses and complications called chronic sequelae. These sequelae can occur in any part of the body, such as the joints, nervous system, kidneys, or heart.

Rates of Infection Tell Part of the Story

Of the nine pathogens, *Salmonella* (nontyphoid) had the highest rate of infection for adults age 60 and older (10.8 cases per 100,000 people); *Campylobacter* had the second highest rate (9.7 cases per 100,000 people). These findings are not surprising as *Campylobacter* and *Salmonella* cause far more total illnesses each year in the United States than the other seven FoodNet pathogens.

Although younger individuals usually face far higher infection rates from these pathogens, older adults are more likely to have some of the more severe complications. For example, many studies have found that Guillain-Barré syndrome (GBS) has a bimodal age distribution with the highest peak for people older than 50 and that older patients are more likely than younger patients to require a ventilator and to have a poor prognosis. Other studies suggest that the elderly are far more susceptible to death from *Salmonella* infections than the general population.

E. coli O157:H7 has the third-highest rate of infection for older adults, 1.8 cases per 100,000 people. Some studies suggest that nursing home residents and other elderly individuals appear to be particularly vulnerable to fatal *E. coli* O157:H7 infections.

Therefore, analyzing the rates of infection among the elderly is only part of the story, as illnesses vary in severity, with some posing higher risks of hospitalization and death. More information is needed to determine the distribution of severity of illness among different age groups.

Elderly Susceptible to Foodborne Illness

According to a study by James Smith, a microbiologist with USDA's Agricultural Research Service, the elderly are more vulnerable to death from gastroenteritis than younger individuals.

Poor nutrition and decreased food consumption, combined with normal age-related decreases in immune system functioning, may weaken older adults' ability to fight foodborne pathogens. A person's immune system functioning decreases with age, and therefore people have decreased resistance to pathogens as they age. Also, decreased contractions that push food through the intestines slow the time it takes to eliminate pathogens from the intestinal tract, allowing more time for toxin formation and damage.

Many Foodborne Illnesses in Older Adults Can Be Prevented

While people can't turn back the clock or stop aging, older adults can take several actions to prevent foodborne illness. They can practice a healthful lifestyle that includes exercising regularly, eating a balanced diet, obtaining regular health care, practicing good food sanitation and handling practices, and paying careful attention to personal hygiene. Additionally, many older adults could benefit from food safety education that would encourage them to reduce risky food handling or food consumption behavior.

Older adults can also benefit from improved food safety practices of their caregivers. Many older people rely on family members or home health care workers to prepare food for them.

Section 23.4

The Hidden Dangers of Eating Alone

In this fast-paced world, few families make time to eat together anymore. And because eating alone—and on the go—is becoming more common, nutrition usually suffers.

That may be especially true for seniors. Cooking for one person can be harder because they have to scale down recipes, and it's also not as much fun. Instead of stimulating dinner conversation, the television becomes the other person at the table.

"Unfortunately a lot of meal choices turn out to be what's quick and easy to obtain," explains Anne Linge, a dietician at the University of Washington Medical Center in Seattle.

While many seniors are very active, others don't have the energy or ability to prepare meals for themselves. Some may have never set foot in the kitchen, or they're no longer physically able to prepare complex meals.

After her grandmother lost a considerable amount of weight in just a few months, Gretchen Kenney insisted that she move in with her and her husband, David, in Shoreline, Washington.

"She lost like 40 pounds, she just stopped eating," Kenney explains. "Part of it was her health, her arthritis; she couldn't get around very easily. She was just depressed and didn't want to eat."

After moving in with the Kenneys, her grandmother slowly put some of that weight back on.

"I make sure that she gets a much better balance," Kenney says. "Given what she wants, she would be happy with sweets and carbohydrates. She will ask for vegetables mostly because she thinks she should have them."

Inadequate nutrition can lead to a weakening of the immune system, increasing the risk of illness or infections, or contributing to mental confusion. And continued malnutrition could lead to depression, which in turn could lead to a loss of appetite—a vicious cycle.

For the elderly, other factors can contribute to malnutrition, including lack of money to buy adequate food, or transportation to the grocery store.

Linge had a client who lived directly across the street from a grocery store—but on the third floor. "She was trapped in her building because of her physical abilities and she couldn't get what she needed," Linge says. "So, when you think about your parents and their needs, think not only do they have enough income to purchase what they need, but, secondly, is shopping something they are able to do?"

Ask your loved one if they would prefer that you bring in groceries for them to cook, or that you cook for them. Be sure to ask them if they are having difficulty with chewing or swallowing, if food tastes too bland, or if they've lost their appetite (it could be because of medications they may be taking, or possibly depression, which can have serious consequences). Also, check their refrigerator and see what kinds of food are in there, and whether any have passed the expiration date.

To alleviate the burden of cooking for one, grocery store delis have a wide variety of nutritious, precooked foods, such as roasted chicken and salads with raw vegetables. A whole chicken can last a senior for several meals (but it's best not to keep it for more than three or four days; after that, it may spoil). Buy a package of vegetables or meat already cut up for stir-fry, or a premade meatloaf that just needs to go in the oven. If they think food is too bland, enhance the flavor with olive oil, vinegars, garlic, or spices (but not salt). Cinnamon, cloves, ginger, and turmeric are also good for the digestion.

Getting together with other people—whether seniors or not—can make cooking and eating more fun.

"Sometimes seniors have been really creative and have gotten together with other seniors in their neighborhood or their building and said 'Let's get together and today I'll make the meal and tomorrow you'll make the meal,' " Linge says.

Finding a neighborhood hangout is also a good idea. "There are cafes in any community where seniors tend to gather. They will have their regulars in there who will be in there almost daily," Linge says. "Even if you're a party of one, you can see other people."

Living in a retirement home or assisted living community may help some seniors eat better.

"It makes a huge difference when you get residents sitting at a table together," explains gerontologist Ashley Kraft, the "Life's Neighborhood" director at Aegis at Northgate in Seattle, an assisted living facility with Alzheimer's and dementia care. "It brings back the memories of eating with your family. What happens, especially with dementia, is they forget about the things we take for granted, knowing that we're hungry, knowing that we're thirsty, or they don't know how to explain that feeling."

Little tricks can help make mealtime for your loved one more enjoyable:

- Make sure they have a comfortable place to eat; set out a nice placemat and linen napkin, or fresh flowers.

- Have a picnic in the park.

- Find a neighbor or friend for your loved one to eat with on a regular basis—have them take turns cooking the meal or cook together.

- Start (or have your loved one start) a potluck dinner club.

- If finances are not an issue, hire a personal chef to create a week's worth of meals for the fridge and freezer, or contact a gourmet meal delivery service.

- Have your loved one join a mall walker program (they often have breakfast with others in the group after their walks).

- Have breakfast for dinner, or dinner for breakfast.

- When cooking, make extra, then freeze in single servings. Make sure to label not only what it is, but cooking instructions as well, so no one has to go hunting for cooking or reheating instructions later.

- Keep a list of what's in the freezer or fridge on the refrigerator door; it's easier to plan a meal when your loved one knows what she has.

- Encourage your loved one to eat congregate meals at the local senior center.

- Sign up for elderly programs like Meals on Wheels (www. mowaa.org).

- If your loved one has trouble chewing, puree several pieces of fruit, and add a little protein powder, for a shake full of vitamins, minerals, and fiber. Make more than one serving and put the rest in the freezer for later.

While many people may not eat as well when eating alone as they would sitting down at a family meal, there are many options to ensure adequate nutrition. Whether by finding friends to eat with, using easy-to-prepare recipes, or making a change in the living situation, your loved one can still stay healthy with your help and encouragement.

Part Four

Lifestyle and Nutrition

Chapter 24

Nutrition Statistics in America

Chapter Contents

Section 24.1

Americans' Attitudes toward Food Safety, Nutrition, and Health

Excerpted from International Food Information Council 2010 *Food & Health Survey: Consumer Attitudes Toward Food Safety, Nutrition, and Health.* © 2010 International Food Information Council (www.foodinsight.org). Reprinted with permission.

The International Food Information Council Foundation's 2010 Food and Health Survey takes an extensive look at what Americans are doing regarding their eating and health habits and food safety practices.

When it comes to calories consumed versus calories burned, most Americans (58%) do not make an effort to balance the two; a large majority of people (77%) are not meeting the U.S. Department of Health and Human Services' *Physical Activity Guidelines.*

The 2010 *Food and Health Survey: Consumer Attitudes toward Food Safety, Nutrition, and Health,* commissioned by the International Food Information Council Foundation, is the fifth annual national quantitative study designed to gain insights from consumers on important food safety, nutrition, and health-related topics. The research provides the opportunity to gain insight on how consumers view their own diets, their efforts to improve them, how they balance diet and exercise, and their actions when it comes to food safety practices.

There is now more of a need than ever to understand consumers' perceptions of nutrition and food safety issues. The 2010 *Dietary Guidelines for Americans* will target, for the first time, an overweight and obese American population and advocate a "total diet" approach. There also are ongoing initiatives to address childhood obesity from the White House to Main Street, including First Lady Michelle Obama's Let's Move initiative. Landmark health care legislation was signed into law requiring calorie counts at restaurant chains. And, there is pending food safety legislation before the U.S. Congress.

While the *Food and Health Survey* highlights that many different messages about the importance of a healthful lifestyle are being heard, the survey also shows disconnects in consumers' awareness of the relationship between diet, physical activity, and calories. Although weight loss and physical activity are top of mind with Americans, the survey provides valuable insights into consumer beliefs and behaviors with regards to food safety, safe food handling, and consumer food shopping preferences, among other topics.

This survey offers the important voice and insights of the consumer for the health professionals, government officials, educators, and other interested individuals who seek to improve the lives of Americans.

The following are key findings from 2010 with comparisons to results from the 2006 through the 2009 editions of the *Food and Health Survey*.

Overall health status: Americans' perceptions of their health status remains steady from previous years with 38% indicating their health is "excellent" or "very good." Although there was no significant change from year to year, Americans' degree of satisfaction with their health status remains relatively high with 57% indicating "extremely satisfied" or "somewhat satisfied."

Weight: Americans' concern with their weight status remains unchanged since last year and continues to be a strong factor influencing the decision to make dietary changes and remain physically active. Most Americans (70%) say they are concerned about their weight status, and the vast majority (77%) is trying to lose or maintain their weight. When asked what actions they are taking, most Americans say they are changing the amount of food they eat (69%); changing the type of foods they eat (63%); and engaging in physical activity (60%). Further, 65% of Americans report weight loss as a top driver for improving the healthfulness of their diet; 16% report improving their diet to maintain weight. Americans are more singularly focused on making dietary changes for losing weight, rather than a variety of other motivators, as has been true in the past. In addition, losing or maintaining their weight is the top motivator (35%) for Americans who are physically active.

Diet and physical activity: Two-thirds of Americans (64%) report making changes to improve the healthfulness of their diet. The primary driver for making these changes is "to lose weight" (65%). Other drivers for making dietary changes have significantly decreased since previous years, including "to improve overall well-being" (59% vs. 64% in 2009) and "to improve physical health" (56% vs. 64% in 2008). The specific types of dietary changes they most often report are changing the type of food they eat (76%), changing the amount of food they eat (70%), and changing how often they eat (44%).

Americans' reports of their physical activity levels show that, on average, 63% are physically active, and 68% of those who are physically active report being "moderately" or "vigorously" active three to five days a week. However, among those who are active, slightly more than half (56%) do not include any strength training sessions. Further, a large majority of Americans (77%) are not meeting the U.S. Department of Health and Human Services' *Physical Activity Guidelines.*

Calorie and energy balance: Few Americans (12%) can accurately estimate the number of calories they should consume in a day for a person their age, height, weight, and physical activity. Of those who say they are trying to lose or maintain weight, only 19% say they are keeping track of calories. Additionally, almost half of Americans do not know how many calories they burn in a day (43%) or offer inaccurate estimates (35% say 1,000 calories or less). When it comes to calories consumed versus calories burned, most Americans (58%) do not make an effort to balance the two.

Dietary fats: Americans are confused about the differences among dietary fats. While Americans who have "heard" of these various types of dietary fats are reducing their consumption of saturated and trans fats (64% are trying to consume less trans fats and saturated fats), less than half (43%) state they consume more omega-3 fatty acids, and only a quarter (26%) state that they are consuming more omega-6 fatty acids.

Americans also seem to be less focused on dietary fat when looking at the Nutrition Facts panel. When looking at the Nutrition Facts panel listing of dietary fats, Americans are less frequently focusing on: total fat (62% vs. 69% in 2009); saturated fat (52% vs. 58% in 2008); trans fat (52% vs. 59% in 2008); and calories from fat (51% vs. 57% in 2007).

Carbohydrates and sugars: Americans who have "heard" of the various types of carbohydrates and sugars are trying to consume more fiber (72%) and whole grains (73%) in their diets but remain confused about the benefits of consuming more complex carbohydrates. Americans generally agree with the statement that "moderate amounts of sugar can be part of an overall healthful diet"; however, this sentiment declined to 58% from 66% in 2009.

Protein: New to this year's survey were questions about protein. Close to half of Americans say they are trying to consume more protein. Moreover, Americans are twice as likely to say protein is found in animal sources (56%) vs. plant sources (28%). The majority of Americans (68%) believe protein helps build muscle.

Sodium: Another new topic to this year's survey was sodium. More than half of Americans (53%) are concerned with the amount of sodium in their diet. Six in 10 Americans regularly purchase reduced/lower sodium foods. Among those that do purchase reduced/lower sodium foods, the most cited items include canned soup (58%), snacks (48%), and canned vegetables (41%).

Low-calorie sweeteners: Nearly 4 in 10 Americans (38%) agree that low-calorie/artificial sweeteners can play a role in weight loss or weight management, and one-third of Americans (34%) also agree that low-calorie/artificial sweeteners can reduce the calorie content of foods. Consistent with these data, one-third of Americans (32%) say they consume low-calorie/artificial sweeteners to help with calorie management.

Caffeine: Nearly three-quarters of Americans (72%) report consuming caffeine in moderation this year, significantly more than in 2009 (66%). There are also significantly fewer Americans (10% vs. 16% in 2009) who say they have either eliminated caffeine from their diet or say they consume more than the average person (18% in 2010 vs. 22% in 2008). Those who say they consume caffeine in moderation are more likely to perceive their health as "very good" or "excellent."

Food additives: The majority of Americans (61%) agree with at least two out of five statements provided regarding food additive facts or benefits. Those with the highest percent agreement include: "Food additives extend the freshness of food/act as a preservative" (57%), "Food additives can add color to food products" (54%), and "Food additives can help keep or improve the flavor of food products" (47%).

Food safety: For the past three years, consumer confidence in the safety of the U.S. food supply has remained steady with nearly half of Americans (47%) rating themselves as confident in the safety of the U.S. food supply. Those not confident fell significantly (down to 18% from 24% in 2009), and those who are neither confident nor unconfident increased to 35% from 26% in 2009.

As in previous years, we see consistency in consumers' beliefs that food safety is primarily the responsibility of government (74%) and industry (70%). Overall, approximately one-third of Americans (31%) see food safety as a shared responsibility among five or more stakeholder groups including farmers/producers, retailers, and themselves.

Safe food handling: While still high, there continues to be a decline in basic consumer food safety practices such as washing hands with soap and water (89% vs. 92% in 2008). These same declines are also relevant in microwave food safety practices, where 69% vs. 79%

in 2008 of Americans follow all the cooking instructions. Although a significant number of Americans (84%) use their microwave to prepare packaged products such as soup, popcorn, and frozen meals where microwave cooking instructions are clearly indicated, an even larger number of Americans (92%) cite the main reason for using the microwave is to reheat leftovers, foods, and/or beverages.

Consumer information sources and purchasing influences: In addition to information gathered on the Nutrition Facts panel and the food label, consumers were asked about their awareness and use of the U.S. Department of Agriculture's MyPyramid food guidance system. [MyPyramid was replaced by MyPlate (www.choosemyplate.gov) on June 2, 2011.] While 85% of Americans say they are aware of MyPyramid, only 29% of individuals report having used MyPyramid in some way.

Consistent with previous years, taste remains the biggest influence on purchasing decisions (86%), followed by price, healthfulness (58%), and convenience (56%). The importance of price continues to have a large impact on consumers' food and beverage purchasing decisions (73% in 2010 vs. 64% in 2006).

Food labeling: Similar to previous years, Americans say they are actively using the Nutrition Facts panel (68%), the expiration date (66%), and, increasingly, the brand name (50% vs. 40% in 2008) and allergen labeling (11% vs. 6% in 2008). Among consumers who use the Nutrition Facts panel, they rank calories as the top piece of information they use (74%), followed by sodium content (63% vs. 56% in 2009). Fewer Americans, however, are looking at total fat content (62% vs. 69% in 2009) and sugars (62% vs. 68% in 2008).

Food purchasing influences: The vast majority of Americans (88%) conduct the bulk of their food shopping at a supermarket/grocery store. Roughly three-quarters of Americans are satisfied with the healthfulness of products offered at their supermarket/grocery store (73%) and warehouse membership club (80%).

The full survey findings and webcasts are available on the International Food Information Council Foundation's website: www .foodinsight.org.

About the International Food Information Council Foundation

The International Food Information Council Foundation is dedicated to the mission of effectively communicating science-based information on health, food safety, and nutrition for the public good.

Additional information on the Foundation is available on the "About" section of our website: www.foodinsight.org.

Section 24.2

Hunger and Food Insecurity

Excerpted from *Journal of the American Dietetic Association*, Volume 110, Issue 9, pp 1368–1377, September 2010. Position of the American Dietetic Association: Food Insecurity in the United States. © 2010 American Dietetic Association. Reprinted with permission from Elsevier.

Food Insecurity Is Prevalent in the United States

According to the most recent national estimates, 85.4% of U.S. households were food secure throughout 2008. However, 14.6% of households (17.1 million), representing 49.1 million individuals, experienced food insecurity sometime during the year due to resource constraints. Of all U.S. households, 8.9% of all households (10.4 million households) had low food security, representing 31.8 million individuals. Coping strategies used by these households to avoid very low food security included:

- eating less varied diets;

- participating in federal food and nutrition assistance programs; and

- obtaining emergency food from community food pantries, emergency kitchens, and shelters.

Yet, 5.7% of all households (6.7 million households), representing 17.3 million individuals, had experienced very low food security. In most households, children, especially younger children, were protected from hunger by older members of the households, especially the mother. Overall, 1.1 million children lived in households classified as very low food security among children (1.5% of the children in the nation).

Consistent with previous years' estimates, households at risk for food insecurity during 2008 included:

- households with incomes below the income-to-poverty ratio (<1.00, 42.2% of households; <1.30, 39% of households; <1.85, 33.9% of households);

- households with children and headed by a single woman (37.2% of households) or man (27.6% of households);

- households headed by a black non-Hispanic (25.7% of households) or Hispanic (26.9% of households); and

- households located in principal cities (17.7% of households). (Principal cities are "incorporated areas of the largest cities in each metropolitan area.")

Households with older adults have rates of food insecurity less than the national average (8.1% for households with older adults; 8.8% for households with older adults living alone). As the number of older adults increases in the United States, continuing to monitor and further understand food insecurity in this segment of the population is important. Households receiving food from emergency food providers, including pantries (e.g., food pantries and food shelves), kitchens (e.g., soup kitchens and emergency dining rooms), and shelters (e.g., emergency shelters and homeless shelters), appear to be particularly vulnerable to food insecurity. Although the national estimates probably underestimate participation due to sampling strategies utilized, about 4.1% of U.S. households (4.8 million), representing 8.8 million adults and 4.5 million children, obtained food from pantries at least once in 2008, and 0.5% of households (623,000) ate at least one meal at a kitchen. Of those households reporting use of a pantry in the past 12 months, 46%, 28%, and 26% reported that this had occurred only in 1 or 2 months, some months (but not every month), and almost every month, respectively. Almost 70% of food insecure households, however, did not use a pantry, despite knowing of availability of one in their community.

The most recent Feeding America (formerly America's Second Harvest) study published in 2010 reported that only 24.5% of households using either pantries, kitchens, or shelters were food secure (high food security or marginal food security). Whereas 75.5% were food insecure, with 44.3% and 34.2% of all households being characterized as having low food security and very low food security, respectively. Similar to previous years, according to the most recent national estimates of food insecurity in the United States:

- about 31% of households using pantries were food secure (high food security, marginal food security); yet, of those, 55% were classified as having marginal food security and were 10 times as likely to have used a pantry and 5 times as likely to have eaten at a emergency kitchen as households classified as high food security (those with no indicators of food insecurity);

• food pantry and emergency kitchen use was strongly associated with food insecurity, with food insecure households being 13 and 14 times more likely than their food secure counterparts to have obtained food from a pantry or kitchen, respectively; and

• compared to usage nationally (4.1%), pantry use was higher among households with incomes below the poverty line (17%), with children (5.6%), headed by a single woman with children (11.5%), classified as non-Hispanic black (8.1%) or Hispanic (5.7%), and located in principal cities (4.8%).

Important caveats to interpreting food security assessment measures used for the annual estimates include that questions are posed to respondents regarding the previous 12 months. Therefore, those experiencing food insecurity any time during the previous year are classified as food insecure. Consequently, the daily rates of food insecurity are substantially less than the annual rates. On average, it is estimated that 0.9% to 1.2% of households (1.1 to 1.4 million households) experience very low food security each day. In addition, experiencing very low food security and the associated reduced food intake and disrupted eating patterns appear to be episodic, rather than chronic, in nature.

The causes of food insecurity must be understood before it can be eradicated. Poverty, high housing and utility costs, unemployment, medical and health costs, mental health problems, lack of education, transportation costs, and substance abuse are cited as factors contributing to food insecurity in American cities. Smoking also appears to be associated with food insecurity, according to the National Health and Nutrition Examination Survey, 1999–2002, a nationally representative sample of households with children.

Rose [Economic determinants and dietary consequences of food insecurity in the United States. *J Nutr.* 1999;129(suppl): 517S–520S] noted that food insecurity is often triggered by an event that stresses the household budget—losing a job or assistance benefits, including Supplemental Nutrition Assistance Program (SNAP) benefits, or gaining a household member. Overall, food insecure households must often choose between buying food and buying or paying for other items or needs, including medication, healthful housing conditions, and utility costs for heating or cooling. Among households using food pantries and other emergency food programs, many reported choosing between buying food and medical care/medication (31.6%), rent/mortgage (35%), or utilities/ heating (41.5%). Cook and colleagues [Cook JT, Frank DA, Levenson SM, Neault NB, Heeren T, Black MM, Berkowitz C, Casey PH, Meyers AF, Cutts DB, Chilton M. Child food insecurity increases risks posed by household food insecurity to young children's health. *J Nutr.* 2006;136:1073–6] developed a measure of household energy security, "access to enough of the kinds of energy needed [to heat/cool home and operate lighting/appliances] for a healthy and safe life in the geographic area." Overall, household and child food insecurity was associated with household energy insecurity, as well as poor health, hospitalizations, and developmental risks among infants and toddlers.

Immediate and long-range interventions targeting the causes of food insecurity will undoubtedly assist in reducing rates of food insecurity. Adequate funding for and increased use of food and nutrition assistance programs, as well as innovative programs to promote and support economic self-sufficiency, is paramount. Registered dietitians (RDs) and dietetic technicians, registered (DTRs), can encourage clients to access existing programs providing food and nutrition assistance, social services, and job training as an immediate intervention. RDs and DTRs can also partner with key stakeholders in the community to build local food systems and reduce hunger.

Food Insecurity Is Related to Nutrition and Non-Nutrition Outcomes

Food insecurity is a high priority for public health action, especially in view of its potential negative effect on the nation from public health and economic perspectives. As summarized by Nord and Prell [Struggling to feed the family: What does it mean to be food insecure? *Amber Waves.* 2007;5:32–39], "it is clear that food insecurity is part of a complex of potentially serious health and developmental conditions." Overall, it can have grave consequences, including physical impairments related to insufficient food, psychological issues due to lack of access to food, and sociofamilial disturbances. As previously reviewed, food insecurity is associated with:

- inadequate intake of key nutrients; poor physical and mental health in adults and depression in women;
- overweight and weight gain (especially among women from marginal and low food security households);

- adverse health outcomes for infants and toddlers;

- behavior problems in preschool-aged children;

- lower educational achievement in kindergarteners; and

- depressive disorder and suicidal symptoms in adolescents.

The relationship of food insecurity to nutrition and non-nutrition-related outcomes will be the primary focus of this section.

Dietary Intake in Children and Adults

Several studies have demonstrated a relationship between food insecurity and less-than-optimal food and nutrient intake, as well as risk for nutrient deficiencies among some life course groups. Although children are typically protected from very low food security in the United States, evidence suggests that food insecurity or insufficiency may be associated with lower dietary quality in children, especially older children (and adults).

Food insufficiency has been associated with decreased consumption of vegetables, particularly nutrient-rich dark green vegetables, among U.S. children. In contrast, Lorson and colleagues [Lorson BA, Melgar-Quinonez HR, Taylor CA. Correlates of fruit and vegetable intakes in US children. *J Am Diet Assoc.* 2009;109:474–8] found that total fruit and vegetable intakes of all U.S. children were at less than recommended levels and did not vary among children from fully food-secure, marginally food-secure, low food-secure, and very-low food-secure households. Compared to their food secure counterparts, however, the proportion of french fries consumed by children and adolescents living in food insecure households made up a greater proportion of total vegetable intake. Widome and colleagues [Widome R, Neumark-Sztainer D, Hannan PJ, Haines J, Story M. Eating when there is not enough to eat: Eating behaviors and perceptions of food among food-insecure youths. *Am J Public Health.* 2009;99:822–8] focused on diet quality and food insecurity among middle and high school youth. They found that, compared to food secure youth, food insecure youth consumed a greater percentage of energy from fat, ate fewer family meals and breakfasts, had less food availability at home, and perceived greater barriers to eating a healthful diet. Therefore, the authors suggested that interventions aimed at eliminating barriers to healthful eating would be prudent.

Poor nutrition outcomes, including inadequate intakes of key nutrients, among food insecure adults and older adults have been previously reported in nationally representative samples. Olson [Food insecurity in women: A recipe for unhealthy trade-offs. *Top Clin Nutr.* 2005;20:321–8] reviewed food insecurity in women and emphasized that the role of women in managing family feeding makes them vulnerable to the negative consequences of food insecurity, with fruits and vegetables being sacrificed initially in the face of approaching food insecurity. Women may modify their dietary intake to spare other family members, especially children, from experiencing nutrient deprivation. Nonetheless, in U.S. adults, energy intakes did not differ between food secure and food insecure adults. Rather, meal and snack behaviors differed, with food insecure adults consuming fewer (but larger) meals and more snacks, which may compensate for the reduced meal frequency. This study underscores the importance of focusing on meal and snack behaviors, rather than only total energy, when monitoring diet quality of food insecure adults.

The literature demonstrates that individuals residing in households lacking access to food may consume diets deficient in particular food groups and nutrients, increasing the risk of poor health, chronic disease development, and other non-nutrition-related outcomes, if not immediately, in the long term. Continuing to document the dietary outcomes of food insecurity is paramount, as is development of appropriate interventions and provision of innovative food and nutrition education by RDs and DTRs, including collaborative, community-based education programs. Since gardening interventions have the potential to enhance produce availability and intake, one example of a potential community-based program is gardening education in collaboration with a master gardener or county extension educator to increase household produce availability. Adequate funding for and increased use of food and nutrition assistance programs, including those providing nutrition education, is particularly important to improve the dietary outcomes related to food insecurity. In addition, developing community partnerships and networks that build local food systems are crucial. Examples include partnerships in local communities with emergency food and feeding programs, farmers' markets, community gardens, and farm-to-school programs. In the short term, to improve community food security, maximizing access to and use of existing food and nutrition assistance programs is vital.

Other Nutrition and Non-Nutrition Outcomes

Collectively, the literature demonstrates that food insecurity has negative nutrition and non-nutrition outcomes and underscores the potential negative implications of food insecurity on the health of citizens and residents of the United States and U.S. health care costs. Health status, chronic disease incidence and risk, diabetes, overweight and obesity, school performance, and mental health are all related to food insecurity. Food insecurity is a preventable health threat. Therefore, it is imperative to document outcomes of food insecurity through collaborative research projects across the life course. Development of appropriate interventions, especially for households with youth, and provision of innovative food and nutrition education by RDs and DTRs and adequate funding for food and nutrition assistance programs is also vital.

Child/Adolescent Health, Development, and Other Outcomes

Food insecurity is associated with adverse health, growth, and development outcomes among children aged 0 to 18 years. In addition, maternal food insecurity has been shown to be associated with increased risk of certain birth defects. For children, food insecurity/insufficiency is associated with poor health. Very low food security among children further increases the odds of poor health and is associated with more frequent hospitalizations among young children. Children of immigrant mothers are especially prone to this negative outcome. Infants and toddlers from food insecure households have also been shown to be at developmental risk and at risk for iron deficiency and iron deficiency anemia, especially among ethnic minorities. Compared to those from food secure households, children and adolescents in food insecure households are also more likely to exhibit behavioral and psychological problems, including suicide risk in adolescents, as well as poorer academic performance and achievement.

Adult Health and Chronic Disease Risk and Development

Among adults, food insecurity/insufficiency is associated with poor physical and mental health status, as well as depression in women and risk for and incidence of chronic diseases, including diabetes. In U.S. adults, food insecurity appears to be associated with diabetes incidence, independent of body mass index. Diabetes and chronic disease management is also associated with food insecurity. Finally, human immunodeficiency virus infection and poorer human immunodeficiency virus infection management/treatment outcomes have been associated with food insecurity.

Child and Adult Overweight and Obesity

For children, studies exploring the relationship between food insecurity and childhood obesity have used a variety of data sets and methods, yielding mixed results—a positive, negative, or no relationship. Although additional research should further explore the trends, most recently, a study by Gunderson and Kreider [Bounding the effects of food insecurity on children's health outcomes. *J Health Econ.* 2009;28:971–83] found food security to be positively associated with a healthful weight in a nationally representative sample of U.S. children (National Health and Nutrition Examination Survey, 2001–2006).

For adults, research continues to support that food insecurity is associated with overweight and obesity, especially among women from households experiencing marginal food security or low food security. Possible causes of this phenomenon include a binge-like eating pattern or overeating when food is available and consumption of low-quality diets of empty-energy, high-fat, and sugary foods. As with children, additional research is needed to further clarify the relationship of food insecurity and weight status in adults.

Chapter 25

Smart Supermarket Shopping

Chapter Contents

Section 25.1

Planning for Healthy Food Shopping

"Shopping, Cooking, and Meal Planning," National Agricultural Library,
Food and Nutrition Information Center, U.S. Department of Agriculture
(www.nutrition.gov), September 1, 2010.

We have the power of choice to decide which foods to buy at the grocery store. Making the healthiest food choices when shopping and eating out is a key to consuming a well-balanced diet.

Guidelines for a Healthy You

Healthy food choices are important for good health and well-being. Eating well means eating a variety of nutrient-packed foods and beverages from the food groups of ChooseMyPlate.gov and staying within your calorie needs. This, combined with choosing foods low in saturated and trans fats, cholesterol, added sugars, and salt (sodium), will help ensure you are eating a healthy diet while helping maintain a healthy weight. If you choose to drink alcoholic beverages, do so sensibly and in moderation.

Basic Healthy Shopping Skills

Know Your Store

Grocery stores have thousands of products, with most food items grouped together to make your decision making easier. Many grocery stores have sections where foods are shelved much like the food groups of MyPlate.

The MyPlate food groups put foods with similar nutritional value together. These groups are the following:

- Fruits
- Vegetables
- Grains
- Milk (calcium-rich foods)

- Meat and Beans (protein-rich foods)

Don't forget that your local farmers market is a great place for finding healthy foods. Find a farmers market in your state at apps.ams .usda.gov/FarmersMarkets.

Bring a List

And stick to it! Healthy decisions start at home. Planning ahead can improve your health while saving you time and money. Before shopping, decide which foods you need and the quantity that will last until your next shopping trip.

Consider creating a shopping list based on the MyPlate food groups to include a variety of healthy food choices. Think about your menu ideas when adding items to your list. Write your list to match the groups to the layout of your store.

Have everyone in your family make suggestions for the shopping list. Kids (and adults too!) are more willing to try new foods when they help to pick them.

Table 25.1. Locations of Food Groups in the Grocery Store

Food Group	Typical Store Location(s)	Best Choices
Fruits	Produce aisle, canned goods, freezer aisle, salad bar	Variety! Fresh, frozen, canned, and dried fruits
Vegetables	Produce aisle, canned goods, freezer aisle, salad bar, pasta, rice, and bean aisle	Variety! Fresh, frozen, and canned (especially dark green and orange); dry beans and peas
Grains	Bakery, bread aisle, pasta and rice aisle, cereal aisle	Whole grains for at least half of choices
Milk, yogurt, and cheese (calcium-rich foods)	Dairy case, refrigerated aisle	Nonfat and low-fat milk, yogurt, low-fat and fat-free cheeses
Meat and beans, fish, poultry, eggs, soy, and nuts (protein foods)	Deli meat and poultry case, seafood counter, egg case, canned goods, salad bar	Lean meats, skinless poultry, fish, legumes (dried beans and peas), nuts

Use the Facts

The Nutrition Facts, that is! The Nutrition Facts panel on the food label is your guide to making healthy choices. Using the Nutrition Facts panel is important when shopping to be able to compare foods before you buy.

What are the facts? When reading the Nutrition Facts panel, use the % Daily Value (DV) column when possible: 5%DV or less is low, 20%DV or more is high.

Keep These Low

- Saturated fats

- Trans fats

- Cholesterol

- Sodium

Look for More of These

- Fiber

- Vitamins A, C, and E

- Calcium, potassium, magnesium, and iron

Enjoy!

Enjoy food shopping while exploring different foods and learning about their Nutrition Facts. Healthy choices can make a healthy you!

Try Recipes and Tips for Healthy, Thrifty Meals (at www.cnpp.usda.gov/Publications/FoodPlans/MiscPubs/FoodPlansRecipeBook.pdf) for ideas on making healthful food choices and meal preparation with sample shopping lists.

Visit Fruits and Veggies—More Matters (at apps.nccd.cdc.gov/dnparecipe/recipesearch.aspx) to find delicious fruit and vegetable recipes for any meal.

Check Family Meals—Fast, Healthful! (at www.fns.usda.gov/tn/Resources/Nibbles/family_meals.pdf) for tips on how to create speedy meals that are good for you.

Section 25.2

Making Healthy Food Choices

"Grocery Shopping," reprinted with permission from www.heart.org.
© 2010 American Heart Association, Inc.

While it's generally healthier and cheaper to buy groceries at the store and prepare your meals at home, sometimes the sheer number of food choices at the supermarket can seem overwhelming. Here are some tips to help you be heart-smart at the grocery store and choose good-for-you foods.

Now, let's go shopping...

Vegetables and Fruits

Be sure to buy and eat plenty of fresh or frozen fruits and vegetables. Fruits and vegetables that are deeply colored throughout—such as spinach, carrots, peaches, and berries—tend to be higher in vitamins and minerals than others, such as potatoes and corn.

When fresh foods aren't available, choose frozen or canned vegetables and fruits in water without added sugars, saturated and trans fat, or salt.

Buy more fruits and vegetables that are good sources of fiber, including beans, peas, oranges, bananas, strawberries, and apples.

Stock up on raw vegetables for snacks such as carrot and celery sticks, broccoli, cherry tomatoes, and cauliflower.

For desserts, buy fresh or canned fruits (in water without added sugars), dried fruit (without added sugars), and gelatin that contains fruit, instead of baked goods and sweets.

Don't buy lots of fruit juice. It doesn't provide the fiber whole fruit does and it's not as good at satisfying hunger.

Milk, Cheese, Butter, and Eggs

Select fat-free (skim) or low-fat (1%) milk.

Avoid milk that contains added flavorings such as vanilla, chocolate, or strawberry. They usually have added sugars and calories.

Choose fat-free, low-fat, or reduced-fat cheeses.

Use egg whites or egg substitutes instead of egg yolks. (Substitute two egg whites for each egg yolk in recipes that call for eggs.)

Choose soft margarines that contain "0 grams trans fat" instead of buying butter. (These margarines usually come in tubs.)

Don't buy a lot of butter, cream, and ice cream. Save those for special occasions and, even then, limit how much you eat. These foods have more saturated fat than whole milk.

Watch out for the saturated and/or partially hydrogenated fats hidden in casseroles, bakery goods, desserts, and other foods. Read the Nutrition Facts label to determine the saturated fat, trans fat, and cholesterol content of foods you're considering.

Meat, Poultry, Fish, and Nuts

Buy and prepare more fish. You should eat one serving of grilled or baked fish at least twice a week. (A serving is roughly the size of a checkbook.) Good examples of fish to buy include salmon, trout, and herring.

Choose lemon juice and spices to eat with fish. Don't add cream sauces.

Stay away from fried fish. It's usually high in fat—often trans fat.

Choose cuts of red meat and pork labeled "loin" and "round"; they usually have the least fat.

Buy "choice" or "select" grades of beef rather than "prime," and be sure to trim off the fat before cooking.

When buying or eating poultry, choose the leaner light meat (breasts) rather than the fattier dark meat (legs and thighs). Try the skinless version or remove the skin yourself.

Select more meat substitutes such as dried beans, peas, lentils, or tofu (soybean curd) and use them as entrees or in salads and soups. A one-cup serving of cooked beans, peas, lentils, or tofu can replace a two-ounce serving of meat, poultry, or fish.

Pick up nuts and seeds, which are good sources of protein and polyunsaturated and monounsaturated fats—but remember, they tend to be high in calories, so eat them in moderation.

Bread and Baked Goods

Choose whole-grain, high-fiber breads, such as those containing whole wheat, oats, oatmeal, whole rye, whole-grain corn, and buckwheat. Choose breads and other foods that list whole grains as the first item in the ingredient list.

Limit the amount of bakery products you purchase, including dough-nuts, pies, cakes, and cookies. Look instead for fat-free or low-fat and low-sodium varieties of crackers, snack chips, cookies, and cakes.

Remember that most store-baked goods are made with egg yolks, saturated fats, and/or trans fats. (Read the Nutrition Facts label to determine the saturated fat, trans fat, and cholesterol content.) Check for store-baked goods that are made with polyunsaturated or mono-unsaturated oils, skim or reduced-fat milk, and egg whites—or make your own.

Instead of buying a raisin bran muffin, buy a loaf of raisin bread and enjoy a slice for breakfast or lunch.

Oils, Dressings, and Shortening

Buy and use fats and oils in limited amounts.

When you must use oils for cooking, baking, or in dressings or spreads, choose the ones lowest in saturated fats, trans fats, and cholesterol—including canola oil, corn oil, olive oil, safflower oil, sesame oil, soybean oil, and sunflower oil.

Stay away from palm oil, palm kernel oil, coconut oil, and cocoa butter. Even though they are vegetable oils and have no cholesterol, they're high in saturated fats.

Buy a nonstick pan or use nonstick vegetable spray when cooking.

Choose reduced-fat, low-fat, light, or fat-free salad dressings (if you need to limit your calories) to use with salads, for dips, or as marinades.

Section 25.3

Are There Benefits to Purchasing Organic Food?

Even the most casual food shoppers have probably noticed the increased quantity and variety of organic foods available in regular grocery stores. Once the specialty of health food stores, organic foods are spreading from specialty aisles to shelves throughout the big food stores.

Maybe you're wondering what all the fuss is about. Are organic foods healthier? Are they safer? Are they worth the extra money if they cost more than conventional foods? How do they taste?

And what about those labels touting foods as "sustainable," "natural," "free-range," "grass-fed," or "fair trade"? What do they mean, and are those foods organic, too?

Read on for a crash course in organic and other environmentally friendly foods.

Defining "Organic"

If a food is labeled "organic," what does that mean? To meet the organic standards set by the U.S. Department of Agriculture (USDA), an organic food is one that is grown without:

- pesticides;
- fertilizers made with synthetic ingredients or sewage sludge;
- herbicides;
- antibiotics;
- bioengineering;

- hormones;

- ionizing radiation.

Organic animal products—meat, poultry, eggs, and dairy foods—come from animals that are fed 100% organic feed products, receive no antibiotics or growth hormones, and have access to the outdoors.

If a product is labeled "organic," it means that a government-approved certifier has inspected the farm where it was produced to ensure that the farmer followed all the rules necessary to meet the USDA's organic standards. Farmers who produce organic foods use renewable resources that conserve the soil and water for future generations. And any company that handled or processed that food on its way to the grocery store must be certified organic, too.

Foods labeled "organic" can be either:

- **100% organic** (they're completely organic or made of all organic ingredients) or

- **organic** (they're at least 95% organic).

If you see "made with organic ingredients" on a label, it means the food contains at least 70% organic ingredients, but can't have the "organic" seal on its packaging.

Bioengineered Foods

A GMO (genetically modified organism)—also sometimes called a GEO (genetically engineered organism)—is a food that has been altered genetically. This involves taking genes from one species of plant and inserting them into another—for example, the gene from a wild potato that is resistant to potato blight was transferred to a potato variety grown for food.

Sustainable Foods

Another term you might hear in conjunction with organic and natural foods is "sustainable." This movement encourages eating foods grown locally by sustainable agricultural methods—that is, using food-growing techniques that don't harm the environment, are seasonal, and preserve agricultural land. Sustainable practices also are humane to animals, pay growers fairly, and support local farming communities by distributing their food through farmers markets and other venues.

Again, "sustainable" and "organic" don't always mean the same thing. An organic tomato you buy, for example, might not adhere to sustainable principles if it was grown organically but shipped across the country to your market. And some produce you find at your local stand might not have been grown organically.

There's a growing trend among health-conscious consumers to buy food that is both sustainable and organic whenever possible.

You Might Also See

- **Bird friendly or shade grown:** When you see this on coffee, it means it was grown under trees that provide shade for the coffee and a habitat for migratory birds. Coffee grown out in the open under the hot sun is cheaper but requires more pesticides and chemical fertilizers to grow.

- **Cage-free or free range:** Seen on eggs or poultry products, these terms can be misleading or unreliable. "Cage-free" implies that birds were not housed in cages, but is not a guarantee that they had access to the outdoors—or even are able to roam freely—and the "cage-free" label isn't verified by any third party. To be considered "free-range" producers must demonstrate poultry has been allowed open-air access. The USDA has no requirements as to the amount of time spent outdoors, nor the size or quality of the outside range.

- **Grass-fed/open pasture:** "Grass-fed" on a label signifies that the livestock received a diet of natural forage outdoors, but sometimes cows are fed grass while indoors or in a pen or only for the first few months of their lives. So "grass-fed" can—but doesn't always— mean "pasture-raised" or "open pasture." Pasture-raised animals roam freely outdoors where they can eat the grasses and other plants that their bodies are best suited to digest.

- **Fair trade certified:** If you see this on coffee, chocolate, tea, rice, or sugar, it means that the farmers received fair prices for their products.

- **Marine Stewardship Council:** If you see this on your package of fish sticks or Alaskan salmon, it means the seafood was caught without endangering the species or harming the local ecosystem.

Natural Foods

Natural foods are foods that are minimally processed and remain as close as possible to their whole, original state. Natural foods don't have to adhere to the same rigorous standards organic foods do. However, the term "natural" generally means a product has no artificial ingredients or preservatives and that meat or poultry is minimally processed and free of artificial ingredients.

Natural foods can be organic, but not all are—some natural foods, for instance, may have been produced on a farm that has not been certified organic. If you want to be sure that what you're eating is organic, look for the "organic" labeling, which means they've been certified as meeting the USDA's standards.

Getting More Information

Keeping track of all these terms and their meanings can be confusing. To make labels more consistent and understandable, the USDA is now developing standards for labels like grass-fed, pasture-raised, and others that will be subject to USDA inspection.

Also, many individual food producers, dairies, farms, and orchards have websites you can visit to find out more about their standards. You also can find ratings and other label information from reputable consumer groups online.

Is Organic Food Healthier?

The USDA does not claim that organic foods are safer or more nutritious than those produced conventionally, but organic foods can be part of a healthy diet. Whether they are much better for you than conventional food is still up for debate. One benefit of organic food is that it is pesticide free, which is definitely better for the environment. It's probably better for you as well, though many people argue that the pesticide residue on foods is too small to cause health problems.

Even with organic products, though, be sure to follow the safe handling recommendations for all foods:

- Thoroughly wash all produce, and if the skin still isn't clean, peel it off.

- Organically raised and processed meat can harbor bacteria and should be handled the same as regular meat products—follow kitchen cleanliness rules and cook meats to the proper temperature: 180° F for poultry, 160° F for beef.

Where to Buy Organic Foods

It wasn't so long ago that people who wanted to buy primarily organic foods had to turn to their local food co-ops or settle for a few items in their grocery store. Co-ops and local farmstands are great sources for natural and organic foods. But anyone looking for conventionally grown foods and other items will have to make another stop.

These days, though, it's easy to find a well-rounded selection of organic products. Most groceries offer organic produce, juices, cereals, baby food, dairy products, and more. And many stores are 100% organic or natural—if you don't have one in your neighborhood, there's likely to be one a short drive away.

If you can't find a decent selection of organic foods where you shop, talk to the store manager. The more requests a store gets for natural selections, the more likely it is to stock them.

So the next time you see a tempting treat that's labeled "organic," you may want to give it a try—it might be your first step toward a style of shopping and eating that's good for you and the planet.

Chapter 26

Healthy Vegetarianism

Can following a vegetarian diet help you lose weight? It depends. Research does seem to indicate that obesity is less common among vegetarians than their carnivorous counterparts. However, the studies that have examined this issue are often designed in such a way that it is difficult to separate "diet" from other lifestyle behaviors common among vegetarians. That is, forsaking meat is not the only thing separating vegetarians from meat eaters; vegetarians also tend to be more physically active, drink less alcohol, and eat less fat.

When it comes to weight management, the bottom line is calories. Meat eating or not, one must balance the calories they consume with the calories they expend in physical activity. It may, however, be easier to achieve that elusive energy "balance" with a diet rich in vegetables, fruits, and whole grains. Moreover, research suggests that vegetarian diets are associated with a reduced risk of chronic disease. Since improved health is presumably the goal of body weight control, a vegetarian diet might serve a dual purpose of helping you both look and feel your best.

Types of Vegetarianism

Generally speaking, a vegetarian is someone who eats a predominately plant-based diet and excludes meat, fish, and poultry, and any

"Weighing in on Vegetarian Diets," by Katherine Beals, Ph.D., R.D., FACSM. Reprinted with permission of the American College of Sports Medicine, ACSM Fit Society ® Page, Summer 2004, pp 3–4. © 2004 American College of Sports Medicine (www.acsm.org). Reviewed by David A. Cooke, MD, FACP, January 2011.

products containing these foods. Nonetheless, in practice there are varying degrees of animal product restriction as the following descriptions demonstrate:

- **Pesco vegetarian:** Consumes fish and may or may not also consume dairy products and eggs

- **Lacto-ovo vegetarian:** Consumes dairy products and eggs

- **Lacto vegetarian:** Consumes dairy products

- **Vegan:** Consumes only grains, vegetables, fruits, legumes, nuts, and seeds; may also avoid products made from or with animal products (e.g., cosmetics, wool, leather, etc.)

Who Is Practicing Vegetarianism and Why?

According to a 2003 National Harris Poll sponsored by the Vegetarian Resource Group, 2.8% of the U.S. adult population (approximately 5.7 million adults) reported that they never ate meat, poultry, or fish/seafood, while 1.8% reported following a vegan diet. This particular poll also found that vegetarians were most likely to be female between 25–34 years of age, live in the western U.S., and have a college education.

Although vegetarians often cite a concern for animal welfare as fundamental to their decision to consume a plant-based diet, it is often not the only reason. Other common reasons for following a vegetarian diet include health considerations, concern for the environment, economic motivations, world hunger issues, and religious beliefs.

Are Vegetarians Healthier?

There is a growing appreciation for the health benefits of a plant-based diet. A number of health organizations including the American Cancer Society, the American Heart Association, the National Institutes of Health, and the American Academy recommend a diet based on a variety of whole grains, fruits, and vegetables to reduce the risk of major chronic diseases. Research generally indicates that those who follow vegetarian diets enjoy a lower risk of cardiovascular disease, hypertension, type 2 diabetes, cancer (particularly cancers of the gastrointestinal tract), renal disease, and obesity.

Will a Vegetarian Diet Help Me Lose Weight?

Weight loss occurs when you consume fewer calories than you expend (or expend more calories than you consume). This state of "negative energy balance," as dietitians like to call it, may be easier to achieve on a vegetarian diet. However, even plant foods can be high in calories, so it is still necessary to choose your plant foods wisely. Fresh fruits and vegetables are low in calories and fat, yet high in water content and fiber; thus, they tend to fill you up with fewer calories. On the other hand, fruit and vegetable juices and dried fruits are higher in calorie content and generally less filling, so it is easier to overeat these foods and exceed your daily calorie allotment. Similarly, whole grain breads, cereals, rice, and pasta tend to be more filling than the respective refined versions of these foods due to the fiber content. Nuts, while high in protein, iron, and zinc, are also high in calories and should be consumed sparingly by the vegetarian wishing to whittle his or her waistline.

The lacto-ovo and lacto vegetarian interested in weight loss needs to be mindful of the fat and calorie content of many "whole" and even "reduced-fat" dairy and egg products. Selecting non-fat or low-fat versions of milk, yogurt, and cheese will go a long way towards reducing calories. Similarly, using egg substitutes or egg whites will significantly lower fat and, therefore, calories.

Nutritional Considerations for the (Dieting) Vegetarian

Plant-based diets offer a number of nutritional advantages over those that are meat laden, including lower levels of saturated fat, cholesterol, and animal protein, along with higher levels of fiber and antioxidants such as vitamins C and E, carotenoids, and phytochemicals. Nonetheless, dieting vegetarians, particularly vegans, may be at risk for inadequate intakes of certain nutrients. These nutrients, along with suggestions for ensuring adequate intake, include:

- **Protein:** In general, plant foods can provide adequate levels of amino acids to meet protein requirements. However, because the quality of plant proteins varies (e.g., the protein quality of cereals is generally lower than that of soy), protein requirements may be somewhat higher for vegans. Moreover, research indicates that a state of negative energy balance (such as when one is dieting and loses weight) tends to increase protein requirements. Thus, the dieting vegetarian may have somewhat higher protein requirements than the nondieting vegetarian or meat eater. An intake of 1.3–1.8 g/kg [grams per kilogram] of protein per day should readily meet the dieting vegetarian's elevated requirements. In addition, choosing protein-rich plant foods such as nuts, seeds, legumes, and soy will help the dieting vegetarian meet his or her protein needs.

- **Iron:** Plant foods generally contain significantly less iron than animal products. Moreover, the iron in plant foods is nonheme, which is less readily absorbed than heme-iron found in animal products. Plant foods also contain a variety of factors that can inhibit the absorption of nonheme iron such as fiber and phytates. Fortunately, there are also substances in plant foods that can enhance the absorption of non-heme iron such as vitamin C and various organic acids. Some food preparation techniques can also enhance the availability of non-heme iron such as soaking and sprouting beans, grains, and seeds. Similarly, cooking plant foods in an iron skillet can increase the iron content by actually leeching some iron into the food. Plant foods that are high in iron content are listed in Table 26.1.

- **Zinc:** As was true for iron, plant foods are generally poor sources of zinc. In addition, the phytates found in many plant foods also inhibit zinc absorption. Thus, zinc requirements for vegans may exceed the current RDA [recommended daily allowance]. Plant foods that are high in zinc content are listed Table 26.1.

- **Essential fatty acids:** There are certain fatty acids that the body cannot synthesize and, thus, we must get them from our food. These include linoleic (or omega 6) and alpha-linolenic (or omega 3). Whereas vegetarian diets are generally rich in omega 6 fatty acids (i.e., those found in vegetable oils), they are often low in omega 3 fatty acids (typically found in seafood). In addition, dieting vegetarians may restrict fat intake, further limiting their intake of essential fatty acids. Omega 3 fatty acids play key roles in brain development and retinal function and, thus, are particularly important during early developmental periods (i.e., the last trimester of gestation and early infancy). In addition, research has shown that diets rich in omega 3 fatty acids are associated with a reduction in risk factors for heart disease (e.g., decreased LDL [low-density lipoprotein] cholesterol and triglyceride levels) and stroke (decreased platelet aggregation and blood pressure). In addition to seafood, good sources of omega 3 fatty acids include flaxseed and flaxseed oil, walnuts and walnut oil, and soybeans.

Living Life the Vegetarian "Weigh"

Plant-based diets can be nutritionally adequate and have been shown to be beneficial in the prevention and treatment of chronic diseases. Moreover, if designed correctly they can promote energy balance and aid in weight control. As with any dietary regimen, the key to designing a healthful vegetarian diet is making appropriate food choices. Table 26.2 presents a sample of vegetarian websites offering recipes, cooking techniques, and additional information on vegetarian diets. Armed with these tools any aspiring vegetarian can easily make the transition to a meat-free diet!

Table 26.1. Plant Foods Rich in Iron and Zinc

Food Source	Iron (mg)	Zinc (mg)
Soybeans, cooked (1/2 cup)	4.4	1.0
Tofu, firm (1/2 cup)	6.6	1.0
Black beans (1/2 cup)	1.2	1.0
Garbanzo beans (1/2 cup)	1.9	1.3
Lentils (1/2 cup)	3.3	1.2
Navy beans (1/2 cup)	2.3	2.3
Almonds (1/4 cup)	2.1	1.2
Pumpkin seeds, dried (1/4 cup)	5.2	2.6
Oatmeal, instant, fortified, cooked (1/2 cup)	4.2	0.7
Cereal, ready-to-eat, fortified (1 oz)	2.1–18	0.7–15
Mushrooms, cooked (1/2 cup)	1.4	0.7
Veggie burgers, fortified (1 oz)	0.5–1.0	1.2–2.3

Table 26.2. Vegetarian Websites

General Information

Loma Linda University Vegetarian Nutrition and Health Letter:
http://llu.edu/llu/vegetarian/vegnews

Food and Nutrition Information Center—Vegetarian Information:
http://nal.usda.gov/fnic/pubs/bibs/gen/vegetarian.htm

Vegetarian Nutrition Dietetic Practice Group of the American Dietetic Association: http://www.vegetariannutrition.net

Vegetarian Resource Group: http://www.vrg.org

Vegan.com: information by Virginia Messina, MPH, RD:
http://vegrd.vegan.com

Recipes and Cooking Tips

Vegetarian Recipes from AllRecipes.com:
http://www.vegetarianrecipe.com

VegWeb: http://www.vegweb.com

Chapter 27

Healthy Eating at Home

Chapter Contents

Section 27.1

The Importance of Family Meals

Family meals are making a comeback. Shared family meals are more likely to be nutritious, and kids who eat regularly with their families are less likely to snack on unhealthy foods and more likely to eat fruits, vegetables, and whole grains.

Teens who take part in regular family meals are less likely to smoke, drink alcohol, or use marijuana and other drugs, and are more likely to have healthier diets as adults, studies have shown.

Beyond health and nutrition, family meals provide a valuable opportunity to reconnect. This becomes even more important as kids get older.

Boost Your Mealtime Mood

Sometimes, it might seem like drudgery to be cooking dinner, especially if you've had a long day. Try to appreciate the opportunity for a family meal. It's so nice to eat together, and not on the run. So sit down, relax, and enjoy your time together.

Making Family Meals Happen

It can be a big challenge to find the time to plan, prepare, and share family meals, then be relaxed enough to enjoy them.

Try these three steps to schedule family meals and make them enjoyable for everyone who pulls up a chair.

1. Plan

To plan more family meals, look over the calendar to choose a time when everyone can be there.

Figure out which obstacles are getting in the way of more family meals—busy schedules, no supplies in the house, no time to cook. Ask for the family's help and ideas on how these roadblocks can be removed. For instance, figure out a way to get groceries purchased for a family meal. Or if time to cook is the problem, try doing some prep work on weekends or even completely preparing a dish ahead of time and putting it in the freezer.

2. Prepare

Once you have all your supplies on hand, involve the kids in preparations. Recruiting younger kids can mean a little extra work, but it's often worth it. Simple tasks such as putting plates on the table, tossing the salad, pouring a beverage, folding the napkins, or being a "taster" are appropriate jobs for preschoolers and school-age kids. Older kids may be able to pitch in even more, such as getting ingredients, washing produce, mixing and stirring, and serving. If you have teens around, consider assigning them a night to cook, with you as the helper.

If kids help out, set a good example by saying please and thanks for their help. Being upbeat and pleasant as you prepare the meal can rub off on your kids. If you're grumbling about the task at hand, chances are they will too. But if the atmosphere is light, you're showing them how the family can work together and enjoy the fruits of its labor. Tell them, "Mmm, something smells delicious!"

3. Enjoy

Even if you're thinking of all you must accomplish after dinner's done (doing dishes, making lunches, etc.), try not to focus on that during dinner. Make your time at the table pleasant and a chance for everyone to decompress from the day and enjoy being together as a family.

They may be starving, but have your kids wait until everyone is seated before digging in. Create a moment of calm before the meal begins, so the cook can shift gears. It also presents a chance to say grace, thank the cook, wish everyone a good meal, or raise a glass of milk and toast each other. You're setting the mood and modeling good manners and patience.

Family meals are a good time to teach civilized behavior that kids also can use at restaurants and others' houses, so establish rules about staying seated, passing items instead of grabbing them, putting napkins on laps, and not talking with your mouth full. You can gently remind when they break the rules, but try to keep tension and discipline at a minimum during mealtime. The focus should remain on making your kids feel nurtured, connected, and part of the family.

Keep the interactions positive and let the conversation flow. Ask your kids about their days and tell them about yours. Give everyone a chance to talk.

Need some conversation starters? Here are a few:

- If you could have any food for dinner tomorrow night, what would it be?

- Who can guess how many potatoes I used to make that bowl of mashed potatoes?

- What's the most delicious food on the table?

- If you opened a restaurant, what kind would it be?

- Who's the best cook you know? (We hope they say it's you!)

Section 27.2

Healthy Cooking and Food Substitutions

"Healthier Preparation Methods for Cooking," reprinted with permission from www.heart.org. © 2010 American Heart Association, Inc.

When you prepare and cook meals at home, you have better control over the nutritional content and the overall healthfulness of the foods you eat. (You can also save money.) Here are some tips for a sensible home kitchen:

Using Healthier Methods of Food Preparation

- Stock up on heart-healthy cookbooks and recipes for cooking ideas.

- Use "choice" or "select" grades of beef rather than "prime," and be sure to trim the fat off the edges before cooking.

- Use cuts of red meat and pork labeled "loin" and "round," as they usually have the least fat.

- With poultry, use the leaner light meat (breasts) instead of the fattier dark meat (legs and thighs), and be sure to remove the skin.

- Make recipes or egg dishes with egg whites, instead of egg yolks. Substitute two egg whites for each egg yolk.

- For recipes that require dairy products, try low-fat or fat-free versions of milk, yogurt, and cheese.

- Use reduced-fat, low-fat, light, or no-fat salad dressings (if you need to limit your calories) on salads, for dips, or as marinades.

- Use and prepare foods that contain little or no salt.

Cooking with Healthier Seasonings

- Avoid using prepackaged seasoning mixes because they often contain a lot of salt. Use fresh herbs whenever possible. Grind herbs with a mortar and pestle for the freshest and fullest flavor.

- Add dried herbs such as thyme, rosemary, and marjoram to dishes for a more pungent flavor—but use them sparingly because they're powerful.

- Use vinegar or citrus juice as wonderful flavor enhancers—but add them at the last moment. Vinegar is great on vegetables, such as greens; and citrus works well on fruits, such as melons.

- Use dry mustard for a zesty flavor when you're cooking, or mix it with water to make a very sharp condiment.

- To add a little more "bite" to your dishes, add some fresh hot peppers. Remove the membrane and seeds first, then finely chop them up. A small amount goes a long way.

- Some vegetables and fruits, such as mushrooms, tomatoes, chili peppers, cherries, cranberries, and currants, have a more intense flavor when dried than when fresh. Add them when you want a burst of flavor.

Preparing and Cooking Foods with Oils

- Use liquid vegetable oils or nonfat cooking sprays whenever possible.

- Whether cooking or making dressings, use the oils that are lowest in saturated fats, *trans* fats, and cholesterol—such as canola oil, corn oil, olive oil, safflower oil, sesame oil, soybean oil, and sunflower oil—but use them sparingly, because they contain 120 calories per tablespoon.

- Stay away from coconut oil, palm oil, and palm kernel oil. Even though they are vegetable oils and have no cholesterol, they are high in saturated fats.

Alternative Cooking Methods to Frying

Instead of frying foods—which adds unnecessary fats and calories— use cooking methods that add little or no fat, like these:

- **Stir-frying:** Use a wok to cook vegetables, poultry, or seafood in vegetable stock, wine, or a small amount of oil. Avoid high-sodium (salt) seasonings like teriyaki and soy sauce.

- **Roasting:** Use a rack in the pan so the meat or poultry doesn't sit in its own fat drippings. Instead of basting with pan drippings, use fat-free liquids like wine, tomato juice, or lemon juice. When making gravy from the drippings, chill first then use a gravy strainer or skim ladle to remove the fat.

- **Grilling and broiling:** Use a rack so the fat drips away from the food.

- **Baking:** Bake foods in covered cookware with a little extra liquid.

- **Poaching:** Cook chicken or fish by immersing it in simmering liquid.

- **Sautéing:** Use a pan made with nonstick metal or a coated, non-stick surface, so you will need to use little or no oil when cooking. Use a nonstick vegetable spray to brown or sauté foods; or, as an alternative, use a small amount of broth or wine, or a tiny bit of vegetable oil rubbed onto the pan with a paper towel.

- **Steaming:** Steam vegetables in a basket over simmering water. They'll retain more flavors and won't need any salt.

Section 27.3

Fun Family Recipes and Tips

This section excerpted from "Fun Family Recipes and Tips," National
Heart, Lung, and Blood Institute (www.nhlbi.nih.gov), 2010.

Food doesn't have to be high in fat to be interesting and delicious.
Get the whole family to help slice, dice, and learn how to put fat and
calories on the kitchen chopping block. You'd be surprised how easy
heart-healthy cooking and snacking can be.

Healthy Family Snacks

- Put sliced apples, berries, or whole-grain cereal on top of low-fat
  plain yogurt.

- Put a slice of low-fat or fat-free cheese on whole-grain crackers.

- Make a whole-wheat pita pocket with hummus, lettuce, tomato,
  and cucumber.

- Pop some low-fat popcorn.

- Microwave or toast a soft tortilla with low-fat cheese, sliced peppers, and mushrooms to make a mini-burrito or quesadilla.

- Blend low-fat milk with a banana or strawberries and some ice
  for a smoothie.

Heart-Healthy Cooking Tips

- Cook with low-fat methods such as baking, broiling, boiling, or
  microwaving rather than frying.

- Choose low-fat or fat-free dairy products, salad dressings, mayonnaise, and other condiments.

- Serve fruit, instead of cookies or ice cream, for dessert.

- Add salsa to baked potatoes, instead of butter or sour cream.

- Eat fruits canned in their own juice instead of syrup.

327

- Remove skin from poultry and discard before cooking.
- Cool soups and gravies and skim off fat before reheating to serve.
- Use the microwave because it's fast and adds no fat or calories.

Table 27.1. Healthy Baking and Cooking Substitutions

Instead of	Substitute
1 cup cream	1 cup evaporated fat-free milk
1 cup butter, margarine, or oil	1/2 cup apple butter or applesauce
1 egg	2 egg whites or 1/4 cup egg substitute
Pastry dough	Graham cracker crumb crust
Butter, margarine, or vegetable oil for sautéing	Cooking spray, chicken broth, or a small amount of olive oil
Bacon	Lean turkey bacon
Ground beef	Extra lean ground beef or ground turkey breast
Sour cream	Fat-free sour cream
1 cup chocolate chips	1/4–1/2 cup mini chocolate chips
1 cup sugar	3/4 cup sugar (this works with nearly everything except yeast breads)
1 cup mayonnaise	1 cup reduced-fat or fat-free mayonnaise
1 cup whole milk	1 cup fat-free milk
1 cup cream cheese	1/2 cup ricotta cheese pureed with 1/2 cup fat-free cream cheese
Oil and vinegar dressing with 3 parts oil to 1 part vinegar	1 part olive oil + 1 part vinegar (preferably a flavored vinegar, such as balsamic) + 1 part orange juice
Unsweetened baking chocolate (1 ounce)	3 tablespoons unsweetened cocoa powder + 1 tablespoon vegetable oil or margarine

Note: Substitute the ingredients in YOUR own favorite recipes to lower the amounts of fat, added sugar, and calories.

Section 27.4

Safe Food Preparation and Handling

This section excerpted from "To Your Health! Food Safety for Seniors," U.S. Food and Drug Administration (www.fda.gov), September 2006. Reviewed by David A. Cooke, MD, FACP, January 2011.

Americans enjoy one of the safest, most healthful food supplies in the world. However, preventing the growth of dangerous microorganisms in food is the key to reducing the millions of illnesses and thousands of deaths each year.

This section will help you learn more about what many of us call "food poisoning"—the experts call it foodborne illness.

Modern Food Safety

It used to be that food was produced close to where people lived. Many people shopped daily and prepared and ate their food at home. Eating in restaurants was saved for special occasions. Today, food in your local grocery store comes from all over the world. And nearly 50% of the money we spend on food goes to buy food that others prepare, like "carry out" and restaurant meals.

Another thing that has changed is our awareness and knowledge of illnesses that can be caused by harmful bacteria in food:

- Through science, we have discovered new and dangerous bacteria and viruses that can be found in food—bacteria we didn't even know about years ago.

- Science has also helped us identify illnesses that can be caused by bacteria and viruses in food—illnesses we didn't recognize before. Today, for instance, we realize that some illnesses, like some kinds of arthritis, can be traced to foodborne illness.

- One of the other things that we know today is that some people can be more susceptible to getting sick from bacteria in food.

Why Some People Face Special Risks

Some people are more likely to get sick from harmful bacteria that can be found in food. And once they are sick, they face the risk of more serious health problems, even death.

A variety of people may face these special risks—pregnant women and young children, people with chronic illnesses and weakened immune systems, and older adults, including people over 65.

Recognizing Foodborne Illness

It can be difficult for people to recognize when harmful bacteria in food have made them sick. For instance, it's hard to tell if food is unsafe because you can't see, smell, or taste the bacteria it may contain.

Sometimes people think their foodborne illness was caused by their last meal. In fact, there is a wide range of time between eating food with harmful bacteria and the onset of illness. Usually foodborne bacteria take 1 to 3 days to cause illness. But you could become sick anytime from 20 minutes to 6 weeks after eating some foods with dangerous bacteria. It depends on a variety of factors, including the type of bacteria in the food.

Sometimes foodborne illness is confused with other types of illness. If you get foodborne illness, you might be sick to your stomach, vomit, or have diarrhea. Or symptoms could be flu-like with a fever and headache and body aches. The best thing to do is check with your doctor. And if you become ill after eating out, also call your local health department so they can investigate.

Foodborne illness can be dangerous but is often easy to prevent. By following the basic rules of food safety, you can help prevent foodborne illness for yourself and others.

Food Safety at Home

Just follow four basic rules—clean, separate, cook, and chill—and you will Fight BAC!® (bacteria that can cause foodborne illness.) Fight BAC! is a national education campaign designed to teach everyone about food safety. Keep these Fight BAC! rules in mind. Tell your friends and family and grandchildren to join the team and get them to be "BAC-Fighters" too.

Clean: Wash Hands and Surfaces Often

Bacteria can be present throughout the kitchen, including on cutting boards, utensils, sponges, and counter tops.

- Wash your hands with warm water and soap before and after handling food and after using the bathroom, changing diapers, or handling pets.

- Wash your cutting boards, dishes, utensils, and countertops with hot water and soap after preparing each food item and before you go on to the next food. Periodically, kitchen sanitizers (including a solution of one tablespoon of unscented, liquid chlorine bleach to one gallon of water) can be used for added protection.

- Once cutting boards (including plastic, nonporous, acrylic, and wooden boards) become excessively worn or develop hard-to-clean grooves, you should replace them.

- Consider using paper towels to clean up kitchen surfaces. If you use cloth towels, wash them often in the hot cycle of your washing machine.

- Rinse raw produce in water. Don't use soap or other detergents. If necessary—and appropriate—use a small vegetable brush to remove surface dirt.

Separate: Don't Cross-Contaminate

Cross-contamination is the scientific word for how bacteria can be spread from one food product to another. This is especially true when handling raw meat, poultry, and seafood, so keep these foods and their juices away from foods that aren't going to be cooked.

- Separate raw meat, poultry, and seafood from other foods in your grocery-shopping cart and in your refrigerator.

- If possible, use a different cutting board for raw meat, poultry, and seafood products.

- Always wash cutting boards, dishes, and utensils with hot, soapy water after they come in contact with raw meat, poultry, seafood, eggs, and unwashed fresh produce.

- Place cooked food on a clean plate. If you put cooked food on the unwashed plate that held raw food (like meat, poultry, or seafood), bacteria from the raw food could contaminate your cooked food.

Cook: Cook to Proper Temperatures

Food safety experts agree that foods are safely cooked when they are heated for a long enough time and at a high enough temperature to kill the harmful bacteria that cause foodborne illness.

- Use a clean food thermometer, which measures the internal temperature of cooked foods, to make sure meat, poultry, and other foods are safely cooked all the way through.

- Cook beef, veal, and lamb roasts and steaks to at least 145° F. Cook all poultry to a safe minimum internal temperature of 165° F or to higher temperatures according to personal preference.

- Cook ground beef, where bacteria can spread during processing, to at least 160° F. Check the temperature with a food thermometer.

- Cook eggs until the yolk and white are firm. Don't use recipes in which eggs remain raw or only partially cooked.

- Fish should be opaque and flake easily with a fork.

- When cooking in a microwave oven, make sure there are no cold spots in food where bacteria can survive. To do this, cover food, stir, and rotate the dish by hand once or twice during cooking. (Unless you have a turntable in the microwave.) Use a food thermometer to make sure foods have reached a safe internal temperature.

- If you are reheating food, leftovers should be heated to 165° F. Bring sauces, soup, and gravy to a boil.

Cooking food—especially raw meat, poultry, fish, and eggs—to a safe minimum internal temperature kills harmful bacteria. Thoroughly cook food as follows:

Ground Products
- Beef, veal, lamb, pork: 160° F
- Chicken, turkey: 165° F

Beef, Veal, Lamb Roasts, and Steaks
- Medium-rare: 145° F
- Medium: 160° F
- Well-done: 170° F

Pork
- Chops, roast, ribs
  - Medium: 160° F
  - Well-done: 170° F

- Ham, fully cooked: 140° F
- Ham, fresh: 160° F
- Sausage, fresh: 160° F

Poultry (Turkey and Chicken)

- Whole bird: at least 165° F
- Breast: at least 165° F
- Legs and thighs: at least 165° F
- Stuffing (cooked separately): 165° F

Eggs and Fish

- Fried, poached: yolk and white are firm
- Casseroles: 160° F
- Sauces, custards: 160° F
- Fish: flakes with a fork

Chill: Did You Know?

At room temperature, bacteria in food can double every 20 minutes. The more bacteria there are, the greater the chance you could become sick.

So refrigerate foods quickly because cold temperatures keep most harmful bacteria from multiplying. A lot of people think it will harm their refrigerator to put hot food inside—it's not true. It won't harm your refrigerator and it will keep your food—and you—safe.

Set your home refrigerator to 40° F or below and the freezer unit to 0° F or below. Check the temperature occasionally with an appliance thermometer.

Then, follow these steps:

- Refrigerate or freeze perishables, prepared food, and leftovers within two hours.
- Divide large amounts of leftovers into shallow containers for quick cooling in the refrigerator.

Safe Thawing

Never thaw foods at room temperature. You can safely thaw food in the refrigerator. Four to five pounds takes 24 hours to thaw.

Table 27.2. Refrigerator and Freezer Storage Chart

Food	Refrigerator (40° F)	Freezer (0° F)
Eggs		
Fresh, in shell	4–5 weeks	Don't freeze
Hard cooked	1 week	Doesn't freeze well
Egg substitutes, opened	3 days	Don't freeze
Egg substitutes, unopened	10 days	1 year
Dairy Products		
Milk	1 week	3 months
Cottage cheese	1 week	Doesn't freeze well
Yogurt	1–2 weeks	1–2 months
Commercial mayonnaise (refrigerate after opening)	2 months	Don't freeze
Vegetables	Raw	Blanched/cooked
Beans, green or waxed	3–4 days	8 months
Carrots	2 weeks	10–12 months
Celery	1–2 weeks	10–12 months
Lettuce, leaf	3–7 days	Don't freeze
Lettuce, iceberg	1–2 weeks	Don't freeze
Spinach	1–2 days	10–12 months
Squash, summer	4–5 days	10–12 months
Squash, winter	2 weeks	10–12 months
Tomatoes	2–3 days	2 months
Deli Foods		
Entrees, cold or hot	3–4 days	2–3 months
Store–prepared or homemade salads	3–5 days	Don't freeze
Hot Dogs and Luncheon Meats		
Hot dogs, opened package	1 week	
Hot dogs, unopened package	2 weeks	1–2 months in freezer wrap
Lunch meats, opened	3–5 days	1–2 months
Lunch meats, unopened	2 weeks	1–2 months
TV Dinners/Frozen Casseroles		
Keep frozen until ready to serve		3–4 months

Table 27.2. *continued*

Food	Refrigerator (40° F)	Freezer (0° F)
Fresh Meat		
Beef steaks, roasts	3–5 days	6–12 months
Pork chops, roasts	3–5 days	4–6 months
Lamb chops, roasts	3–5 days	6–9 months
Veal roast	3–5 days	4–6 months
Fresh Poultry		
Chicken or turkey, whole	1–2 days	1 year
Chicken or turkey pieces	1–2 days	9 months
Fresh Fish		
Lean fish (cod, flounder, etc.)	1–2 days	6 months
Fatty fish (salmon, etc.)	1–2 days	2–3 months
Ham		
Canned ham (label says "keep refrigerated")	6–9 months	Don't freeze
Ham, fully cooked (half and slices)	3–5 days	1–2 months
Bacon and Sausage		
Bacon	1 week	1 month
Sausage, raw (pork, beef, or turkey)	1–2 days	1–2 months
Precooked smoked breakfast links/patties	1 week	1–2 months
Leftovers		
Cooked meat, meat dishes, egg dishes, soups, stews, and vegetables	3–4 days	2–3 months
Gravy and meat broth	1–2 days	2–3 months
Cooked poultry and fish	3–4 days	4–6 months

Fresh Produce

The quality of certain perishable fresh fruits and vegetables (such as strawberries, lettuce, herbs, and mushrooms) can be maintained best by storing in the refrigerator. If you are uncertain whether an item should be refrigerated to maintain quality, ask your grocer. All produce purchased precut or peeled should be refrigerated. Produce cut or peeled at home should be refrigerated within two hours. Any cut or peeled produce that is left at room temperature for more than two hours should be discarded.

You can also thaw food outside the refrigerator by immersing in cold water. Change the water every half hour to keep the water cold. Cook immediately after thawing.

You can thaw food in the microwave, but if you do, be sure to continue cooking right away.

- Marinate foods in the refrigerator.

- Don't pack the refrigerator too full. Cold air must circulate to keep food safe.

Eating Out, Bringing In

Let's face it. Sometimes it's just easier and more enjoyable to let someone else do the cooking. All of these options, however, do have food safety implications that you need to be aware of.

Bringing In: Complete Meals to Go and Home-Delivered Meals

When you want to eat at home but don't feel like cooking or aren't able to, where do you turn?

- Many convenience foods, including complete meals to go, are increasingly popular.

- Purchased from grocery stores, deli stores, or restaurants, some meals are hot and some are cold.

- Ordering home-delivered meals from restaurants or restaurant-delivery services is an option many consumers like to take advantage of.

- And, of course, for those who qualify, there are programs like Meals on Wheels that provide a ready-prepared meal each day.

Hot or cold ready-prepared meals are perishable and can cause illness when mishandled. Proper handling is essential to ensure the food is safe.

The Two-Hour Rule

Harmful bacteria can multiply in the "Danger Zone" (between 40° F and 140° F). So remember the two-hour rule. Discard any perishable foods left at room temperature longer than two hours. When temperatures are above 90° F, discard food after one hour!

When you purchase hot cooked food, keep it hot. Eat and enjoy your food within two hours to prevent harmful bacteria from multiplying.

If you are not eating within two hours—and you want to keep your food hot—keep your food in the oven set at a high enough temperature to keep the food at or above 140° F. (Use a food thermometer to check the temperature.) Side dishes, like stuffing, must also stay hot in the oven. Covering food will help keep it moist.

However, your cooked food will taste better if you don't try to keep it in the oven for too long. For best taste, refrigerate the food and then reheat when you are ready to eat. Here's how:

- Divide meat or poultry into small portions to refrigerate or freeze.

- Refrigerate or freeze gravy, potatoes, and other vegetables in shallow containers.

- Remove stuffing from whole cooked poultry and refrigerate.

Cold foods should be eaten within two hours or refrigerated or frozen for eating at another time.

Reheating

You may wish to reheat your meal, whether it was purchased hot and then refrigerated or purchased cold initially.

- Heat the food thoroughly to 165° F.

- Bring gravy to a rolling boil.

- If heating in a microwave oven, cover food and rotate the dish so the food heats evenly and doesn't leave "cold spots" that could harbor bacteria.

Eating Out

Whether you're eating out at a restaurant or a fast food diner, it can be both a safe and enjoyable experience. All food service establishments are required to follow food safety guidelines set by state and local health departments. But you can also take actions to ensure your food's safety. Keep these Fight BAC!® rules in mind: clean, cook, chill.

Clean: When you go out to eat, look at how clean things are before you even sit down. If it's not up to your standards, you might want to eat somewhere else.

Cook: No matter where you eat out, always order your food cooked thoroughly to a safe internal temperature. Remember that foods like meat, poultry, fish, and eggs need to be cooked thoroughly to kill harmful bacteria. When you're served a hot meal, make sure it's served to you piping hot and thoroughly cooked, and if it's not, send it back.

Don't eat undercooked or raw foods, such as raw oysters or raw or undercooked eggs. Undercooked or raw eggs can be a hidden hazard in some foods like Caesar salad, custards, and some sauces. If these foods are made with commercially pasteurized eggs, however, they are safe. If you are unsure about the ingredients in a particular dish, ask before ordering it.

Chill: It seems like meal portions are getting bigger and bigger these days. A lot of people are packing up these leftovers to eat later. Care must be taken when handling these leftovers. If you will not be arriving home within two hours of being served (one hour if temperatures are above 90° F), it is safer to leave the leftovers at the restaurant.

Also, remember that the inside of a car can get very warm. Bacteria may grow rapidly, so it is always safer to go directly home after eating and put your leftovers in the refrigerator.

Chapter 28

Healthy Eating Out

Chapter Contents

Section 28.1

Tips for Eating Out

This section excerpted from "Tips for Eating Healthy When Eating Out," ChooseMyPlate.gov, U.S. Department of Agriculture (www.choosemyplate .gov), May 27, 2011, and "Tipsheet: Eating Healthy Ethnic Food," National Heart, Lung, and Blood Institute (www.nhlbi.nih.gov), August 2005.

Tips for Eating Healthy when Eating Out

- As a beverage choice, ask for water or order fat-free or low-fat milk, unsweetened tea, or other drinks without added sugars.

- Ask for whole-wheat bread for sandwiches.

- In a restaurant, start your meal with a salad packed with veggies to help control hunger and feel satisfied sooner.

- Ask for salad dressing to be served on the side. Then use only as much as you want.

- Choose main dishes that include vegetables, such as stir-fries, kebobs, or pasta with a tomato sauce.

- Order steamed, grilled, or broiled dishes instead of those that are fried or sautéed.

- Choose a "small" or "medium" portion. This includes main dishes, side dishes, and beverages.

- Order an item from the menu instead heading for the "all-you-can-eat" buffet.

- If main portions at a restaurant are larger than you want, try one of these strategies to keep from overeating:

  - Order an appetizer-sized portion or a side dish instead of an entrée.

  - Share a main dish with a friend.

  - If you can chill the extra food right away, take leftovers home in a doggy bag.

- When your food is delivered, set aside or pack half of it to go immediately.

- Resign from the "clean your plate club"—when you've eaten enough, leave the rest.

- Follow these tips to keep your meal moderate in calories, fat, and sugars:

  - Ask for salad dressing to be served on the side so you can add only as much as you want.

  - Order foods that do not have creamy sauces or gravies.

  - Add little or no butter to your food.

  - Choose fruits for dessert most often.

- On long commutes or shopping trips, pack some fresh fruit, cut-up vegetables, low-fat string cheese sticks, or a handful of un-salted nuts to help you avoid stopping for sweet or fatty snacks.

Eating Healthy Ethnic Food

Trying different ethnic cuisines to give yourself a taste treat is possible while counting calories and fat. Many ethnic cuisines offer lots of low-fat, low-calorie choices.

So if you want to eat healthy and still have lots of different choices, take a taste adventure with ethnic foods. Here's a sample of healthy food choices (lower in calories and fat) and terms to look for when making your selection:

Chinese

- Zheng (steamed)
- Kao (roasted)
- Steamed rice
- Jum (poached)
- Shao (barbecued)
- Dishes without monosodium glutamate (MSG) added

Italian

- Red sauces
- Piccata (lemon)
- Crushed tomatoes
- Grilled
- Primavera (no cream)
- Sun-dried tomatoes
- Lightly sautéed

341

Mexican

- Spicy chicken
- Salsa or picante

- Rice and black beans
- Soft corn tortillas

Section 28.2

Making Healthy Fast Food Choices

"Healthy Fast Food: Tips for Making Healthier Fast Food Choices" by Maya W. Paul and Lawrence Robinson. © 2010 Helpguide.org. All rights reserved. Reprinted with permission. Helpguide provides a detailed list of references and resources for this article, including links to related Helpguide topics and information from other websites. For a complete list of these resources, including information about finding healthy fast food and coping with special dietary needs, go to http://helpguide.org/life/fast_food_nutrition.htm.

Fast food is cheap, convenient, filling, and to many of us it tastes good. If you are eating out, a fast food restaurant is often the cheapest option, but unfortunately not a healthy one. Eating just one fast food meal can pack enough calories, sodium, and fat for an entire day or more. Eating fast food on a regular basis can lead to a host of different health problems, both physical and psychological.

Still, in a bad economy the quick-and-cheap temptation can often be hard to resist. As an informed customer, though, you can make healthier choices and still enjoy the price and convenience of fast food restaurants.

When Is It Healthy to Eat Fast Food?

The short answer is: rarely. Typically, fast food is low in nutrition and high in trans fat, saturated fat, sodium, and calories. Some examples:

- One sack of hash bites or potato snackers from White Castle, for example, contains 10 grams of very unhealthy trans fat. The American Heart Association recommends we consume less than 2 grams of trans fat per day. So in one side order, you've just eaten more than five days' worth of heart-busting trans fat!

- A single meal of a Double Whopper with cheese, a medium order of fries, and an apple pie from Burger King contains more saturated fat than the American Heart Association recommends we consume in two days.

Moderation becomes the key. It's okay to indulge a craving for french fries every now and then, but to stay healthy you can't make it a regular habit. Finding a healthy, well-balanced meal in most fast food restaurants can be a challenge, but there are always choices you can make that are healthier than others.

Learning to Make Healthier Choices at Fast Food Restaurants

Making healthier choices at fast food restaurants is easier if you prepare ahead by checking guides that show you the nutritional content of meal choices at your favorite restaurants. Free downloadable guides help you evaluate your options. If you have a special dietary concern, such as diabetes, heart health, or weight loss, the websites of national nonprofits provide useful advice. You can also choose to patronize restaurants that focus on natural, high quality food.

If you don't prepare ahead of time, common sense guidelines help to make your meal healthier. For example, a seemingly healthy salad can be a diet minefield when smothered in high-fat dressing and fried toppings, so choose a salad with fresh veggies, grilled toppings, and a lighter dressing. Portion control is also important, as many fast food restaurants serve enough food for several meals in the guise of a single serving.

Tips for Making Healthy Choices at Fast Food Restaurants

- **Make careful menu selections**. Pay attention to the descriptions on the menu. Dishes labeled deep-fried, pan-fried, basted, batter-dipped, breaded, creamy, crispy, scalloped, Alfredo, au gratin, or in cream sauce are usually high in calories, unhealthy fats, or sodium. Order items with more vegetables and choose leaner meats.

- **Drink water with your meal.** Soda is a huge source of hidden calories. One 32-oz Big Gulp with regular cola packs about 425 calories, so one Big Gulp can quickly gulp up a big portion of your daily calorie intake. Try adding a little lemon to your water or ordering unsweetened iced tea.

343

- **"Undress" your food.** When choosing items, be aware of calorie- and fat-packed salad dressings, spreads, cheese, sour cream, etc. For example, ask for a grilled chicken sandwich without the mayonnaise. You can ask for a packet of ketchup or mustard and add it yourself, controlling how much you put on your sandwich.

- **Special order.** Many menu items would be healthy if it weren't for the way they were prepared. Ask for your vegetables and main dishes to be served without the sauces. Ask for olive oil and vinegar for your salads or order the dressing "on the side" and spoon only a small amount on at a time. If your food is fried or cooked in oil or butter, ask to have it broiled or steamed.

- **Eat mindfully.** Pay attention to what you eat and savor each bite. Chew your food more thoroughly and avoid eating on the run. Being mindful also means stopping before you are full. It takes time for our bodies to register that we have eaten. Mindful eating relaxes you, so you digest better, and makes you feel more satisfied.

Tips for What to AVOID at Fast Food Restaurants

- **Supersized portions.** An average fast food meal can run to 1,000 calories or more, so choose a smaller portion size, order a side salad instead of fries, and don't supersize anything. At a typical restaurant, a single serving provides enough for two meals. Take half home or divide the portion with a dining partner.

- **Salt.** Fast food restaurant food tends to be very high in sodium, a major contributor to high blood pressure. Don't add insult to injury by adding more salt.

- **Bacon.** It's always tempting to add bacon to sandwiches and salads for extra flavor, but bacon has very few nutrients and is high in fat and calories. Instead, try ordering extra pickles, onions, lettuce, tomatoes, or mustard to add flavor without the fat.

- **Buffets**—even seemingly healthy ones like salad bars. You'll likely overeat to get your money's worth. If you do choose buffet dining, opt for fresh fruits, salads with olive oil and vinegar or low-fat dressings, broiled entrees, and steamed vegetables. Resist the temptation to go for seconds, or wait at least 20 minutes after eating to make sure you're really still hungry before going back for more.

Watch your fast food sodium intake: High salt/sodium intake is a major contributor to cardiovascular disease. The American Heart Association recommends that adults stay under 1,500 mg of sodium per day, and never take in more than 2,300 mg a day. A study by the New York City Health Department surveyed 6,580 meals bought at fast-food restaurant chains and found that:

- about 57% of the meals exceeded the 1,500-mg daily sodium level;

- fried chicken outlets including KFC and Popeye's were the worst offenders, with 83% of meals exceeding 1,500 mg of sodium and 55% of the meals surpassing 2,300 mg of sodium;

- at only one of the 11 chains included in the study, Au Bon Pain, did more than 7% of meals contain less than 600 mg, the FDA's "healthy" sodium level for meals. But even there, 46% of meals had 1,500 mg or more of sodium;

- even those eating lower calorie meals were likely to exceed their daily sodium limit within a single meal.

Source: MedPage Today [www.medpagetoday.com/PrimaryCare/DietNutrition/19771]

Guides Can Help You Make Healthier Meal Choices

Many fast food chains post nutritional information on their websites. Unfortunately, these lists are often confusing and hard to use. Instead you can go to other websites that provide health and nutrition information, but in easier to follow formats. Some even publish comparison downloadable guides or inexpensive pocket guides. Learn how to make a healthier meal selection at your favorite restaurant:

- **HealthyDiningFinder.com** allows you to search for restaurants offering a selection of healthier menu options and view the nutrition data for selected items. You can search for area restaurants or a specific restaurant.

- **Stop&Go Fast Food Nutrition Guide [www.fastfoodbook. com]:** This guide is particularly convenient and easy to use. Look up any of the major chain restaurants and find out how to make healthier choices.

Guides for Your Individual Needs

There are many websites geared toward how to make healthy choices at restaurants depending on your specific dietary needs, whether it is for diabetes, cancer, heart disease, or weight management. For more information, see helpguide.org/life/fast_food_nutrition.htm#related.

Healthier Fast Food at Burger Chains

Figuring out healthier options at your favorite fast food burger chain can be tricky. A typical meal at a burger joint consists of a "sandwich," some fries, and a drink, which can quickly come in at over 1,700 calories for something like Burger King's Triple Whopper with a large fries and a 16-oz. soda. A better option would be a regular single patty burger, small fries, and water, which is about 500 calories.

Alternatively you may enjoy a veggie burger smothered in grilled onion and mushrooms. Or if you want a large beef burger, then skip the fries and soda and have a side salad and water instead.

The Big Burger Chains

Less Healthy Choices

1. Double-patty hamburger with cheese, mayo, special sauce, and bacon

2. Fried chicken sandwich

3. Fried fish sandwich

4. Salad with toppings such as bacon, cheese, and ranch dressing

5. Breakfast burrito with steak

6. French fries

7. Milkshake

8. Chicken "nuggets" or tenders

9. Adding cheese, extra mayo, and special sauces

Healthier Choices

1. Regular, single-patty hamburger without mayo or cheese

2. Grilled chicken sandwich

3. Veggie burger

4. Garden salad with grilled chicken and low-fat dressing

5. Egg on a muffin

6. Baked potato or a side salad

7.   Yogurt parfait

8.   Grilled chicken strips

9.   Limiting cheese, mayo, and special sauces

For a healthier fast food option at a burger restaurant try:

- **McDonald's Hamburger:** 260 calories, 9 g fat (3.5 g saturated fat)

- **Wendy's Jr. Hamburger:** 280 calories, 9 g fat (3.5 g saturated fat)

Healthier Fast Food at Fried Chicken Chains

Although certain chains have been advertising "no trans fats" in their food, the fact is that fried chicken can pack quite a fattening punch. According to the restaurant's nutrition info, just a single Extra Crispy Chicken breast at KFC has a whopping 440 calories, 27 g of fat, and 970 mg of sodium. A healthier choice is the drumstick, which has 160 calories, 10 g of fat, and 370 mg of sodium. Alternatively, if you like the breast meat, take off the skin and it becomes a healthy choice at 140 calories, 2 g of fat, and 520 mg of sodium.

Some tips for making smarter choices at fast food chicken restaurants:

The Big Fried Chicken Chains

Less Healthy Choices

1.   Fried chicken, original or extra-crispy

2.   Teriyaki wings or popcorn chicken

3.   Caesar salad

4.   Chicken and biscuit "bowl"

5.   Adding extra gravy and sauces

Healthier Choices

1.   Skinless chicken breast without breading

2.   Honey BBQ chicken sandwich

3.   Garden salad

4.   Mashed potatoes

5.   Limiting gravy and sauces

For a healthier fast food option at a fried chicken restaurant try:

- **KFC Original Recipe Chicken Breast (with breading and skin removed) and a side of green beans:** 190 calories, 4.5 g fat (1.5 g saturated fat)

Healthy Fast Food: Mexican Chains

Fast food chains that specialize in tacos or burritos can be caloric minefields or they can be a good option for finding healthy fast food. Rice, beans, salsa, and a few slices of fresh avocado can make a very healthy meal. But adding cheese, sour cream, and tortilla chips can turn even a good meal unhealthy. Be sure to also remember portion control since these types of restaurants can have enormous menu items (eat half and take the rest for another meal).

Several chains, like Taco Bell and Baja Fresh, have "healthy" menu options that feature less fat and fresher ingredients.

The Big Taco Chains

Less Healthy Choices

1. Crispy shell chicken taco

2. Refried beans

3. Steak chalupa

4. Crunch wraps or gordita-type burritos

5. Nachos with refried beans

6. Adding sour cream or cheese

Healthier Choices

1. Grilled chicken soft taco

2. Black beans

3. Shrimp ensalada

4. Grilled "fresco" style steak burrito

5. Veggie and bean burrito

6. Limiting sour cream or cheese

For a healthier fast food option at a Mexican restaurant try:

- **Taco Bell Taco Salad (without the shell, sour cream, or cheese):** 330 calories, 13 g fat (5 g saturated fat)

Healthy Fast Food: Sub Sandwich Chains

Americans love all types of sandwiches: hot, cold, wrapped, foot long. Usually eaten with a salad instead of fries. The ads promote the health benefits of sandwich shops. Easier said than done … studies have found that many people tend to eat more calories per meal at a sub shop than at McDonald's. This may be because people feel so virtuous eating "healthy" like the ads promise that they reward themselves with chips, sodas, or extra condiments.

You can make healthier choices at a deli or sub shop but you need to use some common sense.

Subs, Sandwich, and Deli Choices

Less Healthy Choices

1.   Foot-long sub

2.   High-fat meat such as ham, tuna salad, bacon, meatballs, or steak

3.   The "normal" amount of higher-fat (cheddar, American) cheese

4.   Adding mayo and special sauces

5.   Keeping the sub "as is" with all toppings

6.   Choosing white bread or "wraps" which are often higher in fat than normal bread

Healthier Choices

1.   Six-inch sub

2.   Lean meat (roast beef, chicken breast, lean ham) or veggies

3.   One or two slices of lower-fat cheese (Swiss or mozzarella)

4.   Adding low-fat dressing or mustard instead of mayo

5.   Adding extra veggie toppings

6.   Choosing whole-grain bread or taking the top slice off your sub and eating it open-faced

For a healthier fast food option at a sub sandwich restaurant try:

- **Subway Six-Inch Roast Beef Sub (on whole wheat bread with veggies, no mayo):** 290 calories, 5 g fat (2 g saturated fat)

Healthy Asian Food

Asian cultures tend to eat very healthfully, with an emphasis on veggies, and with meat used as a "condiment" rather than being the focus of the meal. Unfortunately, Americanized versions of these ethnic foods tend to be much higher in fat and calories—so caution is needed. But here's a great tip for all Asian restaurants—use the chopsticks! You'll eat more slowly, since you can't grasp as much food with them at one time as you can with your normal fork and knife.

Asian Food Choices

Less Healthy Choices

1. Fried egg rolls, spare ribs, tempura
2. Battered or deep-fried dishes (sweet and sour pork, General Tso's chicken)
3. Deep-fried tofu
4. Coconut milk, sweet and sour sauce, regular soy sauce
5. Fried rice
6. Salads with fried or crispy noodles

Healthier Choices

1. Egg drop, miso, wonton, or hot and sour soup
2. Stir-fried, steamed, roasted, or broiled entrees (shrimp chow mein, chop suey)
3. Steamed or baked tofu
4. Sauces such as ponzu, rice-wine vinegar, wasabi, ginger, and low-sodium soy sauce
5. Steamed brown rice
6. Edamame, cucumber salad, stir-fried veggies

For a healthier fast food option at a Chinese restaurant try:

- **Panda Express Tangy Shrimp with a side of mixed veggies:** 260 calories, 7.5 g fat (1.5 g saturated fat)

Healthy Italian Fast Food

The anti-carbohydrate revolution has given Italian food a bad rap, but Italian is actually one of the easiest types of cuisine to make healthy. Stay away from fried, oily, or overly buttery, as well as thick-crust menu items, and you can keep your diet goals intact.

Watch out for the following terms, which are common culprits of high fat and calories: alfredo, carbonara, saltimbocca, parmigiana, lasagna, manicotti, stuffed (all have heavy amounts of cream and cheese). Generally Italian places have lots of veggies in their kitchen so it's easy to ask to have extra veggies added to your meal.

Italian and Pizza Restaurant Choices

Less Healthy Choices

1. Thick-crust or butter-crust pizza with extra cheese and meat toppings

2. Garlic bread

3. Antipasto with meat

4. Pasta with cream or butter-based sauce

5. Entree with side of pasta

6. Fried ("frito") dishes

Healthier Choices

1. Thin-crust pizza with half the cheese and extra veggies

2. Plain rolls or breadsticks

3. Antipasto with vegetables

4. Pasta with tomato sauce and veggies

5. Entree with side of veggies

6. Grilled ("griglia") dishes

For a healthier fast food option at a pizza restaurant try:

- **Pizza Hut Fit 'N Delicious Chicken & Veggie Pizza (2 slices):** 208 calories, 9 g fat (4 g saturated fat)

Chains with Natural, High-Quality Fast Food

Whether you choose to eat fast food at a McDonald's, a Subway, or a local deli, there are always menu choices that are healthier than others. However, some fast food restaurants offer a greater variety of healthy menu choices than others. In a recent survey of the 100 largest fast food chains in America, *Health* magazine compiled a list of the healthiest fast food restaurants. The top five were:

Panera Bread provides a wide variety of healthy menu options, half-sized portions, and organic chicken. Plenty of healthy choices on the kids' menu, too, but avoid the sticky buns on display at the counter.

Jason's Deli uses organic ingredients and encourages portion control by offering smaller meals at a discounted price. Beware of the sodium content of their sandwiches, though.

Au Bon Pain serves healthy, low-calorie soups, salads, and sandwiches using whole grains and organic chicken. Nutritional information is posted at each restaurant, so it's a good idea to check the sodium content before ordering.

Noodles and Company cooks noodle bowls using healthy soybean oil, fresh vegetables, and organic meat and tofu. The desserts, however, are much less healthy.

Corner Bakery and Café offers healthy breakfast choices, plus healthy salads, sandwiches, and soup. Check their website for nutritional information first, though, as it's not available in the restaurants.

Chapter 29

Sports Nutrition

Chapter Contents

Section 29.1

Nutrition for Athletes

"Nutrition: Who Needs It? If You're an Athlete, You Do!" by Jane LeBlond, MS, and Katherine Beals, Ph.D., R.D., FACSM. Reprinted with permission of the American College of Sports Medicine, ACSM Fit Society® Page, Winter 2007, pp 5–6. © 2007 American College of Sports Medicine (www.acsm.org).

Carbohydrates, protein, and fat are all needed to fuel performance, repair and build lean muscle tissue, and protect against injury and illness. The Dietary Reference Intakes for normal adults specify a diet of 45% to 65% of total calories from carbohydrates, 10% to 35% protein, and 20% to 35% fat.

Many athletes wonder if these same recommendations apply to them or if they require a separate set of unique recommendations. The answer is yes and no. These ranges are broad enough to encompass the needs of most athletes. Nonetheless, many sport dietitians prefer to tailor carbohydrate, protein, and even fat recommendations to an athlete's body weight, thereby creating an absolute amount (i.e., a specific number of grams) as opposed to a relative amount (i.e., percent of total calories). Here are some general guidelines for formulating carbohydrate, protein, and fat recommendations for athletes.

Carbohydrates

Carbohydrates are the body's primary source of energy, and are stored in the muscle and liver as glycogen. These glycogen stores provide fuel during moderate to intense exercise, and provide the brain with energy to focus and concentrate. Carbohydrate recommendations for athletes are typically formulated based on the athlete's body weight. Elite athletes (those in high-training college athletics, or professional or Olympic athletics) require 7 to 10 grams per kilogram of body weight (approximately 3 to 5 grams per pound). For most recreational athletes, 5 to 8 grams of carbohydrate per kilogram (approximately 2 to 3 grams per pound) per day is enough to replace and maintain muscle glycogen stores used during a workout or game. For example, a 150-pound runner training for a 10K would need to take in between

300 and 450 grams of carbohydrates per day. Good sources of carbohydrates include fruits and fruit juices, rice, cereals, potatoes, pasta, and bread. Choosing whole grains like oatmeal and brown rice will add fiber, B vitamins, and a little protein to your meal, while helping you feel full for longer.

Grams of Carbohydrate per Food Source

- 1 medium banana: 27 g
- 1 cup orange juice: 26 g
- 1 cup brown rice: 45 g
- 1 cup oatmeal: 25 g
- 1 medium potato: 32 g
- 1 cup pasta: 40 g
- 2 pieces whole wheat bread: 26 g

Carbohydrates also serve a critical role in exercise recovery. Eating or drinking a high-carbohydrate snack within an hour of exercising speeds recovery and prepares you for your next exercise session. Pack along a piece of fruit, some orange juice, or a granola bar when exercising away from home so you can refuel as soon after your workout as possible.

Protein

Protein has many important functions in the body. In addition to building muscle and connective tissue, it supports the immune system and is used to make enzymes and hormones involved in energy metabolism. Protein requirements for athletes are higher than those of sedentary individuals, but not high enough to require protein supplements or shakes. Because of protein's relationship to lean body mass, protein requirements for athletes are formulated based on body weight. Most athletes need between 1.2–1.7 grams of protein per kilogram of body weight per day (approximately 0.5–0.75 grams per pound) for muscle repair and maintenance. For example, a 175-pound body builder lifting weights four to five days per week would require about 1.4 grams of protein per kilogram body weight, or about 111 grams of protein per day. Watch out, though—eating more protein won't build muscle faster. In fact, just the opposite could happen—excess protein may contribute to increased body fat. The reason? The body has a limit as to how much protein it needs, and if you exceed that limit, the excess protein will be converted to fat and stored on the body! Moreover, animal protein is also high in saturated fat and cholesterol; too much could lead to elevated blood lipid levels and increased heart disease risk. There is currently some disagreement over what the upper limit to protein intake is, but the bulk of the research suggests consuming no more than 1.8–2.0 grams of protein per kilogram body weight per day. Good sources of protein are eggs, fish, lean meats, and low-fat or non-fat dairy products. In addition, including more plant sources of protein in your diet, such as soy, beans, and legumes, may be beneficial as they are very low fat, have no cholesterol, and are rich in folate and fiber.

Grams of Protein per Food Source

- 1 egg: 6 g
- 4 oz steak: 30 g
- 1 cup soy milk: 7 g
- 1/2 cup refried beans: 7 g
- 1/2 can tuna: 20 g
- 1/2 cup cottage cheese: 13 g
- 1 oz almonds: 6 g

Fat

Athletes often avoid dietary fats in an effort to keep body weight down, but some fats are actually good for us and have an important place in an athlete's diet. Saturated fat, which is mostly found in animal products and fried foods, and trans fats, which are found in processed baked goods and snack foods, both increase cholesterol and raise your risk of heart disease. However, unsaturated fats, especially the omega-3 fatty acids found in fish, can actually protect against chronic disease. These fats have been shown to help reduce inflammation, repair cell damage, and supply fat-soluble vitamins. Fat is also a valuable source of energy during prolonged physical activity of low-to-moderate intensity (i.e., greater than three hours). Athletes should aim to consume about one gram of fat per kilogram body weight (approximately 0.45 grams per pound) per day. For example, a 115-pound swimmer should consume about 50 g of fat per day. Good sources of healthy unsaturated fats include avocados, nuts, fish, and vegetable oils. Cold-water fish like salmon are the best source of omega-3 fats, but smaller amounts are also found in walnuts.

Fat Types in Food Sources

- 1/2 medium avocado: 11 g, unsaturated fat
- 1 Tbsp walnuts: 4 g, unsaturated fat and omega-3

- 2 Tbsp peanut butter: 16 g, unsaturated fat
- 1 Tbsp olive oil: 13 g, unsaturated fat
- 4 oz salmon: 15 g, unsaturated fat and omega-3

Putting It All Together

Meeting your nutritional needs as an athlete doesn't mean you need to stock up on special foods or supplements. Instead, choose nutrient-rich foods and include carbohydrates, proteins, and fats at every meal. Add two to three snacks between meals to supply a little extra protein and carbohydrate, and you'll be energized and ready for your next workout!

Section 29.2

Performance-Enhancing Sports Supplements

"Supplements," © 2006 Iowa State University Extension (www.extension.iastate.edu). Reprinted with permission. Reviewed by David A. Cooke, MD, FACP, January 2011.

Athletes are known to use substances, commonly dietary supplements, to improve performance. These are referred to as ergogenic aids. Athletes have used ergogenic aids since ancient times. Ancient Greek Olympians ate mushrooms to increase their chances to win the laurel wreath, and Aztec athletes ate human hearts. The ergogenic aid industry is massive, and most sporting magazines contain advertisements for new "revolutionary" ergogenic aids that are sold as dietary supplements. The world of sports is a competitive business. Athletes fear that others are taking something that will give them an advantage. This means that many athletes will try out new substances and supplements on the off chance that it will give them the edge over other competitors. Forgotten in the push to excel are the unknown dangers of unproven substances and the temptations for misuse and abuse. Dietary supplements can be harmful as well as useful.

What Are Supplements?

Prior to 1994, the term "dietary supplement" referred to products made of one or more of the essential nutrients, such as vitamins, minerals, and protein. Congress passed the Dietary Supplement Health and Education Act (DSHEA) in 1994, which expanded the definition so that dietary supplements now include herbs, or other botanicals (except tobacco), and any dietary substance that can be used to supplement the diet.

This has led to many new dietary supplements, for example:

- herbs and other botanicals;

- amino acids;

- extracts from animal glands;

- fibers such as psyllium and guar gum;

- compounds not generally recognized as foods or nutrients such as enzymes and hormone-like compounds.

This new definition has meant that many substances that the FDA [Food and Drug Administration] formerly classified as drugs or unapproved food additives have become readily available as dietary supplements. Thousands of dietary supplements are on the market. Many contain vitamins and minerals to supplement the amounts of these nutrients we get from the foods we eat. There are also many products on the market that contain other substances like high-potency free amino acids, botanicals, enzymes, herbs, animal extracts, bioflavonoids, and synthetically manufactured pro-hormones melatonin and dehydroepiandrosterone (DHEA), which exert drug-like effects on the body.

Supplement Standards/Regulations

The FDA's review of the safety and effectiveness of these products is significantly less than for drugs and foods. Be cautious about using any supplement that claims to treat, prevent, or cure a serious disease. The FDA has approved only a few claims for labeling, based on a review of the scientific evidence (for example, claims about folic acid and a decreased risk of neural tube birth defects). A recent court case prevents the FDA from regulating health claims on dietary supplement labels. Read carefully and think critically about the claims you see on the packages.

Supplement manufacturers do not have to prove that their products are safe! In the past, supplement manufacturers had to prove to the FDA that their products were safe. Under current law, however, it has become the responsibility of the FDA to prove that a supplement is unsafe. With the high number of new supplements coming onto the market and the limited resources of the FDA, it is very likely that a product could cause harm before the FDA can take action. In addition, even after the FDA has declared a supplement unsafe, they then have to prove that the supplement is unsafe in the court of law.

Some dietary supplements may be harmful under some conditions. For example, many herbal products and other "natural" supplements have real and powerful pharmacological effects that can cause harmful reactions in some people or can cause dangerous interactions with prescribed or over-the-counter medicines. It does not necessarily mean that supplements marketed as "natural" are safe and without side effects.

Because of the lack of regulation with dietary supplements, athletes run the risk of consuming a dietary supplement that is contaminated. Steroid contamination, such as anandrolone and testosterone, has been documented. An athlete WILL test positive for drug use if they consume a dietary supplement containing banned substances such as anandrolone and testosterone. Some substances that could be present in the supplements are banned by the NCAA (see the list of banned drug classes at www.ncaa.org/wps/wcm/connect/public/NCAA/Student-Athlete+Experience/NCAA+banned+drugs+list). Consuming them will jeopardize your eligibility. Visit the Gatorade® Sport Science Institute (at www.gssiweb.com/Article_List.aspx?topicid=2&subtopicid=111) for more information.

Protein Supplements

The list of protein supplements on the market is never ending. Protein supplements promise anything from increased strength, energy, muscle mass, weight loss, staying fit, and obtaining lean slender bodies. Today you can hardly find a gym where protein supplements are not being used or sold. But are these supplements really beneficial, and who should take them? What are the long-term effects?

For years, research studies have been studying their effects on muscle strength and performance. The results of the different studies are conflicting with little to no data supporting the proclaimed benefits of protein supplements.

Currently, only creatine has been shown to benefit high-intensity, short-duration exercise. However, a few other supplements including amino acids and beta-hydroxy-beta-methylbutyrate (HMB) have shown promise in some studies. More research is necessary to examine their effects on performance and health.

Amino Acids

The athlete's protein source needs to provide the essential amino acids (those not synthesized in the body), since non-essential amino acids can by made by the body when needed. The essential amino acids can easily be obtained from the diet by consuming quality proteins such as egg, chicken, red meats, fish, or milk, etc., thus supplementation is not necessary.

If supplemental amino acids are needed, the key to obtaining benefits from amino acids is the timing of consumption. Amino acids should be consumed either immediately prior to exercise, or during the recovery period one to two hours after exercise. A consumption of 0.1 g of essential amino acids per kilogram of body weight is recommended.

Remember: The amount of protein that the body can utilize is limited. Large protein consumption in one setting that exceeds the body's requirement will be converted into fat. It will NOT increase muscle mass.

HMB

HMB is derived from an amino acid called leucine. HMB is believed to prevent muscle loss with intensive resistive training. Considering muscle breakdown always occurs with exercise, preventing this breakdown preserves and increases muscle mass. However, more research is necessary to verify the effects of this supplement.

Creatine

What Is Creatine?

Discovered in 1832, creatine is a food constituent derived from animals. The compound is primarily found in skeletal muscle and is synthesized in the body and transported to muscle tissues. In muscles, creatine is used in short bouts of intense energy production in the form of creatine-phosphate. The end-product energy release from creatine-phosphate is creatinine, which is excreted by the kidneys in the urine.

Creatine in the Body

Creatine is synthesized in the liver, the kidneys, and the pancreas. After production, it is transported in the blood to body tissues. The creatine transporter is limited in the amount of creatine it can transport. This means that even if a person consumes more creatine, the body has a maximum amount it can use.

Creatine in the Diet

Although creatine is synthesized in the body, it can be obtained from dietary intake and creatine supplementation. A good food source of creatine includes muscle meat, where 1.1 kg (about 2 1/2 pounds) of beef provides 5 g of creatine. A typical American diet, containing some meat, provides approximately 1 g of creatine daily. Creatine obtained from the diet can either be utilized as energy, or be stored in the body. For example, a 70-kg adult man can store approximately 120 g of creatine.

Role in Exercise

Oral creatine supplementation increases muscle creatine-phosphate, which can enhance performance during repeated bouts of high-intensity exercise. The benefit of creatine supplementation for high-intensity and short-duration exercise has been shown to be greater than low-intensity and long-duration exercise.

Creatine Supplementation

Creatine is supplemented to improve muscle power output primarily in high-intensity and short-duration exercise. However, creatine has also been used to prevent breakdown of muscle mass during immobilization. In other words, it may prevent muscle wasting when a person is injured and/or unable to exercise.

Creatine supplementation involves a loading phase and a maintenance phase. For the best results, a loading of about 20 g of creatine monohydrate for four to five days is recommended. Thereafter, to maintain desirable levels of creatine, 3 g of creatine monohydrate per day should be consumed. The response to the supplementation varies depending on individual need. However, the best response will be seen the first three days of ingestion.

Table 29.1. Effects and Benefits of Creatine

Effect of Creatine	Potential Benefit
More power	Perform more exercise repetitions
More strength	Perform more exercise repetitions and enhance activities of daily living performance
More lean mass	Functional recovery
Less oxidative stress	Long-term cellular protection

Side Effects

Scientists are not sure whether long-term creatine supplementation is harmful to humans. Research on long-term safety has been initiated, but currently no severe health implications have been identified. However, water retention and decreased urine production have been reported to cause weight gain with creatine supplementation. Other side effects reported are muscle cramps, headaches, diarrhea, and gastrointestinal pain.

Table 29.2. Ergogenic Aids

Ergogenic Aid	Proposed Action	What Research Says	Side Effects
Androstenedione	Steroid hormone that increases testosterone levels	No documented benefits	Major
Caffeine	Increases fat metabolism, thus sparing glucose and glycogen stores; stimulates the central nervous system	Supports	Mild
Carbohydrates	An important energy source for muscles	Supports	Mild at high doses
Creatine	Delays fatigue and improves performance during high, intense bursts of exercise; builds muscle mass	Supports; however, there is limited data on long-term use	Mild
DHEA [dehydroepiandrosterone]	Increases amount of steroids produced in the body	No benefit in healthy athletes	May be dangerous
HMB	Prevents muscle breakdown, speeds up muscle repair, and increases lean body mass	Limited; some strength benefits	None
Protein	Helps build muscle and improves muscle repair	Supports; high force outputs from their muscles, such as sprinters and weight lifters, need extra protein to ensure muscle maintenance	None

Speculations that creatine supplementation could lead to kidney failure have not been proven. Clinical trials have shown no adverse effects of low-dose (1.5 g), long-term (one to five years) creatine supplementation on renal function. However, high doses for a prolonged period of time will increase the stress on the kidneys.

Conclusions on Creatine

- Creatine supplementation has only been shown to be beneficial in those sports/exercise of short duration, high intensity.

Table 29.2. *continued*

Ergogenic Aid	Proposed Action	What Research Says	Side Effects
Pycnogenol	Boosts antioxidant levels, enhances recovery	Supports, dietary sources offer same benefit	None
Tryptophan	Increases athletic endurance; decreases pain perception	No definite results; no benefit in trained athletes	Potentially dangerous
Vitamin B 6 (pyridoxine)	Increases growth of muscle and decreases anxiety	No benefit unless individual has deficiency	Mild at high doses
Vitamin B12 (cobalamin)	Increases growth of muscle	No benefit unless individual has deficiency	None
Vitamin C	Acts as an antioxidant; increases energy production and aerobic reactions	No benefit unless individual has deficiency	Mild at high doses
Vitamin E	Acts as an antioxidant; increases aerobic capacity	No definite results	Mild
Zinc	Increases muscle mass and aerobic capacity	Few studies; mostly negative	Mild

Source: Ahrendt DM. Ergogenic aids: Counseling the athlete. *American Family Physician.* 2001;63:913–22.

- Long-term safety of creatine supplementation is unknown.

- Creatine supplements, as other dietary supplements, are not well regulated and could contain contaminants or illegal substances, which could jeopardize an athlete's health and eligibility.

Chapter 30

Alcohol Use

Chapter Contents

Section 30.1

Recommendations for the Consumption of Alcohol

"Dietary Guidelines for Americans 2005, Chapter 9. Alcoholic Beverages,"
U.S. Department of Health and Human Services (www.hhs.gov), July 9, 2008.

The consumption of alcohol can have beneficial or harmful effects depending on the amount consumed, age and other characteristics of the person consuming the alcohol, and specifics of the situation. In 2002, 55% of U.S. adults were current drinkers. Forty-five percent of U.S. adults do not drink any alcohol at all. Abstention is an important option. Fewer Americans consume alcohol today as compared to 50 to 100 years ago.

The hazards of heavy alcohol consumption are well-known and include increased risk of liver cirrhosis, hypertension, cancers of the upper gastrointestinal tract, injury, violence, and death. Moreover, certain individuals who are more susceptible to the harmful effects of alcohol should not drink at all. In addition, alcohol should be avoided by those participating in activities that require attention, skill, and/or coordination.

Alcohol may have beneficial effects when consumed in moderation. The lowest all-cause mortality occurs at an intake of one to two drinks per day. The lowest coronary heart disease mortality also occurs at an intake of one to two drinks per day. Morbidity and mortality are highest among those drinking large amounts of alcohol.

Key Recommendations

- Those who choose to drink alcoholic beverages should do so sensibly and in moderation—defined as the consumption of up to one drink per day for women and up to two drinks per day for men.

- Alcoholic beverages should not be consumed by some individuals, including those who cannot restrict their alcohol intake, women of childbearing age who may become pregnant, pregnant and lactating women, children and adolescents, individuals taking medications that can interact with alcohol, and those with specific medical conditions.

- Alcoholic beverages should be avoided by individuals engaging in activities that require attention, skill, or coordination, such as driving or operating machinery.

Discussion

Alcoholic beverages supply calories but few essential nutrients. As a result, excessive alcohol consumption makes it difficult to ingest sufficient nutrients within an individual's daily calorie allotment and to maintain a healthy weight. Although the consumption of one to two alcoholic beverages per day is not associated with macronutrient or micronutrient deficiencies or with overall dietary quality, heavy drinkers may be at risk of malnutrition if the calories derived from alcohol are substituted for those in nutritious foods.

The majority of American adults consume alcohol. Those who do so should drink alcoholic beverages in moderation. Moderation is defined as the consumption of up to one drink per day for women and up to two drinks per day for men. Twelve fluid ounces of regular beer, 5 fluid ounces of wine, or 1.5 fluid ounces of 80-proof distilled spirits count as one drink for purposes of explaining moderation. This definition of moderation is not intended as an average over several days but rather as the amount consumed on any single day.

The effect of alcohol consumption varies depending on the amount consumed and an individual's characteristics and circumstances. Alcoholic beverages are harmful when consumed in excess. Excess alcohol consumption alters judgment and can lead to dependency or addiction and other serious health problems such as cirrhosis of the liver, inflammation of the pancreas, and damage to the heart and brain. Even less than heavy consumption of alcohol is associated with significant risks. Consuming more than one drink per day for women and two drinks per day for men increases the risk for motor vehicle accidents, other injuries, high blood pressure, stroke, violence, some types of cancer, and suicide. Compared with women who do not drink, women who consume one drink per day appear to have a slightly higher risk of breast cancer.

Studies suggest adverse effects even at moderate alcohol consumption levels in specific situations and individuals. Individuals in some situations should avoid alcohol—those who plan to drive, operate machinery, or take part in other activities that require attention, skill, or coordination. Some people, including children and adolescents, women of childbearing age who may become pregnant, pregnant and lactating women, individuals who cannot restrict alcohol intake, individuals taking medications that can interact with alcohol, and individuals with specific medical conditions should not drink at all. Even moderate drinking during pregnancy may have behavioral or developmental consequences for the baby. Heavy drinking during pregnancy can produce a range of behavioral and psychosocial problems, malformation, and mental retardation in the baby.

Moderate alcohol consumption may have beneficial health effects in some individuals. In middle-aged and older adults, a daily intake of one to two alcoholic beverages per day is associated with the lowest all-cause mortality. More specifically, compared to non-drinkers, adults who consume one to two alcoholic beverages a day appear to have a lower risk of coronary heart disease. In contrast, among younger adults alcohol consumption appears to provide little, if any, health benefit, and alcohol use among young adults is associated with a higher risk of traumatic injury and death. As noted previously, a number of strategies reduce the risk of chronic disease, including a healthful diet, physical activity, avoidance of smoking, and maintenance of a healthy weight. Furthermore, it is not recommended that anyone begin drinking or drink more frequently on the basis of health considerations.

Table 30.1. Calories in Selected Alcoholic Beverages

This table is a guide to estimate the caloric intake from various alcoholic beverages. An example serving volume and the calories in that drink are shown for beer, wine, and distilled spirits. Higher alcohol content (higher percent alcohol or higher proof) and mixing alcohol with other beverages, such as calorically sweetened soft drinks, tonic water, fruit juice, or cream, increases the amount of calories in the beverage. Alcoholic beverages supply calories but few essential nutrients.

Beverage	Approximate Calories per One Fluid Ounce[a]	Example Serving Volume	Approximate Total Calories[b]
Beer (regular)	12	12 oz	144
Beer (light)	9	12 oz	108
White wine	20	5 oz	100
Red wine	21	5 oz	105
Sweet dessert wine	47	3 oz	141
80-proof distilled spirits (gin, rum, vodka, whiskey)	64	1.5 oz	96

a. *Source:* Agricultural Research Service (ARS) Nutrient Database for Standard Reference (SR), Release 17 (www.nal.usda.gov/fnic/foodcomp/index.html). Calories are calculated to the nearest whole number per one fluid ounce.
b. The total calories and alcohol content vary depending on the brand. Moreover, adding mixers to an alcoholic beverage can contribute calories in addition to the calories from the alcohol itself.

Section 30.2

Red Wine and Cancer Prevention

"Red Wine and Cancer Prevention: Fact Sheet," National Cancer Institute (www.cancer.gov), November 27, 2002. Revised by David A. Cooke, MD, FACP, January 2011.

Red wine is a rich source of biologically active phytochemicals, chemicals found in plants. Particular compounds called polyphenols found in red wine—such as catechins and resveratrol—are thought to have antioxidant or anticancer properties.

What are polyphenols and how do they prevent cancer?

Polyphenols are antioxidant compounds found in the skin and seeds of grapes. When wine is made from these grapes, the alcohol produced by the fermentation process dissolves the polyphenols contained in the skin and seeds. Red wine contains more polyphenols than white wine because the making of white wine requires the removal of the skins after the grapes are crushed. The phenols in red wine include catechin, gallic acid, and epicatechin.

Polyphenols have been found to have antioxidant properties. Antioxidants are substances that protect cells from oxidative damage caused by molecules called free radicals. These chemicals can damage important parts of cells, including proteins, membranes, and DNA. Cellular damage caused by free radicals has been implicated in the development of cancer. Research on the antioxidants found in red wine has shown that they may help inhibit the development of certain cancers.

What is resveratrol and how does it prevent cancer?

Resveratrol is a type of polyphenol called a phytoalexin, a class of compounds produced as part of a plant's defense system against disease. It is produced in the plant in response to an invading fungus, stress, injury, infection, or ultraviolet irradiation. Red wine contains high levels of resveratrol, as do grapes, raspberries, peanuts, and other plants.

Resveratrol has been shown to reduce tumor incidence in animals by affecting one or more stages of cancer development. It has been shown to inhibit growth of many types of cancer cells in culture. Evidence also exists that it can reduce inflammation. It also reduces activation of NF kappa B, a protein produced by the body's immune system when it is under attack. This protein affects cancer cell growth and metastasis. Resveratrol is also an antioxidant.

What have red wine studies found?

The cell and animal studies of red wine have examined effects in several cancers, including leukemia and skin, breast, and prostate cancers. Scientists are studying resveratrol to learn more about its cancer preventive activities. Recent evidence from animal studies suggests this anti-inflammatory compound may be an effective chemopreventive agent in three stages of the cancer process: initiation, promotion, and progression.

Research studies published in the *International Journal of Cancer* show that drinking a glass of red wine a day may cut a man's risk of prostate cancer in half and that the protective effect appears to be strongest against the most aggressive forms of the disease. It was also seen that men who consumed four or more four-ounce glasses of red wine per week have a 60% lower incidence of the more aggressive types of prostate cancer.

However, studies of the association between red wine consumption and cancer in humans are in their initial stages. Although consumption of large amounts of alcoholic beverages may increase the risk of some cancers, there is growing evidence that the health benefits of red wine are related to its nonalcoholic components.

Despite these encouraging signs, there is no firm answer as to whether red wine intake reduces your risk of cancer. The vast majority of studies have focused on the effects of red wine on various antioxidants and hormones in the blood. Changes in these levels may affect cancer risk, but this has not been proven. Settling the question will require studies of people who begin drinking red wine and whether health outcomes improve relative to those who do not. Such studies are difficult to perform, very expensive, and need to last many years.

In addition, it remains unclear whether any health benefits of red wine are due to its alcoholic component, nonalcoholic components, or both. A number of studies have concluded red wine's effects are independent of alcohol, while others found that benefits were not seen in non-alcoholic red wine. There is no definitive answer to this question so far.

Section 30.3

Red Wine and Your Heart

"Agent in Red Wine Found to Keep Hearts Young" by Terry Devitt, University of Wisconsin News (www.news.wisc.edu), June 4, 2008. © University of Wisconsin. Reprinted with permission.

How, scientists wonder, do the French get away with a clean bill of heart health despite a diet loaded with saturated fats?

The answer to the so-called "French paradox" may be found in red wine. More specifically, it may reside in small doses of resveratrol, a natural constituent of grapes, pomegranates, red wine, and other foods, according to a new study by an international team of researchers.

Writing this week (June 3 [2008]) in the online, open-access journal *Public Library of Science One*, the researchers report that low doses of resveratrol in the diet of middle-aged mice has a widespread influence on the genetic levers of aging and may confer special protection on the heart.

Specifically, the researchers found that low doses of resveratrol mimic the effects of what is known as caloric restriction—diets with 20%–30% fewer calories than a typical diet—that in numerous studies has been shown to extend lifespan and blunt the effects of aging.

"This brings down the dose of resveratrol toward the consumption reality mode," says senior author Richard Weindruch, a University of Wisconsin [UW]–Madison professor of medicine and a researcher at the William S. Middleton Memorial Veterans Hospital. "At the same time, it plugs into the biology of caloric restriction."

Previous research has shown that resveratrol in high doses extends lifespan in invertebrates and prevents early mortality in mice given a high-fat diet. The new study, conducted by researchers from academia and industry, extends those findings, showing that resveratrol in low doses and beginning in middle age can elicit many of the same benefits as a reduced-calorie diet.

"Resveratrol is active in much lower doses than previously thought and mimics a significant fraction of the profile of caloric restriction at the gene expression level," says Tomas Prolla, a UW–Madison professor of genetics and a senior author of the new report.

371

The group explored the influence of the agent on heart, muscle, and brain by looking for changes in gene expression in those tissues. As animals age, gene expression in the different tissues of the body changes as genes are switched on and off.

In the new study—which compared the genetic crosstalk of animals on a restricted diet with those fed small doses of resveratrol—the similarities were remarkable, explains lead author Jamie Barger of Madison-based LifeGen Technologies. In the heart, for example, there are at least 1,029 genes whose functions change with age, and the organ's function is known to diminish with age. In animals on a restricted diet, 90% of those heart genes experienced altered gene expression profiles, while low doses of resveratrol thwarted age-related change in 92%. The new findings, say the study's authors, were associated with prevention of the decline in heart function associated with aging.

In short, a glass of wine or food or supplements that contain even small doses of resveratrol are likely to represent "a robust intervention in the retardation of cardiac aging," the authors note.

That finding may also explain the remarkable heart health of people who live in some regions of France where diets are soaked in saturated fats but the incidence of heart disease, a major cause of mortality in the United States, is low. In France, meals are traditionally complemented with a glass of red wine.

The new resveratrol study is also important because it suggests that caloric restriction, which has been widely studied in animals from spiders to humans, and resveratrol may govern the same master genetic pathways related to aging.

"There must be a few master biochemical pathways activated in response to caloric restriction, which in turn activate many other pathways," explains Prolla. "And resveratrol seems to activate some of these master pathways as well."

The new findings, according to Weindruch and Prolla, provide strong evidence that resveratrol can improve quality of life through its influence on the different parameters of aging such as cardiac function. However, whether the agent can extend lifespan in ways similar to caloric restriction will require further study, according to the new report's authors.

The work of the Wisconsin team was funded by grants from the National Institutes of Health and DSM Nutritional Products of Basel, Switzerland.

Part Five

Nutrition-Related Health Concerns

Chapter 31

The Western Diet and Metabolic Syndrome

Otherwise-healthy adults who eat two or more servings of meat a day—the equivalent of two burger patties—increase their risk of developing metabolic syndrome by 25% compared with those who eat meat twice a week, according to research published in *Circulation: Journal of the American Heart Association*.

Metabolic syndrome is a cluster of cardiovascular disease and diabetes risk factors including elevated waist circumference, high blood pressure, elevated triglycerides, low levels of high-density lipoprotein (HDL or "good") cholesterol, and high fasting glucose levels. The presence of three or more of the factors increases a person's risk of developing diabetes and cardiovascular disease.

But it's not just meat that adds inches to the waist, increases blood pressure, and lowers HDL—"it's fried foods as well," said Lyn M. Steffen, PhD, MPH, RD, co-author of the study and an associate professor of epidemiology at the University of Minnesota.

Dairy products, by contrast, appeared to offer some protection against metabolic syndrome.

Steffen said that, "Fried foods are typically synonymous with commonly eaten fast foods, so I think it is safe to say that these findings support a link between fast-food consumption and an increase in metabolic risk factors."

"Burgers, Fries, Diet Soda: Metabolic Syndrome Blue-Plate Special," reprinted with permission from www.heart.org. © 2008 American Heart Association, Inc.

375

The findings emerged from an analysis of dietary intake by 9,514 participants in the Atherosclerosis Risk in Communities (ARIC) study. ARIC is a collaborative study funded by the National Heart, Lung, and Blood Institute.

Unlike other researchers who have investigated relationships between nutrients and cardiovascular risk, "we specifically studied food intake. When making recommendations about dietary intake it is easier to do so using the framework of real foods eaten by real people," Steffen said.

Researchers assessed food intake using a 66-item food frequency questionnaire. From those responses, they categorized people by their dietary preferences into a Western-pattern diet or a prudent-pattern diet.

In general, the Western-pattern diet was heavy on refined grains, processed meat, fried foods, red meat, eggs, and soda and light on fish, fruit, vegetables, and whole grain products.

Prudent diet eating patterns, by contrast, favored cruciferous vegetables (e.g., cabbage, radish, and broccoli), carotenoid vegetables (e.g., carrots, pumpkins, red pepper, cabbage, broccoli, and spinach), fruit, fish and seafood, poultry, and whole grains, along with low-fat dairy.

Researchers also assessed associations with individual food items: fried foods, sweetened beverages (regular soda and fruit drinks), diet soda, nuts, and coffee.

After nine years of follow-up, 3,782 (nearly 40%) of the participants had three or more of the risk factors for metabolic syndrome.

At baseline, participants were 45 to 64 years old—ages at which many people gain weight.

Steffen said that weight gain over the years of follow-up might explain some of the cases of metabolic syndrome. But "after adjusting for demographic factors, smoking, physical activity, and energy intake, consumption of a 'Western' dietary pattern was adversely associated with metabolic syndrome," she said.

"One surprising finding was while it didn't increase the risk of metabolic syndrome, there was no evidence of a beneficial effect of consuming a prudent diet either. I had expected to find a beneficial effect because we have seen that in other studies."

When Steffen and colleagues analyzed the results by specific foods, they found that meat, fried foods, and diet soda were all significantly associated with increased risk of metabolic syndrome, but consumption of dairy products was beneficial.

The study did not address the mechanisms involved in the increased risk of metabolic syndrome seen with certain foods, but Steffen speculated that "it may be a fatty acid mechanism since saturated fats are a common link and certainly overweight and obesity are contributing to the development of metabolic syndrome." She also said more research on the relationship between diet soda and its association to metabolic syndrome is needed.

The fact that 60.5% of the ARIC population had metabolic syndrome at the start of the study or developed it during nine years of follow-up is troubling, researchers said.

Steffen said the study's results are clear: Too much meat, fried foods, and diet soda do not add up to a healthy life.

American Heart Association dietary guidelines for healthy Americans age two and older include:

- limit saturated fat, trans fat, cholesterol, and sodium in the diet;
- minimize the intake of food and beverages with added sugars;
- eat a diet rich in vegetables, fruits, and whole-grain foods;
- select fat-free and low-fat dairy;
- eat fish at least twice per week;
- emphasize physical activity and weight control;
- avoid use of and exposure to tobacco products;
- achieve and maintain healthy cholesterol, blood pressure, and blood glucose levels.

Co-authors are Pamela L. Lutsey, MPH, and June Stevens, PhD, MS, RD.

Statements and conclusions of study authors that are published in the American Heart Association scientific journals are solely those of the study authors and do not necessarily reflect association policy or position. The American Heart Association makes no representation or warranty as to their accuracy or reliability.

Chapter 32

Sugar and Added Sweeteners

Chapter Contents

Section 32.1

Questions and Answers about Sugar

"Frequently Asked Questions about Sugar," reprinted with permission from www.heart.org. © 2010 American Heart Association, Inc.

Are all sugars bad?

No, but sugars add calories and zero nutrients to food. Adding a limited amount of sugars to foods that provide important nutrients—such as whole-grain cereal, flavored milk, or yogurt—to improve their taste, especially for children, is a better use of added sugars than nutrient-poor, highly sweetened foods.

How can I tell by looking at a nutrition facts label if a products has added sugars?

Current nutrition labels don't list the amount of added sugars (alone) in a product. It will be important for policy makers, the food industry, and other public health groups to create dialogue regarding how to make assessing added sugars simpler for consumers.

The line for "sugars" you see on a nutrition label includes both added and naturally occurring sugars in the product. Naturally occurring sugars are found in milk (lactose) and fruit (fructose). Any product that contains milk (such as yogurt, milk, cream) or fruit (fresh, dried) contains some natural sugars.

But you can read the ingredient list on a processed food's label to tell if the product contains added sugars. Names for added sugars on labels include:

- brown sugar;
- corn sweetener;
- corn syrup;
- sugar molecules ending in "ose" (dextrose, fructose, glucose, lactose, maltose, sucrose);
- high-fructose corn syrup;

- fruit juice concentrates;

- honey;

- invert sugar;

- malt sugar;

- molasses;

- raw sugar;

- sugar;

- syrup.

What are added sugars?

Added sugars are sugars and syrups that are added to foods or beverages during processing or preparation. They do not include naturally occurring sugars such as those found in milk (lactose) and fruits (fructose).

Added sugars (or added sweeteners) include natural sugars (such as white sugar, brown sugar, and honey) as well as other caloric sweeteners that are chemically manufactured (such as high fructose corn syrup).

What is the difference between added sugars and naturally occurring sugars?

Added sugars include any sugars or caloric sweeteners that are added to a food during processing. Naturally occurring sugars are found naturally in foods such as fruit (fructose) and milk (lactose).

All carbohydrates are made up of units of sugar ("saccharide"). Carbohydrates containing only one unit of sugar (called "monosaccharides") or two units of sugar (called "disaccharides") are known as simple sugars or simple carbohydrates.

Simple sugars are quickly broken down and provide a very fast increase in blood sugar, while complex carbs take longer and cause blood sugar to rise more gradually. Complex carbohydrates are found in foods such as starchy vegetables (corn, potatoes, peas, etc.), breads, cereals, rice, and grains. Complex carbs are broken down into the simple sugars during digestion, which causes them to be processed more slowly in the body.

Why are sugars added to food?

Sugars are often added to food during processing to improve the taste of certain foods.

What does the AHA [American Heart Association] recommend as a limit for daily added sugars intake?

Your daily discretionary calorie allowance consists of calories available after meeting nutrient needs—these calories don't contribute to weight gain. The American Heart Association recommends that no more than half of your daily discretionary calorie allowance come from added sugars. For most American women, this is no more than 100 calories per day and no more than 150 per day for men (or about six teaspoons a day for women and nine teaspoons a day for men). [Under the new MyPlate food guidance system, adopted June 2, 2011, the term "empty calories" has replaced the previously used "discretionary calories."]

Sugar's primary role in the body is to provide energy (calories). To get the nutrients you need, eat a diet that's rich in fruits, vegetables, whole grains, lean meats, fish, poultry, and low-fat or fat-free dairy products. Typically, foods high in added sugars do not have the nutrients the body needs and only contain extra calories.

How many calories are in one teaspoon (tsp) of sugar?

One teaspoon of sugar has about four grams of sugar and 16 calories.

How much added sugars do most Americans consume?

A report from the 2001–04 NHANES (National Health and Nutrition Examination Survey) database showed that Americans get about 22.2 teaspoons of sugar a day or about 355 calories. This number has increased steadily over the past three decades. Teens and men consume the most added sugars.

A major contributor of added sugars to American diets are soft drinks and other sugar-sweetened beverages.

What are discretionary calories?

You have a daily energy need—the amount of calories (or energy units) your body needs to function and provide energy for your activities. Think of it as a budget. You'd organize a real budget with "essentials" (for example, rent and utilities) and "extras" (for example, vacation and entertainment). In a daily calorie budget, the essentials are the minimum number of calories you need to meet your nutrient needs.

Select low-fat and no-sugar-added foods to make good "buys" with your budget. Depending on the foods you choose and the amount of physical activity you do each day, you may have more calories left over for "extras" that can be used on treats like solid fats, added sugars, and alcohol. These are discretionary calories, or calories to be spent at your discretion.

A person's discretionary calorie budget varies depending on how physically active they are and how many calories they need to consume to meet their daily nutrient requirements.

How are the remaining discretionary calories consumed if not as added sugars?

Discretionary calories are in addition to those that supply the nutrients to your body for daily function and activity. Your body does not actually need them to function. Common sources of discretionary calories (in addition to added sugars) are fats, oils, and alcohol. Fats are the most concentrated source of calories.

Discretionary calories can be used to:

- eat additional foods from a food group above your daily recommendation;

- select a higher-calorie form of a food that's higher in fat or contains added sugars (whole milk vs. skim milk or sweetened vs. unsweetened cereal);

- add fats or sweeteners to the leanest versions of foods (for example, sauce, dressing, butter/margarine);

- eat or drink items that are mostly fat, sugar, or alcohol such as candy, cake, beer, wine, or regular soda.

What is energy density and how do added sugars affect it?

Energy density refers to the number of calories (or amount of energy) per serving of a food. Because sugars contain calories (one teaspoon of white sugar has about 16 calories), the more sugar in a food, the more calories, or energy, that food will have.

A similar-sounding term, nutrient density, refers to the amount of nutrients per serving of a food (nutrients are materials a body needs to function healthfully—for example, carbohydrates, proteins, fats, vitamins, and minerals). Foods that are highly nutrient dense are good for your body. Ideal foods are low in energy density (calories) but highly nutrient dense. Foods that are lacking in nutrients are often referred to as "empty calories."

Because added sugars contain calories but no nutrients, they are energy dense and nutrient poor.

To improve the overall quality of Americans' diets, the American Heart Association recommends people consume foods with more nutrients and less calories.

What foods and beverages are the main sources of added sugars in Americans' diets?

Regular soft drinks; sugars and candy; cakes, cookies, pies; fruit drinks (fruitades and fruit punch); dairy desserts and milk products (ice cream, sweetened yogurt, and sweetened milk); and other grains (cinnamon toast and honey-nut waffles).

Does this mean I should avoid all soft drinks and other sugar-sweetened beverages?

You can choose how to spend your discretionary sugars calories.

Regular soft drinks are the number one source of added sugars in Americans' diets. A 12-ounce can of regular soda contains an estimated 130 calories (or eight teaspoons) of added sugars. People who consume lots of sugar-sweetened beverages eat too many sugar calories which can add up quickly and tend to gain weight. Carefully monitor the number of calories you get from sodas and other sources of added sugars.

How can added sugars be used (within the recommended limits) to enhance the quality of people's diets?

Sugars promote enjoyment of meals and snacks. When sugars are added to nutrient-rich foods, such as flavored milks, studies have shown that the quality of children's diets improves and there is no negative impact on their weight.

How do added sugars affect the quality of an individual's diet?

Some studies show that eating large amounts of added sugars is associated with diets low in calcium, vitamin A, iron, and zinc. Also, diets that are high in added sugars are typically low in fiber. This is important because increasing dietary sources of fiber is associated with decreasing energy intake, which can result in weight loss.

Why are "liquid calories" and "solid calories" different?

Some studies suggest that drinking too many calories is even more likely to cause weight gain than calories from solid foods. It is suggested that liquid calories are not as satisfying as calories consumed from solid foods, so people tend to consume more fluid calories to compensate. As a result, reducing liquid calorie intake has a stronger effect on weight loss than reducing solid calories.

Drinking calorie-containing beverages is connected with overweight and obesity. People should carefully monitor the calories they drink and get enough water to maintain proper hydration every day.

What are the American Heart Association's new (January 2010) recommendations for sugar-sweetened beverages?

The American Heart Association recommends that all Americans consume no more than 450 calories (36 oz) per week from sugar-sweetened beverages. The new recommendations are one component in a suite of cardiovascular measurements developed by the American Heart Association to determine if Americans are improving their cardiovascular health by 20% by 2020.

Do the recommendations to limit sugar-sweetened beverages to no more than 450 calories per week apply to children?

This calorie limit is based on a daily 2000-calorie diet. Daily calorie needs and discretionary calorie levels vary for all individuals, including children, so the recommendations for sugar-sweetened beverages for young children will generally be lower due to their lower energy needs. Some older, very active children may require 2,000 calories and for those children, the 450-calorie limit does apply.

This limit is very important, especially in light of the fact that the rate of childhood obesity has increased and sugar-sweetened soft drinks are relatively high in calories for small children. It is essential to help our children eat a healthy diet and achieve and maintain a healthy body weight. The obesity epidemic among children has caused children to experience adult conditions, such as elevated cholesterol and Type 2 diabetes at younger ages.

Is the American Heart Association taking a position for or against certain types of added sugar (e.g., raw sugar, high-fructose corn syrup, and non-nutritive sweeteners)?

The AHA hasn't taken a position on different types of added sugars, but we will continue to assess the science on this topic and any relevance to the impact on cardiovascular disease.

Since diet sodas and other products made of non-nutritive (artificial) sweeteners contain zero calories from added sugar does that mean they can be consumed freely?

You can drink diet sodas in moderation, but they don't give you any nutrition. Balance them with a variety of whole foods and beverages that provide a range of important nutrients.

Section 32.2

The Controversy over High Fructose Corn Syrup

"A Not-So-Sweet Story: High Fructose Corn Syrup,"
© 2008 Obesity Action Coalition (www.obesityaction.org).
Reprinted with permission.

Increasing articles, both scientific and not, have been pointing fingers at this sweetener as a serious contributor to our rising rates of obesity here in the United States. So, what's the story?

If you haven't heard the growing controversy about high fructose corn syrup (HFCS), then you will.

Normal corn syrup is 100% glucose, a simple sugar that is the primary sugar used by humans for energy. When someone refers to your blood sugar, they are referring to your blood glucose.

What is High Fructose Corn Syrup?

HFCS is not the same thing as simple corn syrup. It is made by using an enzyme to convert the glucose to fructose, a different simple sugar. A blend is then made between this new substance and regular corn syrup to create a standardized product with a precise ratio of fructose to glucose. The most common forms of HFCS are HFCS 42 (the common form used in baked goods), which is approximately 42% fructose and 58% glucose, and HFCS 55 (the form used in soft drinks), which is approximately 55% fructose and 45% glucose.

How High Fructose Corn Syrup Evolved

Before 1970, most things in the U.S. that were sweetened were sweetened with cane sugar. Between the mid-70s and the mid-80s, much of the cane sugar used in the U.S. food industry was replaced with HFCS. There are several reasons for this.

One reason is that sugar became more expensive. Because of the laws to encourage the use of our own domestic sugar supplies (such as those from Hawaii), it is very expensive to import cheaper foreign sugar into the U.S. Conversely, because of farm subsidies, the price of corn in our country is artificially low. So sometime in the early 1980s, it became much cheaper for food companies to use HFCS than to keep using cane sugar (it was in 1984 that both Coke and Pepsi made the switch).

High Fructose Corn Syrup—What Is the Link with Obesity?

As people search for a cause for the obesity epidemic, one place they look is changes in dietary habits. HFCS, as a relatively new ingredient in the American diet, and one that is found in many unhealthy foods and caloric drinks, has raised many eyebrows. Research has also looked at the possible connection, resulting in mixed messages.

If there is one connection that is obvious it is this: calorie consumption in the U.S. has climbed steadily for many decades. One major source of "new" calories in the U.S. diet is sweet beverages such as sodas. (U.S. soft drink consumption grew 135% between 1977 and 2001.)

Making the switch between cane sugar and HFCS in soda and other sweetened drinks made them cheaper, allowing for things like "super-sizing" to become possible, and increasing even more the calorie load from these sources.

For this reason, you will find some people who are concerned about obesity trying to make amendments to legislation such as the Farm Bill, with the hope that making corn products more expensive would ultimately reduce the consumption of HFCS-laden drinks.

So what about a scientific link between HFCS and obesity? Several scientific papers published in early 2000 theorized a direct connection between HFCS and obesity. These papers primarily argued along two lines of thought. One was the aforementioned issue of increased consumption and super-sizing. The other is based on the metabolism of fructose.

387

Fructose and Its Role

Fructose is metabolized differently in the body than glucose is. Glucose is transported into the cells of the body by the hormone insulin; fructose is not. Therefore, its ingestion does not stimulate insulin release. This, in turn, means that fructose ingestion does not lead to the insulin-induced rise in leptin. As an increase in insulin and leptin are associated with satiety, some researchers theorized that perhaps ingesting fructose instead of glucose leads people to consume more calories because they do not get the right signals to feel full.

High fructose diets also have been shown to lead to a more direct formation and storage of fat. Additionally, despite not having the same impact on insulin secretion as glucose, fructose ingestion is strongly tied to the development of insulin resistance and Type 2 Diabetes. This appears to occur because ingestion of a high fructose diet leads to more fat production, including increased production of circulation triglycerides (a kind of fat).

Is Soda the Main Culprit in Weight Gain?

As more studies examined soda than any other drink, there is more evidence for a link between obesity and soda. Regardless of what they are sweetened with, drinks of this kind provide no nutritional value and are primarily a source of empty calories.

As noted by Vasanti S. Malik, Matthias B. Schulze, and Frank B. Hu in their article, "Intake of Sugar-Sweetened Beverages and Weight Gain: A Systematic Review":

> "In the U.S., on average, a 12 oz serving (12 oz = 1 can of soda = 1 serving) of soda provides 150 calories and 40–50 grams of sugar in the form of high fructose corn syrup (45 percent glucose and 55 percent fructose), which is equivalent to 10 teaspoons of table sugar. If these calories are added to the typical U.S. diet without reducing intake from other sources, 1 soda per day could lead to a weight gain of 15 lb, or 6.75 kg in 1 year."

In other words, this many extra calories from anything is likely to cause you to gain weight.

How This All Compares

All of this sounds pretty bad for HFCS. But remember, most HFCS is only a little more than half fructose. While it accounts for a lot of calories in the human diet, on average 132 calories/day for each person over the age of two, only 55% of those are fructose calories.

By comparison, normal unsweetened apple juice is about 64% fructose. Studies comparing weight gain from HFCS products and other sweeteners do not really exist. A recent review conducted by the United States Center for Food, Nutrition, and Agriculture Policy found that while overall calories from fructose in the U.S. diet have increased, the ratio of fructose to glucose in the U.S. diet has stayed constant since roughly the 1960s.

Additionally, there is no evidence that weight gain is more likely to occur from the ingestion of foods and drinks sweetened with HFCS as compared to drinks using other caloric sweeteners or naturally caloric drinks such as fruit juice.

What Does This All Mean?

So what do you need to know? Right now, the current evidence does not really indicate that HFCS is any more responsible for obesity than any other sources of sugar. It may be that some of the metabolic issues we have discussed will eventually be shown to be a serious contributor to obesity, but right now, we do not have enough data to say.

What we do know is that consuming sweet drinks, whatever the source, does appear to contribute to weight gain and obesity. A recent systematic review of 30 studies examining the link between sweet beverages and weight found significant evidence that excess calories from soda, fruit drinks, fruit juice, and other drinks all had some association with body weight.

Remember, many sweet drinks are not sold in 12-ounce servings, but in 16, 20, or larger sizes. Until more is known, the best advice for the weight conscious is to try to minimize consumption of sweet, caloric drinks. If you do include caloric beverages in your diet, opting for nutrient-rich drinks like 100% juice or milk instead of sodas or juice-flavored drinks may be wise, as is limiting serving size.

Section 32.3

Artificial Sweeteners and Cancer Risk

"Artificial Sweeteners and Cancer," National Cancer Institute
(www.cancer.gov), August 5, 2009.

What are artificial sweeteners and how are they regulated in the United States?

Artificial sweeteners, also called sugar substitutes, are substances that are used instead of sucrose (table sugar) to sweeten foods and beverages. Because artificial sweeteners are many times sweeter than table sugar, smaller amounts are needed to create the same level of sweetness.

Artificial sweeteners are regulated by the U.S. Food and Drug Administration (FDA). The FDA, like the National Cancer Institute (NCI), is an agency of the Department of Health and Human Services. The FDA regulates food, drugs, medical devices, cosmetics, biologics, and radiation-emitting products. The Food Additives Amendment to the Food, Drug, and Cosmetic Act, which was passed by Congress in 1958, requires the FDA to approve food additives, including artificial sweeteners, before they can be made available for sale in the United States. However, this legislation does not apply to products that are "generally recognized as safe." Such products do not require FDA approval before being marketed.

Is there an association between artificial sweeteners and cancer?

Questions about artificial sweeteners and cancer arose when early studies showed that cyclamate in combination with saccharin caused bladder cancer in laboratory animals. However, results from subsequent carcinogenicity studies (studies that examine whether a substance can cause cancer) of these sweeteners have not provided clear evidence of an association with cancer in humans. Similarly, studies of other FDA-approved sweeteners have not demonstrated clear evidence of an association with cancer in humans.

What have studies shown about a possible association between specific artificial sweeteners and cancer?

Saccharin: Studies in laboratory rats during the early 1970s linked saccharin with the development of bladder cancer. For this reason, Congress mandated that further studies of saccharin be performed and required that all food containing saccharin bear the following warning label: "Use of this product may be hazardous to your health. This product contains saccharin, which has been determined to cause cancer in laboratory animals."

Subsequent studies in rats showed an increased incidence of urinary bladder cancer at high doses of saccharin, especially in male rats. However, mechanistic studies (studies that examine how a substance works in the body) have shown that these results apply only to rats. Human epidemiology studies (studies of patterns, causes, and control of diseases in groups of people) have shown no consistent evidence that saccharin is associated with bladder cancer incidence.

Because the bladder tumors seen in rats are due to a mechanism not relevant to humans and because there is no clear evidence that saccharin causes cancer in humans, saccharin was delisted in 2000 from the U.S. National Toxicology Program's *Report on Carcinogens,* where it had been listed since 1981 as a substance reasonably anticipated to be a human carcinogen (a substance known to cause cancer). More information about the delisting of saccharin is available at ntp.niehs. nih.gov/ntp/roc/eleventh/append/appb.pdf. The delisting led to legislation, which was signed into law on December 21, 2000, repealing the warning label requirement for products containing saccharin.

Aspartame: Aspartame, distributed under several trade names (e.g., NutraSweet® and Equal®), was approved in 1981 by the FDA after numerous tests showed that it did not cause cancer or other adverse effects in laboratory animals. Questions regarding the safety of aspartame were renewed by a 1996 report suggesting that an increase in the number of people with brain tumors between 1975 and 1992 might be associated with the introduction and use of this sweetener in the United States. However, an analysis of then-current NCI statistics showed that the overall incidence of brain and central nervous system cancers began to rise in 1973, eight years prior to the approval of aspartame, and continued to rise until 1985. Moreover, increases in overall brain cancer incidence occurred primarily in people age 70 and older, a group that was not exposed to the highest doses of aspartame since its introduction. These data do not establish a clear link between the consumption of aspartame and the development of brain tumors.

In 2005, a laboratory study found more lymphomas and leukemias in rats fed very high doses of aspartame (equivalent to drinking 8 to 2,083 cans of diet soda daily). However, there were some inconsistencies in the findings. For example, the number of cancer cases did not rise with increasing amounts of aspartame as would be expected.

Subsequently, NCI examined human data from the NIH [National Institutes of Health]-AARP Diet and Health Study of over half a million retirees. Increasing consumption of aspartame-containing beverages was not associated with the development of lymphoma, leukemia, or brain cancer.

Acesulfame potassium, sucralose, and neotame: In addition to saccharin and aspartame, three other artificial sweeteners are currently permitted for use in food in the United States:

- Acesulfame potassium (also known as ACK, Sweet One®, and Sunett®) was approved by the FDA in 1988 for use in specific food and beverage categories, and was later approved as a general purpose sweetener (except in meat and poultry) in 2002.

- Sucralose (also known as Splenda®) was approved by the FDA as a tabletop sweetener in 1998, followed by approval as a general purpose sweetener in 1999.

- Neotame, which is similar to aspartame, was approved by the FDA as a general purpose sweetener (except in meat and poultry) in 2002.

Before approving these sweeteners, the FDA reviewed more than 100 safety studies that were conducted on each sweetener, including studies to assess cancer risk. The results of these studies showed no evidence that these sweeteners cause cancer or pose any other threat to human health.

Cyclamate: Because the findings in rats suggested that cyclamate might increase the risk of bladder cancer in humans, the FDA banned the use of cyclamate in 1969. After reexamination of cyclamate's carcinogenicity and the evaluation of additional data, scientists concluded that cyclamate was not a carcinogen or a co-carcinogen (a substance that enhances the effect of a cancer-causing substance). A food additive petition was filed with the FDA for the reapproval of cyclamate, but this petition is currently being held in abeyance (not actively being considered). The FDA's concerns about cyclamate are not cancer related.

Section 32.4

Artificial Sweeteners and Weight Gain

Artificial Sweeteners Linked to Weight Gain

Cutting the connection between sweets and calories may confuse the body, making it harder to regulate intake.

Want to lose weight? It might help to pour that diet soda down the drain. Researchers have laboratory evidence that the widespread use of no-calorie sweeteners may actually make it harder for people to control their intake and body weight. The findings appear in the February [2008] issue of *Behavioral Neuroscience*, which is published by the American Psychological Association (APA).

Psychologists at Purdue University's Ingestive Behavior Research Center reported that relative to rats that ate yogurt sweetened with glucose (a simple sugar with 15 calories/teaspoon, the same as table sugar), rats given yogurt sweetened with zero-calorie saccharin later consumed more calories, gained more weight, put on more body fat, and didn't make up for it by cutting back later, all at levels of statistical significance.

Authors Susan Swithers, PhD, and Terry Davidson, PhD, surmised that by breaking the connection between a sweet sensation and high-calorie food, the use of saccharin changes the body's ability to regulate intake. That change depends on experience. Problems with self-regulation might explain in part why obesity has risen in parallel with the use of artificial sweeteners. It also might explain why, says Swithers, scientific consensus on human use of artificial sweeteners is inconclusive, with various studies finding evidence of weight loss, weight gain, or little effect. Because people may have different experiences with artificial and natural sweeteners, human studies that don't take into account prior consumption may produce a variety of outcomes.

Three different experiments explored whether saccharin changed lab animals' ability to regulate their intake, using different assessments—the most obvious being caloric intake, weight gain, and compensating by cutting back.

The experimenters also measured changes in core body temperature, a physiological assessment. Normally when we prepare to eat, the metabolic engine revs up. However, rats that had been trained to respond using saccharin (which broke the link between sweetness and calories), relative to rats trained on glucose, showed a smaller rise in core body temperate after eating a novel, sweet-tasting, high-calorie meal. The authors think this blunted response both led to overeating and made it harder to burn off sweet-tasting calories.

"The data clearly indicate that consuming a food sweetened with no-calorie saccharin can lead to greater body-weight gain and adiposity than would consuming the same food sweetened with a higher-calorie sugar," the authors wrote.

The authors acknowledge that this outcome may seem counter-intuitive and might not come as welcome news to human clinical researchers and health-care practitioners, who have long recommended low- or no-calorie sweeteners. What's more, the data come from rats, not humans. However, they noted that their findings match emerging evidence that people who drink more diet drinks are at higher risk for obesity and metabolic syndrome, a collection of medical problems such as abdominal fat, high blood pressure, and insulin resistance that put people at risk for heart disease and diabetes.

Why would a sugar substitute backfire? Swithers and Davidson wrote that sweet foods provide a "salient orosensory stimulus" that strongly predicts someone is about to take in a lot of calories. Ingestive and digestive reflexes gear up for that intake but when false sweetness isn't followed by lots of calories, the system gets confused. Thus, people may eat more or expend less energy than they otherwise would.

The good news, Swithers says, is that people can still count calories to regulate intake and body weight. However, she sympathizes with the dieter's lament that counting calories requires more conscious effort than consuming low-calorie foods.

Swithers adds that based on the lab's hypothesis, other artificial sweeteners such as aspartame, sucralose, and acesulfame K, which also taste sweet but do not predict the delivery of calories, could have similar effects. Finally, although the results are consistent with the idea that humans would show similar effects, human study is required for further demonstration.

Article: "A Role for Sweet Taste: Calorie Predictive Relations in Energy Regulation by Rats," Susan E. Swithers, PhD, and Terry L. Davidson, PhD, Purdue University; *Behavioral Neuroscience*, Vol. 122, No. 1.

Section 32.5

Sugar Substitutes and Caloric Intake

"New Research: Sugar Substitutes Reduce Caloric Intake without Overeating or Hunger," © 2010 Calorie Control Council (www.caloriecontrol.org). Reprinted with permission.

A new study published in the August 2010 journal *Appetite* further demonstrates that people who consume low-calorie sweeteners are able to significantly reduce their caloric intake and do not overeat. In fact, study participants who received the sugar substitutes instead of sugar consumed significantly fewer calories and there was no difference in hunger levels despite having fewer calories overall.

The researchers noted, "In conclusion, participants did not compensate by eating more at either their lunch or dinner meal and reported similar levels of satiety when they consumed lower calorie preloads [pre-meals] containing stevia or aspartame than when they consumed higher calorie preloads containing sucrose."

This study was conducted in both healthy and overweight adults and participants were given a pre-meal containing either sucrose, aspartame, or stevia. Those who received the stevia or aspartame consumed fewer calories overall, did not overeat, and did not report increased feelings of hunger.

"Although the totality of the scientific evidence demonstrates that low-calorie sweeteners and the products that contain them are not related to weight gain, increased hunger, or overeating, there have been recent reports questioning the benefits of low-calorie sweeteners," notes Beth Hubrich, a dietitian with the Calorie Control Council, an international trade association. "When used as part of an overall healthy diet, low-calorie sweeteners and light products can be beneficial tools in helping people control caloric intake and weight."

"This human study, in addition to the many others, serves as a counter to the recent allegations about low-calorie sweetener benefits from epidemiological studies (which cannot show cause and effect) and studies performed in a small number of rats," adds Hubrich.

This study also builds upon a recent 2009 meta-analysis (evaluating 224 studies) published in the *American Journal of Clinical Nutrition* and conducted by [Richard D.] Mattes and [Barry M.] Popkin. These researchers concluded, "A critical review of the literature, addressing the mechanisms by which non-nutritive [low-calorie] sweeteners may promote energy intake, reveals that none are substantiated by the available evidence."

For further information about low-calorie sweeteners (sugar substitutes) and low-calorie, sugar-free foods and beverages, visit www .caloriecontrol.org.

Anton, S. et al. Effects of stevia, aspartame, and sucrose on food intake, satiety, and postprandial glucose and insulin levels. *Appetite*: 55 (2010) 37–43.

Chapter 33

Food Additives
and Irradiation

Chapter Contents

Section 33.1

Additives

For centuries, ingredients have served useful functions in a variety
of foods. Our ancestors used salt to preserve meats and fish, added
herbs and spices to improve the flavor of foods, preserved fruit with
sugar, and pickled cucumbers in a vinegar solution. Today, consumers demand and enjoy a food supply that is flavorful, nutritious, safe,
convenient, colorful, and affordable. Food additives and advances in
technology help make that possible.

There are thousands of ingredients used to make foods. The Food
and Drug Administration (FDA) maintains a list of over 3,000 ingredients in its data base "Everything Added to Food in the United States,"
many of which we use at home every day (e.g., sugar, baking soda, salt,
vanilla, yeast, spices, and colors).

Still, some consumers have concerns about additives because they may
see the long, unfamiliar names and think of them as complex chemical
compounds. In fact, every food we eat—whether a just-picked strawberry
or a homemade cookie—is made up of chemical compounds that determine
flavor, color, texture, and nutrient value. All food additives are carefully
regulated by federal authorities and various international organizations
to ensure that foods are safe to eat and are accurately labeled.

The purpose of this section is to provide helpful background information about food and color additives: what they are, why they are
used in foods, and how they are regulated for safe use.

Why Are Food and Color Ingredients Added to Food?

Additives perform a variety of useful functions in foods that consumers often take for granted. Some additives could be eliminated if
we were willing to grow our own food, harvest and grind it, spend many
hours cooking and canning, or accept increased risks of food spoilage.
But most consumers today rely on the many technological, aesthetic,
and convenient benefits that additives provide.

Following are some reasons why ingredients are added to foods:

1. **To maintain or improve safety and freshness:** Preservatives slow product spoilage caused by mold, air, bacteria, fungi, or yeast. In addition to maintaining the quality of the food, they help control contamination that can cause foodborne illness, including life-threatening botulism. One group of preservatives—antioxidants—prevents fats and oils and the foods containing them from becoming rancid or developing an off flavor. They also prevent cut fresh fruits such as apples from turning brown when exposed to air.

2. **To improve or maintain nutritional value:** Vitamins and minerals (and fiber) are added to many foods to make up for those lacking in a person's diet or lost in processing, or to enhance the nutritional quality of a food. Such fortification and enrichment has helped reduce malnutrition in the U.S. and worldwide. All products containing added nutrients must be appropriately labeled.

3. **Improve taste, texture, and appearance:** Spices, natural and artificial flavors, and sweeteners are added to enhance the taste of food. Food colors maintain or improve appearance. Emulsifiers, stabilizers, and thickeners give foods the texture and consistency consumers expect. Leavening agents allow baked goods to rise during baking. Some additives help control the acidity and alkalinity of foods, while other ingredients help maintain the taste and appeal of foods with reduced fat content.

Types of Food Ingredients

Table 33.1 lists the types of common food ingredients, why they are used, and some examples of the names that can be found on product labels. Some additives are used for more than one purpose.

What Is a Food Additive?

In its broadest sense, a food additive is any substance added to food. Legally, the term refers to "any substance the intended use of which results or may reasonably be expected to result—directly or indirectly—in its becoming a component or otherwise affecting the characteristics of any food." This definition includes any substance used in the production, processing, treatment, packaging, transportation,

Table 33.1. Food Ingredients

Types of Ingredients	What They Do	Examples of Uses	Names Found on Product Labels
Preservatives	Prevent food spoilage from bacteria, molds, fungi, or yeast (antimicrobials); slow or prevent changes in color, flavor, or texture and delay rancidity (antioxidants); maintain freshness	Fruit sauces and jellies, beverages, baked goods, cured meats, oils and margarines, cereals, dressings, snack foods, fruits, and vegetables	Ascorbic acid, citric acid, sodium benzoate, calcium propionate, sodium erythorbate, sodium nitrite, calcium sorbate, potassium sorbate, BHA [butylated hydroxyanisole], BHT [butylated hydroxytoluene], EDTA [ethylenediaminetetraacetic acid], tocopherols (Vitamin E)
Sweeteners	Add sweetness with or without the extra calories	Beverages, baked goods, confections, table-top sugar, substitutes, many processed foods	Sucrose (sugar), glucose, fructose, sorbitol, mannitol, corn syrup, high fructose corn syrup, saccharin, aspartame, sucralose, acesulfame potassium (acesulfame-K), neotame
Color additives	Offset color loss due to exposure to light, air, temperature extremes, moisture, and storage conditions; correct natural variations in color; enhance colors that occur naturally; provide color to colorless and "fun" foods	Many processed foods (candies, snack foods, margarine, cheese, soft drinks, jams/jellies, gelatins, pudding and pie fillings)	FD&C Blue Nos. 1 and 2, FD&C Green No. 3, FD&C Red Nos. 3 and 40, FD&C Yellow No. 5 (tartrazine) and No. 6, Orange B, Citrus Red No. 2, annatto extract, beta-carotene, grape skin extract, cochineal extract or carmine, paprika oleoresin, caramel color, fruit and vegetable juices, saffron (note: Exempt color additives are not required to be declared by name on labels but may be declared simply as colorings or color added)
Flavors and spices	Add specific flavors (natural and synthetic)	Pudding and pie fillings, gelatin, dessert mixes, cake mixes, salad dressings, candies, soft drinks, ice cream, BBQ sauce	Natural flavoring, artificial flavor, and spices
Flavor enhancers	Enhance flavors already present in foods (without providing their own separate flavor)	Many processed foods	Monosodium glutamate (MSG), hydrolyzed soy protein, autolyzed yeast extract, disodium guanylate or inosinate
Fat replacers (and components of formulations used to replace fats)	Provide expected texture and a creamy "mouth-feel" in reduced-fat foods	Baked goods, dressings, frozen desserts, confections, cake and dessert mixes, dairy products	Olestra, cellulose gel, carrageenan, polydextrose, modified food starch, microparticulated egg white protein, guar gum, xanthan gum, whey protein concentrate

Table 33.1. *continued*

Nutrients	Replace vitamins and minerals lost in processing (enrichment), add nutrients that may be lacking in the diet (fortification)	Thiamine hydrochloride, riboflavin (Vitamin B2), niacin, niacinamide, folate or folic acid, beta-carotene, potassium iodide, iron or ferrous sulfate, alpha tocopherols, ascorbic acid, Vitamin D, amino acids (L-tryptophan, L-lysine, L-leucine, L-methionine)
Emulsifiers	Allow smooth mixing of ingredients, prevent separation Keep emulsified products stable, reduce stickiness, control crystallization, keep ingredients dispersed, and help products dissolve more easily	Soy lecithin, mono- and diglycerides, egg yolks, polysorbates, sorbitan monostearate
Stabilizers and thickeners, binders, texturizers	Produce uniform texture, improve "mouth-feel"	Gelatin, pectin, guar gum, carrageenan, xanthan gum, whey
Leavening agents	Promote rising of baked goods	Baking soda, monocalcium phosphate, calcium carbonate
Anti-caking agents	Keep powdered foods free-flowing, prevent moisture absorption	Calcium silicate, iron ammonium citrate, silicon dioxide
Humectants	Retain moisture	Glycerin, sorbitol
Yeast nutrients	Promote growth of yeast	Calcium sulfate, ammonium phosphate
Dough strengtheners and conditioners	Produce more stable dough	Ammonium sulfate, azodicarbonamide, L-cysteine
Firming agents	Maintain crispness and firmness	Calcium chloride, calcium lactate
Enzyme preparations	Modify proteins, polysaccharides, and fats	Enzymes, lactase, papain, rennet, chymosin
Gases	Serve as propellant, aerate, or create carbonation	Carbon dioxide, nitrous oxide

401

or storage of food. The purpose of the legal definition, however, is to impose a premarket approval requirement. Therefore, this definition excludes ingredients whose use is generally recognized as safe (where government approval is not needed), those ingredients approved for use by FDA or the U.S. Department of Agriculture prior to the food additives provisions of law, and color additives and pesticides where other legal premarket approval requirements apply.

Direct food additives are those that are added to a food for a specific purpose in that food. For example, xanthan gum—used in salad dressings, chocolate milk, bakery fillings, puddings, and other foods to add texture—is a direct additive. Most direct additives are identified on the ingredient label of foods.

Indirect food additives are those that become part of the food in trace amounts due to its packaging, storage, or other handling. For instance, minute amounts of packaging substances may find their way into foods during storage. Food packaging manufacturers must prove to the FDA that all materials coming in contact with food are safe before they are permitted for use in such a manner.

What Is a Color Additive?

A color additive is any dye, pigment, or substance which when added or applied to a food, drug, or cosmetic, or to the human body, is capable (alone or through reactions with other substances) of imparting color. FDA is responsible for regulating all color additives to ensure that foods containing color additives are safe to eat, contain only approved ingredients, and are accurately labeled.

Color additives are used in foods for many reasons: 1) to offset color loss due to exposure to light, air, temperature extremes, moisture, and storage conditions; 2) to correct natural variations in color; 3) to enhance colors that occur naturally; and 4) to provide color to colorless and "fun" foods. Without color additives, colas wouldn't be brown, margarine wouldn't be yellow, and mint ice cream wouldn't be green. Color additives are now recognized as an important part of practically all processed foods we eat.

FDA's permitted colors are classified as subject to certification or exempt from certification, both of which are subject to rigorous safety standards prior to their approval and listing for use in foods.

- Certified colors are synthetically produced (or human made) and used widely because they impart an intense, uniform color; are less expensive; and blend more easily to create a variety of hues. There are nine certified color additives approved for use in the

United States (e.g., FD&C Yellow No. 6; see Table 33.1 for complete list). Certified food colors generally do not add undesirable flavors to foods.

- Colors that are exempt from certification include pigments derived from natural sources such as vegetables, minerals, or animals. Nature-derived color additives are typically more expensive than certified colors and may add unintended flavors to foods. Examples of exempt colors include annatto extract (yellow), dehydrated beets (bluish-red to brown), caramel (yellow to tan), beta-carotene (yellow to orange), and grape skin extract (red, green).

How Are Additives Approved for Use in Foods?

Today, food and color additives are more strictly studied, regulated, and monitored than at any other time in history. FDA has the primary legal responsibility for determining their safe use. To market a new direct food additive or color additive for use in food (or before using an additive already approved for one use in another manner not yet approved), a manufacturer or other sponsor must first petition FDA for its approval. These petitions must provide evidence that the substance is safe for the ways in which it will be used. As a result of a 1997 statutory change, indirect additives are approved via a premarket notification process requiring the same data as was previously required by petition.

When evaluating the safety of a substance and whether it should be approved, FDA considers: 1) the composition and properties of the substance, 2) the amount that would typically be consumed, 3) immediate and long-term health effects, and 4) various safety factors. The evaluation determines an appropriate level of use that includes a built-in safety margin—a factor that allows for uncertainty about the levels of consumption that are expected to be harmless. In other words, the levels of use that gain approval are much lower than what would be expected to have any adverse effect.

Because of inherent limitations of science, FDA can never be absolutely certain of the absence of any risk from the use of any substance. Therefore, FDA must determine—based on the best science available—if there is a reasonable certainty of no harm to consumers when an additive is used as proposed.

If an additive is approved, FDA issues regulations that may include the types of foods in which it can be used, the maximum amounts to

403

be used, and how it should be identified on food labels. In 1999, procedures changed so that FDA now consults with USDA [U.S. Department of Agriculture] during the review process for ingredients that are proposed for use in meat and poultry products. Federal officials then monitor the extent of Americans' consumption of the new additive and results of any new research on its safety to ensure its use continues to be within safe limits.

If new evidence suggests that a product already in use may be unsafe, or if consumption levels have changed enough to require another look, federal authorities may prohibit its use or conduct further studies to determine if the use can still be considered safe.

Regulations known as good manufacturing practices (GMP) limit the amount of food ingredients used in foods to the amount necessary to achieve the desired effect.

Under the Food Additives Amendment, two groups of ingredients were exempted from the regulation process.

GROUP I—prior-sanctioned substances—are substances that FDA or USDA had determined safe for use in food prior to the 1958 amendment. Examples are sodium nitrite and potassium nitrite used to preserve luncheon meats.

GROUP II—GRAS (generally recognized as safe) ingredients—are those that are generally recognized by experts as safe, based on their extensive history of use in food before 1958 or based on published scientific evidence. Among the several hundred GRAS substances are salt, sugar, spices, vitamins, and monosodium glutamate (MSG). Manufacturers may also request that FDA review the industry's determination of GRAS status.

Summary

Food ingredients have been used for many years to preserve, flavor, blend, thicken, and color foods and have played an important role in reducing serious nutritional deficiencies among consumers. These ingredients also help ensure the availability of flavorful, nutritious, safe, convenient, colorful, and affordable foods that meet consumer expectations year-round.

Food and color additives are strictly studied, regulated, and monitored. Federal regulations require evidence that each substance is safe at its intended level of use before it may be added to foods. Furthermore, all additives are subject to ongoing safety review as scientific understanding and methods of testing continue to improve. Consumers should feel safe about the foods they eat.

Questions and Answers about Food and Color Additives

Q: How are ingredients listed on a product label?

A: Food manufacturers are required to list all ingredients in the food on the label. On a product label, the ingredients are listed in order of predominance, with the ingredients used in the greatest amount first, followed in descending order by those in smaller amounts. The label must list the names of any FDA-certified color additives (e.g., FD&C Blue No. 1 or the abbreviated name, Blue 1). But some ingredients can be listed collectively as "flavors," "spices," "artificial flavoring," or in the case of color additives exempt from certification (unless otherwise required by regulation), "artificial colors," without naming each one. Declaration of an allergenic ingredient in a collective or single color, flavor, or spice could be accomplished by simply naming the allergenic ingredient in the ingredient list.

Q: What are dyes and lakes in color additives?

A: Certified color additives are categorized as either dyes or lakes. Dyes dissolve in water and are manufactured as powders, granules, liquids, or other special-purpose forms. They can be used in beverages, dry mixes, baked goods, confections, dairy products, pet foods, and a variety of other products. Lakes are the water insoluble form of the dye. Lakes are more stable than dyes and are ideal for coloring products containing fats and oils or items lacking sufficient moisture to dissolve dyes. Typical uses include coated tablets, cake and donut mixes, hard candies, and chewing gums.

Q: Do additives cause childhood hyperactivity?

A: Although this hypothesis was popularized in the 1970s, results from studies on this issue either have been inconclusive, inconsistent, or difficult to interpret due to inadequacies in study design. A Consensus Development Panel of the National Institutes of Health concluded in 1982 that for some children with attention deficit hyperactivity disorder (ADHD) and confirmed food allergy, dietary modification has produced some improvement in behavior. Although the panel said that elimination diets should not be used universally to treat childhood hyperactivity, since there is no scientific evidence to predict which children may benefit, the panel recognized that initiation of a trial of dietary treatment or continuation of a diet in patients whose families and physicians perceive benefits may be warranted. However, a 1997 review published in the *Journal of the American Academy of Child & Adolescent Psychiatry* noted there is minimal evidence of efficacy and extreme difficulty inducing children and adolescents to comply with restricted diets. Thus, dietary treatment should not be recommended, except possibly with a small number of preschool children who may be sensitive to tartrazine, known commonly as FD&C Yellow No. 5 (see following question). In 2007, synthetic certified color additives again came under scrutiny following publication of a study commissioned by the UK Food Standards Agency to investigate whether certain color additives cause hyperactivity in children. Both the FDA and the European Food Safety Authority independently reviewed the results from this study and each has concluded that the study does not substantiate a link between the color additives that were tested and behavioral effects.

Q: What is the difference between natural and artificial ingredients? Is a naturally produced ingredient safer than an artificially manufactured ingredient?

A: Natural ingredients are derived from natural sources (e.g., soybeans and corn provide lecithin to maintain product consistency; beets provide beet powder used as food coloring). Other ingredients are not found in nature and therefore must be synthetically produced as artificial ingredients. Also, some ingredients found in nature can be manufactured artificially and produced more economically, with greater purity and more consistent quality, than their natural counterparts. For example, vitamin C or ascorbic acid may be derived from an orange or produced in a laboratory. Food ingredients are subject to the same strict safety standards regardless of whether they are naturally or artificially derived.

Q: Are certain people sensitive to FD&C Yellow No. 5 in foods?

A: FD&C Yellow No. 5 is used to color beverages, dessert powders, candy, ice cream, custards, and other foods. FDA's Committee on Hypersensitivity to Food Constituents concluded in 1986 that FD&C Yellow No. 5 might cause hives in fewer than one out of 10,000 people. It also concluded that there was no evidence the color additive in food provokes asthma attacks. The law now requires Yellow No. 5 to be identified on the ingredient line. This allows the few who may be sensitive to the color to avoid it.

Q: *Do low-calorie sweeteners cause adverse reactions?*

A: No. Food safety experts generally agree there is no convincing evidence of a cause and effect relationship between these sweeteners and negative health effects in humans. The FDA has monitored consumer complaints of possible adverse reactions for more than 20 years.

For example, in carefully controlled clinical studies, aspartame has not been shown to cause adverse or allergic reactions. However, persons with a rare hereditary disease known as phenylketonuria (PKU) must control their intake of phenylalanine from all sources, including aspartame. Although aspartame contains only a small amount of phenylalanine, labels of aspartame-containing foods and beverages must include a statement advising phenylketonurics of the presence of phenylalanine.

Individuals who have concerns about possible adverse effects from food additives or other substances should contact their physicians.

Q: *How do they add vitamins and minerals to fortified cereals?*

A: Adding nutrients to a cereal can cause taste and color changes in the product. This is especially true with added minerals. Since no one wants cereal that tastes like a vitamin supplement, a variety of techniques are employed in the fortification process. In general, those nutrients that are heat stable (such as vitamins A and E and various minerals) are incorporated into the cereal itself (they're baked right in). Nutrients that are not stable to heat (such as B vitamins) are applied directly to the cereal after all heating steps are completed. Each cereal is unique—some can handle more nutrients than others can. This is one reason why fortification levels are different across all cereals.

Q: *What is the role of modern technology in producing food additives?*

A: Many new techniques are being researched that will allow the production of additives in ways not previously possible. One approach is the use of biotechnology, which can use simple organisms to produce food additives. These additives are the same as food components found in nature. In 1990, FDA approved the first bioengineered enzyme, rennin, which traditionally had been extracted from calves' stomachs for use in making cheese.

407

Section 33.2

Irradiation

This section excerpted from "Food Irradiation" and "Food Safety," U.S. Environmental Protection Agency (www.epa.gov), October 1, 2010.

Food irradiation is a technology for controlling spoilage and eliminating food-borne pathogens, such as *Salmonella*. The result is similar to conventional pasteurization and is often called "cold pasteurization" or "irradiation pasteurization." Like pasteurization, irradiation kills bacteria and other pathogens that could otherwise result in spoilage or food poisoning. The fundamental difference between the two methods is the source of the energy they rely on to destroy the microbes. While conventional pasteurization relies on heat, irradiation relies on the energy of ionizing radiation. The FDA emphasizes that no preservation method is a substitute for safe food handling procedures.

Irradiation of foods must be approved by the FDA. Some applications also require USDA approval. USDA's Food Safety Inspection Service must approve both the process and the facility for irradiation of meat and poultry. USDA's Animal and Plant Health Inspection Service must approve irradiation for plant quarantine protection. FDA approval comes only after extensive testing demonstrates that the proposed dose of irradiation effectively eliminates the pathogen or insect of concern and does not generate toxic or carcinogenic chemicals in the food.

FDA has approved irradiation for several foodstuffs, including spices and herbs, potatoes, pork, poultry and other meats, fruits, and vegetables. It sets the maximum dose based on test results. The USDA may also set a minimum dose to assure effectiveness, for example, to assure the destruction of insects or plants in quarantine control.

How does irradiation kill bacteria?

When ionizing radiation strikes bacteria and other microbes, its high energy breaks chemical bonds in molecules that are vital for cell growth and integrity. As a result, the microbes die, or can no longer multiply and cause illness or spoilage.

Breaking chemical bonds with radiation is known as radiolysis.

How does irradiation affect the food itself?

Ionizing radiation also breaks some of the chemical bonds within the food itself. The effects of chemical changes in foods are varied. Some are desirable, others are not. Examples of some food changes are the following:

- Changes in structure of certain foods too fragile to withstand the irradiation—for example, lettuce and other leafy vegetables turn mushy

- Slowed ripening and maturation in certain fruits and vegetables lengthens shelf life

- Reduction or destruction of some nutrients, such as vitamins, reduces the nutritional value (the effect is comparable to losses in heat pasteurization)

- Alteration of some flavor compounds

- Formation of compounds that were not originally present requires the strict control of radiation levels

- Generation of free radicals, some of which recombine with other ions

These effects are the result of radiolysis. Whether the products of radiolysis in food are all innocent from a human health perspective is still debated. However, years of experience in food irradiation have not demonstrated any identifiable health problems.

How is safety tested?

Safety testing of irradiated foods has taken place since the early 1950s. Irradiated foods have been fed to several species of animals, some up to 40 generations. Additionally, irradiated foods have been evaluated chemically.

The FDA must approve any use of irradiation on food, and the USDA Food Safety Inspection Service must approve the process and the facility if meat and poultry products are involved. USDA's Animal and Plant Health Inspection Service approves use of irradiation for plant quarantine protection.

Several foods have been approved in the United States. The FDA sets the maximum dose permitted on food based on what was petitioned to assure safety. The USDA sets the minimum dose on some foods to assure the desired effects such as destruction of microorganisms or effective insect quarantine control.

Assessing the safety of irradiated foods has involved investigation in the following areas:

- Radiation chemistry
- General toxicology/animal testing
- Nutrition of irradiated foods
- Microbiology of irradiated foods
- Packaging

Can irradiation make food radioactive?

No. Food does not come in contact with radioactive material during food irradiation and cannot be contaminated this way. Radiation that is too energetic, however, can disrupt the energy balance in the nuclei of food atoms, making them unstable (radioactive). This is known as induced radioactivity.

Electron and X-ray beams can be energetic enough to induce radioactivity. To prevent induced radioactivity, FDA limits the energy of the radiation from these sources to less than four mega-electron volts. Radiation from cobalt-60 sources is not energetic enough to induce radioactivity.

What are the alternatives to food irradiation?

There are many traditional methods for preserving foods, such as drying, smoking, salt or sugar curing, and canning. These methods generally alter the flavor and chemical composition of the food. More modern methods, such as heat pasteurization and refrigeration or freezing, as well as freeze drying, are also common. Decisions about which method to use for individual foods and circumstances must weigh feasibility, effectiveness, and cost as well as the chemical changes each method causes in the food. The FDA emphasizes that no preservation method is a substitute for safe food handling procedures.

How do I know if food has been irradiated?

A distinctive logo, the radura, on the labels of packaged or bulk food identifies irradiated food.

410

Chapter 34

Excess Sodium

Lowering Salt in Your Diet

Everyone needs some salt to function. Also known as sodium chloride, salt helps maintain the body's balance of fluids. Salt also functions in many foods as a preservative by helping to prevent spoilage and keeping certain foods safe to eat. But nearly all Americans consume more salt than they need, according to the 2005 *Dietary Guidelines for Americans*.

The natural salt in food accounts for about 10% of total intake, on average, according to the guidelines. The salt we add at the table or while cooking adds another 5% to 10%. About 75% of our total salt intake comes from salt added to processed foods by manufacturers and salt that cooks add to foods at restaurants and other food service establishments.

What are the health effects of too much salt?

In many people, salt contributes to high blood pressure. High blood pressure makes the heart work harder and can lead to heart disease, stroke, heart failure, and kidney disease.

"Lowering Salt in Your Diet," U.S. Food and Drug Administration (www.fda. gov), May 18, 2010, and "Health Facts: Sodium and Potassium," from *Dietary Guidelines for Americans, 2005—Toolkit for Health Professionals,* U.S. Department of Health and Human Services (www.hhs.gov), 2005. Reviewed by David A. Cooke, MD, FACP, January 2011.

What is the daily recommended amount of sodium for adults?

The amount of salt in a food is listed as "sodium" on the Nutrition Facts label that appears on food packaging. The *Dietary Guidelines* recommend that the general population consume no more than 2,300 milligrams (mg) of sodium a day (about a teaspoon of table salt). Dietary recommendations and food labels use sodium rather than salt since it is the sodium component of salt that is most relevant for human health.

Some people are more sensitive to the effects of salt than others. The guidelines also recommend that, in general, individuals with hypertension, blacks, and middle-aged and older adults should limit intake to 1,500 mg of sodium per day.

The exceptions to this guideline are people whose doctors have put them on a diet that requires even less sodium because of a medical condition. Always follow your doctor's recommendation about how much sodium you can have daily.

What steps can I take to lower my salt intake?

- Eat more fresh fruits and vegetables.
- Consume foods that are rich in potassium. Potassium can help blunt the effects of sodium on blood pressure. The recommended intake of potassium for adolescents and adults is 4,700 mg/day. Potassium-rich foods include leafy green vegetables and fruits from vines.
- Flavor food with pepper and other herbs and spices instead of salt.
- Choose unsalted snacks.
- Read food labels and choose foods low in sodium.

How can I tell if a food is low in sodium or high in sodium?

The Nutrition Facts label that appears on food packaging also lists the "% Daily Value" for sodium. Look for the abbreviation "%DV" to find it. Foods listed as 5% or less for sodium are low in sodium. Anything above 20% for sodium is considered high. Try to select foods that provide 5% or less for sodium, per serving.

Are salt substitutes safe?

Many salt substitutes contain potassium chloride and can be used by individuals to replace salt in their diet. There are no known undesirable effects in healthy people who consume a lot of potassium; however, potassium could be harmful to people with certain medical conditions, such as diabetes, kidney disease, and heart disease. Check with your doctor before using salt substitutes.

What is the U.S. Food and Drug Administration (FDA)'s role in regulating salt?

- Salt is regulated by FDA as a "generally recognized as safe" (GRAS) ingredient. A GRAS substance is one that has a long history of safe, common use in foods or that is determined to be safe, for the intended use, based on proven science. These substances need not be approved by FDA prior to being used.

- FDA requires that sodium content be stated on food labels. FDA has implemented several labeling requirements related to sodium content of foods.

- FDA sets criteria for nutrient-content claims that manufacturers make about foods. Examples are "low sodium" and "reduced in sodium."

- FDA has not exercised its regulatory authority to limit the amount of salt added to processed foods; however, the agency is conducting research in this area. In 2005, the Center for Science in the Public Interest submitted a Citizen's Petition to FDA requesting that the agency make changes to the regulatory status of salt, including requiring limits on the amount of salt in processed food. In November 2007, FDA held a public hearing in College Park, Maryland, on the agency's policies regarding salt in food and solicited comments from the public about future regulatory approaches.

Will FDA be regulating salt as recommended by the Institute of Medicine report?

FDA was a sponsor of the Institute of Medicine (IOM) report, "Strategies to Reduce Sodium Intake in the United States," which was released by IOM on April 20, 2010. The IOM committee reviewed and recommended various ways to reduce sodium intake. The strategies recommended included actions by FDA and other government agencies and by food manufacturers, public health professionals, and consumer educators. These recommendations are being carefully reviewed and evaluated by FDA.

413

Sodium and Potassium

Nearly all Americans eat too much salt (sodium). Most of the salt comes from eating processed foods (75%), or adding salt to food while cooking and using the salt shaker at meals (5% to 10%). On average, the more salt a person eats, the higher his or her blood pressure.

Table 34.1. Ranges of Sodium Content for Selected Foods

This table is provided to show the importance of reading the food label to determine the sodium content of food, which can vary by several hundreds of milligrams in similar foods.

Food	Amount	Range of Sodium Content (mg)	% Daily Value (%DV)* for Sodium
Breads, all types	1 oz	95–210	4%–9%
Frozen pizza, plain cheese	4 oz	450–1,200	19%–50%
Frozen vegetables, all types	1/2 c	2–160	0%–7%
Salad dressing, regular fat, all types	2 Tbsp	110–505	5%–21%
Salsa	2 Tbsp	150–240	6%–10%
Soup (tomato), reconstituted	8 oz	700–1,260	29%–53%
Tomato juice	8 oz (~1 c)	340–1,040	14%–43%
Potato chips[a]	1 oz (28.4 g)	120–180	5%–8%
Tortilla chips[a]	1 oz (28.4 g)	105–160	4%–7%
Pretzels[a]	1 oz (28.4 g)	290–560	12%–23%

* % Daily Values (DV) listed in this column are based on the food amounts listed in the table. The DV for sodium is 2,400 mg.
a. All snack foods are regular flavor, salted.

Source: Agriculture Research Service (ARS) Nutrient Database for Standard Reference, Release 17 and recent manufacturers' label data from retail market surveys. Serving sizes were standardized to be comparable among brands within a food. Pizza and bread slices vary in size and weight across brands.
Note: None of the examples provided were labeled low-sodium products.

Eating less salt is an important way to reduce the risk of high blood pressure, which may in turn reduce the risk of heart disease, stroke, congestive heart failure, and kidney damage. To reduce the amount of sodium in your diet, eat less processed food and use less salt while cooking and at the table.

Table 34.2. Potassium Content of Selected Foods

Food, Amount	Potassium (mg)	% Daily Value*	Calories
Sweet potato, baked, 1 potato (146 g)	694	20%	131
Beet greens, cooked, 1/2 c	655	19%	19
Potato, baked, flesh, 1 potato (156 g)	610	17%	145
White beans, canned, 1/2 c	595	17%	153
Yogurt, plain, nonfat, 8-oz container	579	17%	127
Clams, canned, 3 oz	534	15%	126
Yogurt, plain, low-fat, 8-oz container	531	15%	143
Prune juice, 3/4 c	530	15%	136
Carrot juice, 3/4 c	517	14%	71
Halibut, cooked, 3 oz	490	14%	119
Soybeans, green, cooked, 1/2 c	485	14%	127
Tuna, yellowfin, cooked, 3 oz	484	14%	118
Lima beans, cooked, 1/2 c	484	14%	104
Winter squash, cooked, 1/2 c	448	13%	40
Soybeans, mature, cooked, 1/2 c	443	13%	149
Rockfish, Pacific, cooked, 3 oz	442	13%	103
Cod, Pacific, cooked, 3 oz	439	13%	89
Banana, 1 medium	422	12%	105
Spinach, cooked, 1/2 c	419	12%	21
Tomato juice, 3/4 c	417	12%	31
Tomato sauce, 1/2 c	405	12%	39

* % Daily Values (DV) are based on the food amounts listed in the table and FDA's Daily Value for potassium (3,500 mg).

Source: Nutrient values from Agricultural Research Service (ARS) Nutrient Database for Standard Reference, Release 17. Foods are from ARS single nutrient reports, sorted in descending order by nutrient content in terms of common household measures.

Other lifestyle changes may prevent or delay getting high blood pressure and may help lower elevated blood pressure. These include eating more potassium-rich foods, losing excess weight, being more physically active, eating a healthy diet, and limiting alcoholic beverages, if you choose to drink them.

A diet rich in potassium helps to counterbalance some of sodium's harmful effects on blood pressure. Foods that are good sources of potassium are listed in Table 34.2.

You should get no more than 2,300 milligrams of sodium each day. Some people should get less.

Compare sodium content for similar foods. This can really make a difference. Table 34.1 shows you examples of how you can reduce the amount of sodium you eat by choosing another brand of the same food. Use the Nutrition Facts label to select brands that are lower in sodium.

Use the claims on the front of the food package to quickly identify foods that contain less salt or that are a good source of potassium, a nutrient you want to get more of in your daily diet. Examples include "low in sodium," "very low sodium," and "high in potassium."

When buying packaged food, use the Nutrition Facts label to check potassium content. Use the %DV to look for foods that are low in sodium and high in potassium—which counteracts some of sodium's effects on blood pressure. Note that potassium is not always found on the label.

Get Enough Potassium Each Day

Potassium-containing food sources include leafy greens, such as spinach and collards; fruit from vines, such as grapes and blackberries; root vegetables, such as carrots and potatoes; and citrus fruits, such as oranges and grapefruit. More specific examples are listed on Table 34.2. Adults should aim to consume 4,700 milligrams of potassium from food and beverages each day.

Chapter 35

Commercial Beverages

Chapter Contents

Section 35.1

Making Healthy Beverage Choices

"Rethink Your Drink," Centers for Disease Control and Prevention
(www.cdc.gov), January 4, 2011.

When it comes to weight loss, there's no lack of diets promising fast results. There are low-carb diets, high-carb diets, low-fat diets, grapefruit diets, cabbage soup diets, and blood type diets, to name a few. But no matter what diet you may try to lose weight, you must take in fewer calories than your body uses. Most people try to reduce their calorie intake by focusing on food, but another way to cut calories may be to think about what you drink.

What Do You Drink? It Makes More Difference Than You Think!

Calories in drinks are not hidden (they're listed right on the Nutrition Facts label), but many people don't realize just how many calories beverages can contribute to their daily intake. As you can see Table 35.1, calories from drinks can really add up. But there is good news: you have plenty of options for reducing the number of calories in what you drink.

Substituting no- or low-calorie drinks for sugar-sweetened beverages cuts about 650 calories in the example in Table 35.1.

Of course, not everyone drinks the amount of sugar-sweetened beverages shown here. Check Table 35.2 to estimate how many calories you typically take in from beverages.

Milk contains vitamins and other nutrients that contribute to good health, but it also contains calories. Choosing low-fat or fat-free milk is a good way to reduce your calorie intake and still get the nutrients that milk contains.

Calories per Cup (8 oz) of Milk

- Chocolate milk (whole): 208
- Chocolate milk (2% reduced-fat): 190
- Chocolate milk (1% low-fat): 158

Table 35.1. Reducing Calories in Your Drinks

Occasion	Instead of...	Calories	Try...	Calories
Morning coffee shop run	Medium café latte (16 oz) made with whole milk	265	Small café latte (12 oz) made with fat-free milk	125
Lunchtime combo meal	20-oz bottle of nondiet cola with your lunch	227	Bottle of water or diet soda	0
Afternoon break	Sweetened lemon iced tea from the vending machine (16 oz)	180	Sparkling water with natural lemon flavor (not sweetened)	0
Dinnertime	A glass of nondiet ginger ale with your meal (12 oz)	124	Water with a slice of lemon or lime, or seltzer water with a splash of 100% fruit juice	0 calories for the water with fruit slice, or about 30 calories for seltzer water with 2 ounces of 100% orange juice
Total beverage calories		796		125–55

Table 35.2. Calories in Selected Beverages

Type of Beverage	Calories in 12 Ounces	Calories in 20 Ounces
Fruit punch	192	320
100% apple juice	192	300
100% orange juice	168	280
Lemonade	168	280
Regular lemon/lime soda	148	247
Regular cola	136	227
Sweetened lemon iced tea (bottled, not homemade)	135	225
Tonic water	124	207
Regular ginger ale	124	207
Sports drink	99	165
Fitness water	18	36
Unsweetened iced tea	2	3
Diet soda (with aspartame)	0*	0*
Carbonated water (unsweetened)	0	0
Water	0	0

*Some diet soft drinks can contain a small number of calories that are not listed on the Nutrition Facts label.

- Whole milk (unflavored): 150
- 2% reduced-fat milk (unflavored): 120
- 1% low-fat milk (unflavored): 105
- Fat-free milk (unflavored): 90

Learn to Read Nutrition Facts Labels Carefully

Be aware that the Nutrition Facts label on beverage containers may give the calories for only part of the contents. For example, a typical label on a 20-oz bottle lists the number of calories in an 8-oz serving (100) even though the bottle contains 20 ounces, or 2.5 servings. To figure out how many calories are in the whole bottle, you need to multiply the number of calories in one serving by the number of servings in the bottle (100 x 2.5). The entire bottle actually contains 250 calories even though what the label calls a "serving" only contains 100. You need to look closely at the serving size when comparing the calorie content of different beverages.

Sugar by Any Other Name: How to Tell Whether Your Drink Is Sweetened

Sweeteners that add calories to a beverage go by many different names and are not always obvious to someone looking at the ingredients list. Some common caloric sweeteners are listed here. If these appear in the ingredients list of your favorite beverage, you are drinking a sugar-sweetened beverage.

- High-fructose corn syrup
- Fruit juice concentrates
- Sugar
- Corn syrup
- Dextrose
- Fructose
- Honey
- Syrup
- Sucrose

High-Calorie Culprits in Unexpected Places

Coffee drinks and blended fruit smoothies sound innocent enough, but the calories in some of your favorite coffee-shop or smoothie-stand items may surprise you. Check the website or in-store nutrition information of your favorite coffee or smoothie shop to find out how many calories are in different menu items. And when a smoothie or coffee craving kicks in, here are some tips to help minimize the caloric damage:

At the Coffee Shop

- Request that your drink be made with fat-free or low-fat milk instead of whole milk.

- Order the smallest size available.

- Forgo the extra flavoring. The flavor syrups used in coffee shops, like vanilla or hazelnut, are sugar sweetened and will add calories to your drink.

- Skip the whip. The whipped cream on top of coffee drinks adds calories and fat.

- Get back to basics. Order a plain cup of coffee with fat-free milk and artificial sweetener, or drink it black.

At the Smoothie Stand

- Order a child's size if available.

- Ask to see the nutrition information for each type of smoothie and pick the smoothie with the fewest calories.

- Hold the sugar. Many smoothies contain added sugar in addition to the sugar naturally in fruit, juice, or yogurt. Ask that your smoothie be prepared without added sugar: the fruit is naturally sweet.

Better Beverage Choices Made Easy

Now that you know how much difference a drink can make, here are some ways to make smart beverage choices:

- Choose water, diet, or low-calorie beverages instead of sugar-sweetened beverages.

- For a quick, easy, and inexpensive thirst quencher, carry a water bottle and refill it throughout the day.

- Don't "stock the fridge" with sugar-sweetened beverages. Instead, keep a jug or bottles of cold water in the fridge.

- Serve water with meals.

- Make water more exciting by adding slices of lemon, lime, cucumber, or watermelon, or drink sparkling water.

- Add a splash of 100% juice to plain sparkling water for a refreshing, low-calorie drink.

- When you do opt for a sugar-sweetened beverage, go for the small size. Some companies are now selling 8-oz cans and bottles of soda, which contain about 100 calories.

- Be a role model for your friends and family by choosing healthy, low-calorie beverages.

Section 35.2

Energy Drinks, Caffeine, and Health

"Questions and Answers About Energy Drinks and Health,"
© 2009 International Food Information Council (www.foodinsight.org).
Reprinted with permission.

Energy drinks have been increasing in popularity, especially among teens and children. Due to several articles in the media about negative health effects experienced by people who consumed too many energy drinks, some parents and school personnel have become concerned about their growing popularity specifically among teens and children.

However, if you are aware of how much caffeine you are consuming, people of all ages can safely consume energy drinks in moderation. Caffeine is the primary ingredient in most energy drinks and is often blamed for causing the negative health effects some people have experienced after consuming too many energy drinks. However, the majority of the healthy population can safely enjoy moderate amounts of caffeine without experiencing undesirable symptoms.

Staying aware of how much caffeine you are consuming each day from energy drinks, as well as other sources such as coffee, tea, soda, dietary supplements, and medications, is important to stay within moderate, safe intake levels. Learning how to determine the caffeine content of each item, as well as the number of servings per container, will help you to know how to moderate your consumption. You can also help children and teens learn how to moderate their consumption so that they can safely enjoy an energy drink or soda responsibly without risking undesirable symptoms.

The following are some common questions consumers have about energy drinks and how they work to increase feelings of energy, and what you can do to help children and teens consume them in moderation along with a healthful diet.

Q: *What are energy drinks?*

A: The term "energy drink" is a popular term used to refer to some beverages that typically contain caffeine as well as other ingredients, such as taurine, guarana, and B vitamins, for the purpose of providing an extra energy boost. It is not a term that is recognized by the U.S. Food and Drug Administration (FDA) or the U.S. Department of Agriculture (USDA).

Q: *What are the most common ingredients in energy drinks, and what do they do?*

A: Some common ingredients in energy drinks include caffeine, taurine, guarana, ginseng, B vitamins, and L-carnitine. More about what these ingredients are and why they're added to energy drinks is provided here:

Caffeine is included in energy drinks for its potential to improve mental and physical performance and for its taste profile. As it is often the primary ingredient in energy drinks, we will address more questions about caffeine in the following sections.

Taurine is an amino acid that the body makes from the foods we eat. High levels of taurine are present in animal products (beef, pork, lamb, chicken, etc.), while some fish and shellfish contain the highest amounts of taurine (ex., cod, clams, and oysters). Taurine supports neurological development and helps regulate water and mineral salt levels in the blood. It is included in energy drinks because some studies have suggested that it may improve athletic performance. Additionally, some studies propose caffeine and taurine together may improve athletic performance, and perhaps even mental performance. In a report published in 2003, the European Union's Scientific Committee on Foods (now known as the European Food Safety Authority, or EFSA) concluded that studies have not shown a link between taurine consumption and cancer, and that both taurine and its components occur naturally in humans, and are further broken down and excreted by the body.

Guarana is a plant that comes from South America, and guarana-containing drinks and sodas are widely consumed in Brazil. Guarana contains caffeine and is actually denser in caffeine than coffee beans. It is therefore added to energy drinks for the same reason as caffeine—to increase feelings of energy and to improve mental and physical performance.

Guarana content is not typically listed on energy drink labels and adds only a very small amount of caffeine. Guarana is generally recognized as safe (GRAS) in the U.S. as a natural flavoring substance.

Ginseng is an herb that is thought to provide a number of potential benefits, including increasing a sense of well-being and stamina and improving both mental and physical performance. Other potential benefits include improving the health of people recovering from illness, beneficial effects on immunity, and lowering blood glucose levels. However, most of these studies were small or conducted only in laboratory animals; therefore, additional research is needed to confirm these potential health benefits. For more information on Asian ginseng, read the National Institute of Health (NIH)'s "Asian Ginseng Fact Sheet" [at nccam.nih.gov/health/asianginseng].

B vitamins can be found in different foods and help regulate metabolism. Examples of B vitamins include thiamin and cobalamin. These vitamins are often included in energy drinks because they may contribute to the maintenance of mental function. For more information on different types of B vitamins, visit the IFIC [International Food Information Council] "Functional Foods Backgrounder" [at www.foodinsight.org/Resources/Detail.aspx?topic=Background_on_Functional_Foods].

Carnitine is derived from an amino acid and plays a role in energy production in cells, helping metabolism and energy levels. Some believe carnitine may improve athletic performance; however, there is no consistent research to support this theory. Most people get sufficient amounts of carnitine though the body's natural production, and through the foods we eat, without needing a supplement. For more information about carnitine, read the NIH's "Carnitine Fact Sheet" [at ods.od.nih.gov/factsheets/carnitine.asp].

Q: *How does the caffeine in energy drinks increase feelings of energy?*

A: Most energy drinks contain caffeine, which evidence has shown can improve both mental and athletic performance. Several studies have also found that moderate amounts of caffeine can increase alertness. In one study, participants used the words "vigor," "efficiency," "energy," and "clear-headedness" to describe their moods after consuming caffeine. Research has also shown that moderate caffeine consumption has the ability to improve memory and reasoning in sleep-deprived individuals. Additionally, caffeine has been shown to improve endurance if consumed before physical activity. For more information about caffeine and performance, see the IFIC "Caffeine Review" [at www.foodinsight.org/Resources/Detail.aspx?topic=IFIC_ Review_Caffeine_and_Health_Clarifying_the_Controversies_].

Q: How much caffeine do energy drinks typically contain?

A: The caffeine content of energy drinks can vary greatly. A 250 milliliter (mL) energy drink (about 8.5 ounces) can have anywhere from 50–160 mg of caffeine. Comparatively, an average 8-ounce cup of coffee has about 100 mg caffeine, and a 12-ounce soft drink has about 40 mg caffeine. To put this into perspective, moderate caffeine consumption for most individuals, including sensitive populations such as pregnant women and children, is about 300 mg per day. Therefore, on average, one energy drink would fall within moderate consumption levels. For more information on the caffeine content of various foods and beverages, see the IFIC "Caffeine Review."

As caffeine content can vary between energy drinks, you should look up the caffeine content when trying a new energy drink. Most energy drink manufacturers list the caffeine content of the product on the label, or on the official product website. Also, remember to check the label for the proper serving size—one energy drink container may provide more than one serving, and you could potentially double or even triple your caffeine intake if you consume the full container.

Q: Should I be concerned about the amount of caffeine in energy drinks?

A: Like all caffeinated foods and beverages, energy drinks can be consumed safely in moderation. The collective evidence from both scientific reviews and clinical studies concludes that moderate consumption of 300 mg caffeine per day is safe, even for more sensitive members of the population, such as children and pregnant women.

However, some people may be more sensitive to caffeine than others. Some may feel the effects of caffeine after only one serving, whereas others may be less sensitive. Symptoms experienced by some people may include excitement, restlessness, and nervousness. Most people will adjust their consumption based on the amount of caffeine they can consume without feeling any effects.

Although daily consumption of 200 mg to 300 mg of caffeine has been shown through extensive scientific research not to have adverse effects on pregnancy, pregnant women should monitor their caffeine consumption and talk to their ob/gyn and/or health care provider about their caffeine consumption. See the IFIC Foundation brochure, "Healthy

Eating during Pregnancy," for more information [at www.foodinsight.org/Resources/Detail.aspx?topic=Healthy_Eating_During_Pregnancy].

And, although caffeine has not been found to cause chronic high blood pressure or increase the risk of heart disease, individuals with high blood pressure and/or history of heart attack or stroke should consult their physician about their caffeine intake.

Q: What about reports of calls made to Poison Control Centers from people who were supposedly sent to the hospital from consuming energy drinks?

A: There has been some recent concern over calls to Poison Control Centers due to "caffeine intoxication," with media articles citing an increase in consumption of energy drinks by teens and children as the culprit. However, the majority of calls were actually related to people consuming dietary supplements containing caffeine, as opposed to energy drinks. Many of the reported effects occurred when caffeine was combined with other herbal and botanical ingredients and then ingested along with other pharmaceuticals.

Although studies suggest that most of these calls to Poison Control Centers are actually not from consuming energy drinks, if you have children, you should talk to them about practicing moderation in all aspects of their diet and lives, including consuming moderate amounts of caffeinated foods and beverages. These beverages are designed to provide an extra energy boost, which many teens and children should not need, as they are young and naturally energetic. However, having one energy drink for enjoyment from time to time should not harm a healthy individual.

If you have any concerns or have observed symptoms from consuming just a small amount of caffeine, you should see a health care provider for advice before continuing to consume energy drinks and/or other caffeinated beverages. Also, energy drinks should always be consumed responsibly and should not be combined with alcohol.

Q: With the growing popularity of energy drinks among children, should I be concerned about my child consuming energy drinks?

A: Caffeine in moderation is safe for the general healthy population, including children. Research shows that children are no more sensitive to caffeine than adults.

Although caffeine is safe for children to consume, many energy drinks include warnings on the label that state they are not intended for children. As with all treats, practice common sense when giving energy drinks to children—low to moderate amounts every once in a while can be enjoyed as part of an overall healthful diet. One way you can do this is by sharing a container with them, pouring the correct serving (according to the label) into a small glass.

At an early age, most of children's liquids should come from beverages containing important nutrients, such as calcium and Vitamin D, such as low-fat milk and 100% fruit juice. Additionally, talking to your kids about moderation in all foods and beverages, and teaching them how to read food labels for caffeine content and other vitamins and minerals, can help them to make smart decisions as they get older.

Q: Does caffeine cause children to become hyperactive?

A: No. There is no evidence that caffeine is associated with hyperactive behavior. In fact, most well-designed scientific studies show no effects of caffeine on hyperactivity or attention deficit hyperactivity disorder (ADHD) in children.

Q: Is caffeine addictive?

A: No, caffeine is not an addictive substance. Depending on the amount of caffeine ingested, it can be a mild stimulant to the central nervous system. Although caffeine is sometimes casually referred to as "addictive," moderate caffeine consumption is safe and should not be classified with addictive drugs of abuse. People who say they are "addicted" to caffeine are often using the term loosely, like saying they are "addicted" to running, working, or television.

When regular caffeine consumption is stopped abruptly, some individuals may experience mild symptoms such as headache, fatigue, or drowsiness. These effects are usually mild and will subside in a day or two. By gradually reducing caffeine consumption over time, symptoms may be prevented or reduced.

Bottom Line

Energy drinks are safe and can be consumed in moderation along with a healthful diet. Remember to check the number of servings in an energy drink container to determine the total caffeine content, and to include caffeine from other sources, such as soda and coffee, when determining your total for the day. Use common sense and talk to your kids about consuming all foods and beverages, including energy drinks, in moderation.

Chapter 36

The Health Consequences of Nutrition Misinformation

Types of Food and Nutrition Misinformation

Consumers are interested in health and nutrition information but, although 43% of consumers report that they like to hear about new studies, 22% claim to be confused by reports. Unfortunately, it is not always clear how to distinguish accurate food and nutrition information from nutrition misinformation. Accurate food and nutrition information is a result of significant scientific agreement from studies that have withstood peer review and can be replicated. Conversely, food and nutrition misinformation consists of erroneous, incomplete, or misleading science without any scientific basis at all. It can be disseminated naively or with malicious or self-serving intent (to sell products, gain attention, or promote the philosophy of a special-interest group). Food and nutrition misinformation may be harmful to a consumer's health and general well-being and includes food faddism, health fraud, and misdirected claims.

Food fads involve unreasonable or exaggerated beliefs that eating (or not eating) specific foods, nutrient supplements, or combinations of certain foods may cure disease, convey special health benefits, or offer quick weight loss. The *Surgeon General's Report on Nutrition and Health* defines the promotion of these foods as involving "false or misleading health or therapeutic claims." Although food fads can

Excerpted from *Journal of the American Dietetic Association*, Volume 106, Issue 4, pp 601–607, April 2006. Position of the American Dietetic Association: Food and Nutrition Misinformation. © 2006 American Dietetic Association. Reprinted with permission from Elsevier. Reviewed by David A. Cooke, MD, FACP, January 2011.

be exploitative and entrepreneurial, many people who promote these fads may themselves be victims of misinformation and may sincerely believe that they are providing accurate information.

Health fraud shares many of the characteristics of food faddism, except it is always deliberate and done for gain. According to the American Dietetic Association's (ADA's) *Complete Food and Nutrition Guide*, "health fraud means promotion for financial gain, a health remedy that doesn't work—or hasn't yet been proved to work" and that is "promoted to improve health, well-being, or appearance."

Misdirected claims include those that lead consumers to make incorrect inferences or generalizations about the health benefits of food. This type of claim misdirects consumers by leading them to believe that the foods are more healthful than is the case. The Federal Trade Commission has advocated providing adequate disclosures to correct advertising misinterpretations. Such disclosures can be important tools in qualifying misleading impressions from current claims. Such misleading impressions or "health halos" can occur, for example, when a product is advertised as "low in carbohydrates" but is still very high in calories.

Harmful Effects on Health and Economic Status of Consumers

Consumers are increasingly taking charge of their self-care. Although this brings new promise to the role that sound nutrition information can play in one's life, it also makes people more vulnerable to food and nutrition misinformation that can impact their health and economic well-being. Food and nutrition misinformation may be especially detrimental because people spend increasing amounts of money on weight-loss solutions ($43 billion in 2004). Whether it be related to weight loss or aging, people unrealistically look for simple, convenient, low-cost solutions. This leaves them vulnerable to misinformation that promises just such solutions.

Why Is Food and Nutrition Misinformation on the Rise?

The proliferation of functional foods and dietary supplements has led to an explosion of misinformation because the number of these products has outpaced federal regulations. Consumer spending on functional foods, dietary supplements, natural/organic foods, and natural personal care products totaled $168 billion in 2004. This wide range of herbal, botanical, and sports supplements, which comprise over half of the dietary supplement industry, has helped sales increase $13.9 billion in 2004.

The Dietary Supplement Health Education Act of 1994, which established guidelines for health claims and labeling of dietary supplements, shifted the burden of proving the accuracy of claims, safety, and quality to the U.S. Food and Drug Administration. This shift may have unintentionally led to an undeserved, implied level of credibility to food and nutrition misinformation because the federal government has simply not discovered it and reviewed the claim. Although the Food and Drug Administration and the Federal Trade Commission have critical roles in dealing with food and nutrition misinformation, the overwhelming burden placed on them necessitates greater involvement by nutrition professionals.

Short-Term and Long-Term Costs of Food and Nutrition Misinformation

There are both short-term and long-term costs when nutrition information is misinterpreted by the media, by consumers, or by the food and supplement industry. In the short term, physical harm can occur if there are unknown drug–nutrient interactions or toxic components in foods. Physical harm can also occur if the use of products leads individuals to delay or to avoid seeking proper health care, or if it interferes with sound nutrition education and practices. Economic harm can occur when purported remedies, treatments, and cures fail to work and when products are needlessly purchased. Because the burden of proof falls on the federal government, there are fewer safeguards preventing the development of costly and useless products. The cost of health fraud can be estimated to be in the billions of dollars, especially when including the cost of purchasing products that may do no harm but also provide no benefit.

Long-term costs of food and nutrition misinformation also include insidious lingering psychological issues of suspicion and diminished self-efficacy. Nutrition misinformation can lead consumers to lose faith in traditional sources of nutrition information and to provide less attention and credence to the results of new findings. It may even erode their perception of their ability to confidently manage a healthful lifestyle. When food and nutrition misinformation is common, it is much more difficult to gain public trust for future initiatives to improve public health.

Sources of Food and Nutrition Misinformation

Consumers receive nutrition information from a variety of sources. According to the *ADA's Nutrition and You: Trends 2002* survey and data from the Food Marketing Institute, consumers report that they received the majority of their nutrition information from media sources such as magazines (47%), television (34%), books (29%), and newspapers (28%). Other important sources of nutrition information are physicians (31%), the internet (21%), product labels (19%), and friends and family (18%). Only 13% of consumers claimed their nutrition information came directly from dietetics professionals.

Misinterpretation of Scientific Studies in the Media

Scientific progress does not prevent or eliminate food and nutrition misinformation. The media capitalize on preliminary research findings in an effort to enhance audience and readership ratings. Therefore, it becomes important that universities and research groups that release research results to the media use particular caution when presenting their findings.

The International Food Information Council indicated that the most pervasive cause of food and nutrition misinformation related to scientific reporting was the lack of sufficient context for consumers to understand the findings. For instance, when a food or dietary choice was linked to a specific harm or benefit, only 13% of the stories mentioned how much to eat, and only 21% cited the reference. A content analysis of selected nutrition-related news stories reported during 2000 to 2005 found four common forms of inaccuracy, including (a) reporting a correlation as causation, (b) generalizing a study's results to a broader population not represented by the study, (c) exaggerating the size of an effect, and (d) using a single link in a chain of events to make predictions about events in the future. News reports on nutrition rarely provide sufficient context for consumers to interpret the advice given. The stories often fail to note how much more (or less) of a food should be eaten, how often it should be eaten, or to whom the advice applies. Both the news media and researchers must share responsibility for reporting accurate, balanced, and complete information to the public.

Food and Nutrition Misinformation on the Internet

The internet is a rapidly expanding source of food and nutrition information. Forty-six percent of those participating in a 2005 Food Marketing Institute survey said they used the internet on a regular basis. Although people are increasingly relying on the internet for nutrition information, consumers must be informed that the accuracy of information appearing on websites is not governed by any regulatory agency. As a result, sites featuring sound, science-based content coexist with sites containing questionable, inaccurate, or alarming nutrition information promoted by individuals and groups supporting unscientific views. Chat rooms, blogs, discussion lists, and electronic bulletin boards can provide a forum for exchanging inaccurate nutrition information. In fact, this popularization of electronic interaction has resulted in rapid and widespread dissemination of misinformation and "urban health myths." Several health organizations are addressing the proliferation of misinformation on the internet. It is critical, therefore, that dietetics professionals be skeptical of information on the internet, and that they are especially careful to provide accurate, research-supported evidence when contributing to these venues.

For example, the American Medical Association issued guidelines for medical and health information sites on the internet. The Health on the Net Foundation (www.hon.ch) sets ethical standards for website developers and strives to guide health practitioners and consumers to useful and reliable online health information.

Food and Nutrition Misinformation from Industry

Many food companies are diligent about communicating accurate information about their products. In other cases, food and nutrition misinformation may be disseminated by multilevel marketing companies promoting dietary supplements or unproven weight-loss products. These companies claim that their products can prevent or cure disease. Product literature may contain illegal therapeutic claims, or product distributors may supply such information through anecdotes and independently published literature.

Advertising using testimonials also may spread misinformation. People tend to believe information that is endorsed by sports figures, celebrities, teachers, coaches, ministers, legislators, health care workers, media commentators, and others they respect. When public role models give scientifically unfounded testimonials about the benefits of specific nutritional practices, the effects can be far-reaching and potentially harmful. Role models should carefully examine the accuracy and reliability of any food and nutrition information they disseminate and sharpen their skills at making appropriate inferences from scientific reports. When they are uncertain about the scientific merit of nutrition products they are asked to endorse, role models should seek the advice of a qualified dietetics professional, who must be prepared to provide them with science-based information.

Food and Nutrition Misinformation from Friends, Family, and Culture

Some food beliefs rooted in traditional cultures or religions are not supported by scientific evidence. They can be followed as long as they do not result in possible harm and economic exploitation. For example, some Latinos and Asians believe that "hot" foods (some grains, oils, and meats) and "cold" foods (citrus fruits and dairy foods) have health properties that make them appropriate for different occasions. Despite a high level of cross-cultural agreement regarding whether a food is "hot" or "cold," there are different cultural recommendations about which foods are most appropriate to eat under various circumstances. For instance, many Latinos consider pregnancy a "hot" condition and believe that pregnant women should avoid "hot" foods. Conversely, the Chinese believe that pregnancy is a "cold" condition during which the expectant mother should avoid "cold" foods to keep herself in balance for good health. Cultural beliefs may be well intended, but it must be realized that some of the misinformation they contain may lead to undesirable consequences.

Table 36.1. Questions to Ask to Assess the Credibility of Websites

What is the background, credibility, and affiliation of the researchers or sources?

Does the website identify the publisher and any sponsors?

Does the website say who wrote it or how it was approved?

Is the information up-to-date?

Does the information include credible references such as peer-reviewed journals?

Does the information present both perspectives of the issue?

Is the information balanced and state any caveats?

Is the website designed to sell products?

Are there links that provide support or more detail?

Communicating Evidence-Based Nutrition Information

The impact of nutrition information on promoting healthful lifestyles depends on how effectively nutrition messages are communicated to consumers and how well consumers discern science-based advice. Nutrition information must be presented with sufficient context to provide consumers with a broader understanding of the issues and to determine whether it applies to their unique needs.

The Role of Consumers

Consumers need to recognize qualified dietetics professionals as credible resources for food nutrition information who can help consumers make sound decisions that match their personal needs. One important skill is knowing how to access credible information through ADA's website or other reputable websites. Table 36.1 lists questions that consumers should consider when reading nutrition information appearing on websites. Many consumers may not be aware that food

Table 36.2. Ten Red Flags of Junk Science

Recommendations that promise a quick fix.

Dire warnings of danger from a single product or regimen.

Claims that sound too good to be true.

Simplistic conclusions drawn from a complex study.

Recommendations based on a single study.

Dramatic statements that are refuted by reputable scientific organizations.

Lists of "good" and "bad" foods.

Recommendations made to help sell a product.

Recommendations based on studies published without peer review.

Recommendations from studies that ignore individual or group differences.

Table 36.3. Questions to Ask about a Research Report

Was the research done by a credible institution and by qualified researchers?

Is this a preliminary study? Have other studies reached the same conclusions?

Was the research population large enough? Was the study long enough?

Who paid for the study? Might that affect the findings? Is the science valid despite the funding source?

Was the report reviewed by peers?

Does the report avoid absolutes, such as "proves" or "causes"?

Does the report reflect appropriate context (eg, how the research fits into a broader picture of scientific evidence and consumer lifestyles)?

Do the results apply to a certain group of people?

and nutrition misinformation exists. Consumers need to scrutinize product claims and the qualifications of the source providing the food and nutrition information. Additional information can be obtained by contacting local hospitals or universities for local resources and by contacting ADA, whose website not only offers consumers a referral service to registered dietitians but also provides sound nutrition information on timely issues.

Part Six

Nutrition and Weight Control

Chapter 37

The Health Risks of Overweight and Obesity

Chapter Contents

Section 37.1

Health Problems Associated with Weighing Too Much

"Do You Know the Health Risks of Being Overweight?," Weight-Control Information Network, National Institute of Diabetes and Digestive and Kidney Diseases (win.niddk.nih.gov), December 2007.

What Are the Risks to My Health from Being Overweight?

Weighing too much may increase your risk for developing many health problems. If you are overweight or obese, you may be at risk for the following:

- Type 2 diabetes
- Coronary heart disease and stroke
- Metabolic syndrome
- Certain types of cancer
- Sleep apnea
- Osteoarthritis
- Gallbladder disease
- Fatty liver disease
- Pregnancy complications

You may be able to lower your health risks by losing weight, doing regular physical activity, and eating healthfully.

Body Mass Index

Body mass index (BMI) is a tool that is often used to determine whether a person's health is at risk due to his or her weight. BMI is a ratio of your weight to your height. A BMI of 18.5 to 24.9 is considered healthy; a BMI of 25 to 29.9 is considered overweight; and a BMI of 30 or more is considered obese. View a BMI table at win.niddk.nih.gov/publications/health_risks.htm#table.

Waist Circumference

Another way to determine if your weight is placing your health at risk is to measure your waist. Waist measurement does not determine if you are overweight, but it does indicate if you have excess fat in your abdomen. This is important because extra fat around your waist may increase health risks even more than fat elsewhere on your body.

Women with a waist measurement of more than 35 inches and men with a waist measurement of more than 40 inches may have an increased risk for obesity-related diseases.

Type 2 Diabetes

Type 2 diabetes is a disease in which blood sugar levels are above normal. High blood sugar is a major cause of coronary heart disease, kidney disease, stroke, amputation, and blindness. In 2002, diabetes was the sixth leading cause of death in the United States.

Type 2 diabetes is the most common type of diabetes in the United States. This form of diabetes is most often associated with old age, obesity, family history of diabetes, previous history of gestational diabetes, and physical inactivity. The disease is more common among certain ethnic populations.

How is type 2 diabetes linked to overweight?

More than 85% of people with type 2 diabetes are overweight. It is not known exactly why people who are overweight are more likely to develop this disease. It may be that being overweight causes cells to change, making them resistant to the hormone insulin. Insulin carries sugar from blood to the cells, where it is used for energy. When a person is insulin resistant, blood sugar cannot be taken up by the cells, resulting in high blood sugar. In addition, the cells that produce insulin must work extra hard to try to keep blood sugar normal. This may cause these cells to gradually fail.

What can weight loss do?

You may lower your risk for developing type 2 diabetes by losing weight and increasing the amount of physical activity you do. If you have type 2 diabetes, losing weight and becoming more physically active can help you control your blood sugar levels and prevent or delay complications. Losing weight and exercising more may also allow you to reduce the amount of diabetes medication you take. The Diabetes Prevention Program, a large clinical study sponsored by the National Institutes of Health, found that losing just 5% to 7% of your body weight and doing moderate-intensity exercise for 30 minutes a day, five days a week, may prevent or delay the onset of type 2 diabetes. For more information about the Diabetes Prevention Program, visit www.diabetes.niddk.nih.gov/dm/pubs/prevention program/index.htm.

Coronary Heart Disease and Stroke

Coronary heart disease means that the heart and circulation (blood flow) are not functioning normally. Often, the arteries have become hardened and narrowed. If you have coronary heart disease, you may suffer from a heart attack, congestive heart failure, sudden cardiac death, angina (chest pain), or abnormal heart rhythm. In a heart attack, the flow of blood and oxygen to the heart is disrupted, damaging portions of the heart muscle. During a stroke, blood and oxygen do not flow normally to the brain, possibly causing paralysis or death. Coronary heart disease is the leading cause of death in the United States, and stroke is the third leading cause.

How are heart disease and stroke linked to overweight?

People who are overweight are more likely to develop high blood pressure, high levels of triglycerides (blood fats) and LDL [low-density lipoprotein] cholesterol (a fat-like substance often called "bad cholesterol"), and low levels of HDL [high-density lipoprotein] cholesterol ("good cholesterol"). These are all risk factors for heart disease and stroke. In addition, excess body fat—especially abdominal fat—may produce substances that cause inflammation. Inflammation in blood vessels and throughout the body may raise heart disease risk.

What can weight loss do?

Losing 5% to 10% of your weight can lower your chances for developing coronary heart disease or having a stroke. If you weigh 200 pounds, this means losing as little as 10 pounds. Weight loss may improve blood pressure, triglyceride, and cholesterol levels; improve heart function and blood flow; and decrease inflammation throughout the body.

Metabolic Syndrome

The metabolic syndrome is a group of obesity-related risk factors for coronary heart disease and diabetes. A person has the metabolic syndrome if he or she has three or more of the following risk factors:

- **A large waistline:** For men, this means a waist measurement of 40 inches or more. For women, it means a waist measurement of 35 inches or more.

- **High triglycerides or taking medication to treat high triglycerides:** A triglyceride level of 150 mg/dL (milligrams/deciliter) or higher is considered high.

- **Low levels of HDL ("good") cholesterol or taking medications to treat low HDL:** For men, low HDL cholesterol is below 40 mg/dL; for women, it is below 50 mg/dL.

- **High blood pressure or taking medications to treat high blood pressure:** High blood pressure is 130 mmHg (millimeters of mercury) or higher for systolic blood pressure (the top number) or 85 mmHg or higher for diastolic blood pressure (the bottom number).

- **High fasting blood glucose (sugar) or taking medications to treat high blood sugar:** This means a fasting blood sugar of 100 mg/dL or higher.

A person with metabolic syndrome has approximately twice the risk for coronary heart disease and five times the risk for type 2 diabetes. It is estimated that 27% of American adults have the metabolic syndrome.

How is the metabolic syndrome linked to overweight?

The metabolic syndrome is strongly linked to obesity, especially abdominal obesity. Other risk factors are physical inactivity, insulin resistance, genetics, and old age.

Obesity is a risk factor for the metabolic syndrome because it raises blood pressure and triglycerides, lowers good cholesterol, and contributes to insulin resistance. Excess fat around the abdomen carries even higher risks.

What can weight loss do?

It may be possible to prevent the metabolic syndrome with weight management and physical activity. For patients who already have the syndrome, losing weight and being physically active may help prevent or delay the development of diabetes, coronary heart disease, or other complications.

Individuals who are overweight or obese and who have the metabolic syndrome should aim to lose 10% of their body weight and do at least 30 minutes of moderate-intensity physical activity every day. Quitting smoking, eating healthfully, and taking prescription medications for conditions such as high blood pressure or low HDL cholesterol may also be recommended.

Cancer

Cancer occurs when cells in one part of the body, such as the colon, grow abnormally or out of control. The cancerous cells sometimes spread to other parts of the body, such as the liver. Cancer is the second leading cause of death in the United States.

How is cancer linked to overweight?

Being overweight may increase the risk of developing several types of cancer, including cancers of the colon, esophagus, and kidney. Overweight is also linked with uterine and postmenopausal breast cancer in women. Gaining weight during adult life increases the risk for several of these cancers, even if the weight gain does not result in overweight or obesity.

It is not known exactly how being overweight increases cancer risk. It may be that fat cells release hormones that affect cell growth, leading to cancer. Also, eating or physical activity habits that may lead to being overweight may also contribute to cancer risk.

What can weight loss do?

Avoiding weight gain may prevent a rise in cancer risk. Healthy eating and physical activity habits may lower cancer risk. Weight loss may also lower your risk, although studies have been inconclusive.

Sleep Apnea

Sleep apnea is a condition in which a person stops breathing for short periods during the night. A person who has sleep apnea may suffer from daytime sleepiness, difficulty concentrating, and even heart failure.

How is sleep apnea linked to overweight?

The risk for sleep apnea is higher for people who are overweight. A person who is overweight may have more fat stored around his or her neck. This may make the airway smaller. A smaller airway can make breathing difficult, loud (snoring), or stop altogether. In addition, fat stored in the neck and throughout the body may produce substances that cause inflammation. Inflammation in the neck is a risk factor for sleep apnea.

What can weight loss do?

Weight loss usually improves sleep apnea. Weight loss may help to decrease neck size and lessen inflammation.

Osteoarthritis

Osteoarthritis is a common joint disorder that causes the joint bone and cartilage (tissue that protects joints) to wear away. Osteoarthritis most often affects the joints of the knees, hips, and lower back.

How is osteoarthritis linked to overweight?

Extra weight may place extra pressure on joints and cartilage, causing them to wear away. In addition, people with more body fat may have higher blood levels of substances that cause inflammation. Inflammation at the joints may raise the risk for osteoarthritis.

What can weight loss do?

Weight loss of at least 5% of your body weight may decrease stress on your knees, hips, and lower back and lessen inflammation in your body. If you have osteoarthritis, losing weight may help improve your symptoms.

Gallbladder Disease

Gallbladder disease includes gallstones and inflammation or infection of the gallbladder. Gallstones are clusters of solid material that form in the gallbladder. They are made mostly of cholesterol and can cause abdominal pain, especially after consuming fatty foods. The pain may be sharp or dull.

How is gallbladder disease linked to overweight?

People who are overweight have a higher risk for developing gallbladder disease. They may produce more cholesterol (a fat-like substance found in the body), a risk factor for gallstones. Also, people who are overweight may have an enlarged gallbladder, which may not work properly.

What can weight loss do?

Fast weight loss (more than three pounds per week) or large weight loss can actually increase your chance of developing gallstones. Modest, slow weight loss of about one-half to two pounds a week is less likely to cause gallstones. Achieving a healthy weight may lower your risk for developing gallstones.

Fatty Liver Disease

Fatty liver disease occurs when fat builds up in the liver cells and causes injury and inflammation in the liver. It can sometimes lead to severe liver damage, cirrhosis (build-up of scar tissue that blocks proper blood flow in the liver), or even liver failure. Fatty liver disease is like alcoholic liver damage, but it is not caused by alcohol and can occur in people who drink little or no alcohol. You can learn more about fatty liver disease, also known as nonalcoholic steatohepatitis (NASH), from the National Digestive Diseases Information Clearinghouse, at www.digestive.niddk.nih.gov/ddiseases/pubs/nash.

How is fatty liver disease linked to overweight?

People who have diabetes or prediabetes (when blood sugar levels are higher than normal but not yet in the diabetic range) are more likely to have fatty liver disease than people without these conditions. People who are overweight are more likely to develop diabetes. It is not known why some people who are overweight or diabetic get fatty liver disease and others do not.

What can weight loss do?

Losing weight and being physically active can help you control your blood sugar levels. It can also reduce the build-up of fat in your liver and prevent further injury. People with fatty liver disease should avoid drinking alcohol.

Pregnancy Complications

Overweight and obesity raise the risk of pregnancy complications for both mother and baby. Pregnant women who are overweight or obese may have an increased risk for the following:

- Gestational diabetes (high blood sugar during pregnancy)
- Pre-eclampsia (high blood pressure during pregnancy that can cause severe problems for both mother and baby if left untreated)
- Cesarean delivery or complications with cesarean delivery

Babies of overweight or obese mothers have an increased risk of neural tube defects (defects of the brain and spinal cord), stillbirth, prematurity, and being large for gestational age.

How are pregnancy complications linked to overweight?

Pregnant women who are overweight are more likely to develop insulin resistance, high blood sugar, and high blood pressure. (Insulin resistance is when cells do not respond properly to the hormone insulin, which carries blood sugar to cells for energy. It may result in high levels of blood sugar.) Overweight also increases the risks associated with surgery and anesthesia, and severe obesity increases operative time and blood loss.

Some studies have shown that gaining excess weight during pregnancy—even without becoming obese—may increase risks. It is important to consult with your obstetrician or other health care provider about how much weight to gain during pregnancy.

What can weight loss do?

Women who are overweight or obese and who would like to become pregnant should speak with their health care provider about losing weight before becoming pregnant. Prepregnancy weight loss significantly reduces pregnancy complications. Pregnant women who are overweight or obese should speak with their health care provider about limiting gestational weight gain and being physically active during pregnancy.

Losing excess weight after delivery may help women reduce their health risks. If a woman developed gestational diabetes, losing weight will lower her risk of developing diabetes later in life.

How Can I Lower My Health Risks?

To lose weight and keep it off over time, try to make long-term changes in your eating and physical activity habits.

- Choose healthy foods, such as vegetables, fruits, whole grains, and low-fat meat and dairy products more often.

447

- Eat just enough food to satisfy you. Aim for at least 30 minutes of moderate-intensity physical activity, such as walking, on most or all days of the week.

If you are overweight, losing as little as 5% of your body weight may lower your risk for several diseases, including coronary heart disease and type 2 diabetes. If you weigh 200 pounds, this means losing 10 pounds. Slow and steady weight loss of one-half to two pounds per week, and not more than three pounds per week, is the safest way to lose weight.

To lose weight, or to maintain weight loss, you will likely need to do more than 30 minutes of moderate physical activity daily.

Section 37.2

Weight Cycling

"Weight Cycling," Weight-Control Information Network,
National Institute of Diabetes and Digestive and Kidney Diseases
(win.niddk.nih.gov), May 2008.

What is weight cycling?

Weight cycling is the repeated loss and regain of body weight. This sometimes happens to people who go on weight-loss diets. A small cycle may include loss and regain of 5 to 10 pounds. In a large cycle, weight can change by 50 pounds or more.

Is weight cycling harmful to my health?

Experts are not sure if weight cycling leads to health problems. However, some studies suggest a link to high blood pressure, high cholesterol, gallbladder disease, and other problems. One study showed other problems may be linked to weight cycling as well. The study showed that women who weight cycle gain more weight over time than women who do not weight cycle. Binge eating (when a person eats a lot of food while feeling out of control) was also linked to women who weight cycle. The same study showed that women who weight cycle were also less likely to use physical activity to control their weight.

Weight cycling may affect your mental health too. People who weight cycle may feel depressed about their weight. However, weight cycling should not be a reason to "feel like a failure." If you feel down, try to focus on making changes in your eating and physical activity habits. Keeping a good attitude will help you stay focused. In addition, talk with a health care professional about your weight and ways you can manage it. Doing so may help you determine why you weight cycle. Understanding the cause of your weight cycling may help you in the process of lifelong weight management.

How can I manage weight and avoid weight cycling?

Experts recommend different strategies for different people. The goal for everyone is to achieve a healthy weight. This can help prevent the health problems linked to weight cycling.

- People who are not overweight or obese, and have no health problems related to weight, should maintain a stable weight.

- People who are overweight or obese should try to achieve and maintain a modest weight loss. An initial goal of losing 10% of your body weight can help in your efforts to improve overall health.

If you need to lose weight, be ready to make lifelong changes. Healthy eating and physical activity are the keys to your efforts. Focus on making healthful food choices, such as eating more high-fiber foods like fruits and vegetables and cutting down on foods that are high in saturated or trans fats. And make room for physical activity. Studies show that many people who weight cycle do not participate in regular physical activity. Walking, jogging, or other activities can help keep you active and feeling good. To find out more about healthy eating and the amount of physical activity you need, check out MyPlate, the federal government's food guidance system, at www.choosemyplate.gov.

If I weight cycle after a diet, will I gain more weight than I had before the diet? Will I have less muscle?

Studies do not show that fat tissue increases after a weight cycle. Study results do not support decreases in muscle either. Many people simply regain the weight they lost while on the diet—they have the same amount of fat and muscle as they did before the weight cycle.

Some people worry that weight cycling can put more fat around their stomach area. This is important since people who carry extra body weight around this area are more likely to develop type 2 diabetes.

Studies show that people do not have more fat around their stomach after a weight cycle. However, other studies suggest that women who are overweight and have a history of weight cycling have thicker layers of fat around their stomach—compared to women who do not weight cycle. It is not clear how this relates to weight cycling.

If I regain lost weight, will it be even harder to lose it again?

Losing weight after a weight cycle should not be harder. Studies show weight cycling does not affect how fast you burn food energy, which is called your "metabolic rate." This rate slows as we get older, but healthy eating and regular physical activity can still help you achieve a healthy weight.

Is staying overweight healthier than weight cycling?

This is a hard question to answer since experts are not sure whether weight cycling causes health problems. However, experts are sure that if you are overweight, losing weight is a good thing. Being overweight or obese is associated with the following health problems:

- High blood pressure
- Heart disease
- Stroke
- Gallbladder disease
- Fatty liver disease
- Type 2 diabetes
- Certain types of cancer
- Arthritis
- Breathing problems, such as sleep apnea (when breathing stops for short periods during sleep)

Not everyone who is overweight or obese has the same risk for these problems. Risk is affected by several factors: your gender, family history of disease, the amount of extra weight you have, and where fat is located on your body. You can improve your health with a modest weight loss. Losing just 10% of your body weight over six months will help.

Conclusions

Try to eat healthy and get plenty of physical activity. If you go through a weight cycle, do not feel like a failure. Just keep trying your best.

Experts need to learn more about weight cycling. Knowing if it is a cause or effect of poor physical and mental health is important. In the meantime, you can help yourself if you are overweight or obese. Try to eat healthy and get plenty of physical activity.

Chapter 38

Childhood Obesity

Chapter Contents

Section 38.1

Understanding Childhood Obesity

This section excerpted from "Childhood Overweight and Obesity,"
"Consequences," and "Contributing Factors," Centers for Disease Control
and Prevention (www.cdc.gov), October 20, 2009, and March 31, 2010.

Obesity is a serious health concern for children and adolescents.
Results from the 2007–08 National Health and Nutrition Examination Survey (NHANES), using measured heights and weights, indicate
that an estimated 17% of children and adolescents ages 2–19 years
are obese. Between 1976–80 and 1999–2000, the prevalence of obesity
increased. Between 1999–2000 and 2007–08 there was no significant
trend in obesity prevalence.

Among preschool age children 2–5 years of age, obesity increased
from 5% to 10.4% between 1976–80 and 2007–08 and from 6.5% to
19.6% among 6–11 year olds. Among adolescents aged 12–19, obesity
increased from 5% to 18.1% during the same period.

Obese children and adolescents are at risk for health problems during their youth and as adults. For example, during their youth, obese
children and adolescents are more likely to have risk factors associated
with cardiovascular disease (such as high blood pressure, high cholesterol, and type 2 diabetes) than are other children and adolescents.

Obese children and adolescents are more likely to become obese as
adults. For example, one study found that approximately 80% of children
who were overweight at aged 10–15 years were obese adults at age 25
years. Another study found that 25% of obese adults were overweight
as children. The latter study also found that if overweight begins before
8 years of age, obesity in adulthood is likely to be more severe.

Contributing Factors

At the individual level, childhood obesity is the result of an imbalance between the calories a child consumes as food and beverages
and the calories a child uses to support normal growth and development, metabolism, and physical activity. In other words, obesity
results when a child consumes more calories than the child uses. The

imbalance between calories consumed and calories used can result from the influences and interactions of a number of factors, including genetic, behavioral, and environmental factors. It is the interactions among these factors—rather than any single factor—that is thought to cause obesity.

Genetic Factors

Studies indicate that certain genetic characteristics may increase an individual's susceptibility to excess body weight. However, this genetic susceptibility may need to exist in conjunction with contributing environmental and behavioral factors (such as a high-calorie food supply and minimal physical activity) to have a significant effect on weight. Genetic factors alone can play a role in specific cases of obesity. For example, obesity is a clinical feature for rare genetic disorders such as Prader-Willi syndrome. However, the rapid rise in the rates of overweight and obesity in the general population in recent years cannot be attributed solely to genetic factors. The genetic characteristics of the human population have not changed in the last three decades, but the prevalence of obesity has tripled among school-aged children during that time.

Behavioral Factors

Because the factors that contribute to childhood obesity interact with each other, it is not possible to specify one behavior as the "cause" of obesity. However, certain behaviors can be identified as potentially contributing to an energy imbalance and, consequently, to obesity.

- **Energy intake:** Evidence is limited on specific foods or dietary patterns that contribute to excessive energy intake in children and teens. However, large portion sizes for food and beverages, eating meals away from home, frequent snacking on energy-dense foods, and consuming beverages with added sugar are often hypothesized as contributing to excess energy intake of children and teens. In the area of consuming sugar-sweetened drinks, evidence is growing to suggest an association with weight gain in children and adolescents. Consuming sugar-sweetened drinks may be associated with obesity because these drinks are high in calories. Children may not compensate at meals for the calories they have consumed in sugar-sweetened drinks, although this may vary by age. Also, liquid forms of energy may be less satiating than solid forms and lead to higher caloric intake.

- **Physical activity:** Participating in physical activity is important for children and teens as it may have beneficial effects not only on body weight, but also on blood pressure and bone strength. Physically active children are also more likely to remain physically active throughout adolescence and possibly into adulthood. Children may be spending less time engaged in physical activity during school. Daily participation in school physical education among adolescents dropped 14 percentage points over the last 13 years—from 42% in 1991 to 28% in 2003. In addition, less than one-third (28%) of high school students meet currently recommended levels of physical activity.

- **Sedentary behavior:** Children spend a considerable amount of time with media. One study found that time spent watching TV, videos, DVDs, and movies averaged slightly over three hours per day among children aged 8–18 years. Several studies have found a positive association between the time spent viewing television and increased prevalence of obesity in children. Media use, and specifically television viewing, may have the following effects:

  - Displace time children spend in physical activities

  - Contribute to increased energy consumption through excessive snacking and eating meals in front of the TV

  - Influence children to make unhealthy food choices through exposure to food advertisements

  - Lower children's metabolic rate

Environmental Factors

Home, child care, school, and community environments can influence children's behaviors related to food intake and physical activity.

- **Within the home:** Parent-child interactions and the home environment can affect the behaviors of children and youth related to calorie intake and physical activity. Parents are role models for their children, who are likely to develop habits similar to their parents.

- **Within child care:** Almost 80% of children aged five years and younger with working mothers are in child care for 40 hours a week on average. Child care providers are sharing responsibility with parents for children during important developmental years. Child care can be a setting in which healthy eating and physical activity habits are developed.

- **Within schools:** Because the majority of young people aged 5–17 years are enrolled in schools and because of the amount of time that children spend at school each day, schools provide an ideal setting for teaching children and teens to adopt healthy eating and physical activity behaviors. According to the Institute of Medicine (IOM), schools and school districts are, increasingly, implementing innovative programs that focus on improving the nutrition and increasing physical activity of students.

- **Within the community:** The built environment within communities influences access to physical activity opportunities and access to affordable and healthy foods. For example, a lack of sidewalks, safe bike paths, and parks in neighborhoods can discourage children from walking or biking to school as well as from participating in physical activity. Additionally, lack of access to affordable, healthy food choices in neighborhood food markets can be a barrier to purchasing healthy foods.

Consequences

Childhood obesity is associated with various health-related consequences. Obese children and adolescents may experience immediate health consequences and may be at risk for weight-related health problems in adulthood.

Psychosocial Risks

Some consequences of childhood and adolescent obesity are psychosocial. Obese children and adolescents are targets of early and systematic social discrimination. The psychological stress of social stigmatization can cause low self-esteem, which, in turn, can hinder academic and social functioning and persist into adulthood.

Cardiovascular Disease Risks

Obese children and teens have been found to have risk factors for cardiovascular disease (CVD), including high cholesterol levels, high blood pressure, and abnormal glucose tolerance. In a population-based sample of 5- to 17-year-olds, 70% of obese children had at least one CVD risk factor while 39% of obese children had two or more CVD risk factors.

Additional Health Risks

Less common health conditions associated with increased weight include asthma, hepatic steatosis, sleep apnea, and type 2 diabetes.

- Asthma is a disease of the lungs in which the airways become blocked or narrowed, causing breathing difficulty. Studies have identified an association between childhood obesity and asthma.

- Hepatic steatosis is the fatty degeneration of the liver caused by a high concentration of liver enzymes. Weight reduction causes liver enzymes to normalize.

- Sleep apnea is a less common complication of obesity for children and adolescents. Sleep apnea is a sleep-associated breathing disorder defined as the cessation of breathing during sleep that lasts for at least 10 seconds. Sleep apnea is characterized by loud snoring and labored breathing. During sleep apnea, oxygen levels in the blood can fall dramatically. One study estimated that sleep apnea occurs in about 7% of obese children.

- Type 2 diabetes is increasingly being reported among children and adolescents who are obese. While diabetes and glucose intolerance, a precursor of diabetes, are common health effects of adult obesity, only in recent years has type 2 diabetes begun to emerge as a health-related problem among children and adolescents. Onset of diabetes in children and adolescents can result in advanced complications such as CVD and kidney failure.

Section 38.2

Helping Your Overweight Child

This section excerpted from "Tips for Parents—Ideas to Help Children
Maintain a Healthy Weight," Centers for Disease Control and Prevention
(www.cdc.gov), February 15, 2011.

To help your child maintain a healthy weight, balance the calories
your child consumes from foods and beverages with the calories your
child uses through physical activity and normal growth.

Remember that the goal for overweight and obese children and
teens is to reduce the rate of weight gain while allowing normal growth
and development. Children and teens should *not* be placed on a weight-
reduction diet without the consultation of a health care provider.

Balancing Calories: Help Kids Develop Healthy Eating Habits

One part of balancing calories is to eat foods that provide adequate
nutrition and an appropriate number of calories. You can help children
learn to be aware of what they eat by developing healthy eating habits, looking for ways to make favorite dishes healthier, and reducing
calorie-rich temptations.

Encourage Healthy Eating Habits

There's no great secret to healthy eating. Here are some tips to help
your children and family develop healthy eating habits:

- Provide plenty of vegetables, fruits, and whole-grain products.

- Include low-fat or nonfat milk or dairy products.

- Choose lean meats, poultry, fish, lentils, and beans for protein.

- Serve reasonably sized portions.

- Encourage your family to drink lots of water.

- Limit sugar-sweetened beverages.

- Limit consumption of sugar and saturated fat.

457

Remember that small changes every day can lead to a recipe for success!

Look for Ways to Make Favorite Dishes Healthier

The recipes that you may prepare regularly, and that your family enjoys, can be healthier and just as satisfying with just a few changes. For new ideas about how to add more fruits and vegetables to your daily diet check out the recipe database from FruitsandVeggiesMatter. gov. This database enables you to find tasty fruit and vegetable recipes that fit your needs.

Remove Calorie-Rich Temptations

Although everything can be enjoyed in moderation, reducing the calorie-rich temptations of high-fat and high-sugar or salty snacks can also help your children develop healthy eating habits. Instead, only allow your children to eat them sometimes, so that they truly will be treats! Here are examples of easy-to-prepare, low-fat, and low-sugar treats that are 100 calories or less:

- A medium-size apple
- A medium-size banana
- One cup blueberries
- One cup grapes
- One cup carrots, broccoli, or bell peppers with two tablespoons hummus

Balancing Calories: Help Kids Stay Active

Another part of balancing calories is to engage in an appropriate amount of physical activity and avoid too much sedentary time. In addition to being fun for children and teens, regular physical activity has many health benefits, including the following:

- Strengthening bones
- Decreasing blood pressure
- Reducing stress and anxiety
- Increasing self-esteem
- Helping with weight management

Help Kids Stay Active

Children and teens should participate in at least 60 minutes of moderate intensity physical activity most days of the week, preferably daily. Remember that children imitate adults. Start adding physical activity to your own daily routine and encourage your child to join you.

Reduce Sedentary Time

In addition to encouraging physical activity, help children avoid too much sedentary time. Although quiet time for reading and homework is fine, limit the time your children watch television, play video games, or surf the web to no more than two hours per day. Additionally, the American Academy of Pediatrics (AAP) does not recommend television viewing for children age two or younger. Instead, encourage your children to find fun activities to do with family members or on their own that simply involve more activity.

Section 38.3

Childhood Viral Infection May Be a Cause of Obesity

"Childhood Viral Infection May Be a Cause of Obesity" by Scott La Fee, University of California San Diego News Center, September 20, 2010. Reprinted with permission. This University of California at San Diego News Release is based upon the following published manuscript: "Adenovirus 36 and Obesity in Children and Adolescents," Charles Gabbert, Michael Donohue, John Arnold, and Jeffrey B. Schwimmer, *Pediatrics*, Oct 2010; 126: 721–726.

The emerging idea that obesity may have an infectious origin gets new support in a cross-sectional study by University of California [UC], San Diego School of Medicine researchers who found that children exposed to a particular strain of adenovirus were significantly more likely to be obese.

The study will be published in the September 20 [2010] online edition of the journal *Pediatrics*. September is National Childhood Obesity Awareness Month.

Jeffrey B. Schwimmer, MD, associate professor of clinical pediatrics at UC San Diego, and colleagues examined 124 children, ages 8 to 18, for the presence of antibodies specific to adenovirus 36 (AD36), one of more than 50 strains of adenovirus known to infect humans and cause a variety of respiratory, gastrointestinal, and other infections. AD36 is the only human adenovirus currently linked to human obesity.

Slightly more than half of the children in the study (67) were considered obese, based on a body mass index or BMI in the 95th percentile or greater. The researchers detected neutralizing antibodies specific to AD36 in 19 of the children (15%). The majority of these AD36-positive children (78%) were obese, with AD36 antibodies much more frequent in obese children (15 of 67) than in non-obese children (4 of 57).

Children who were AD36-positive weighed almost 50 pounds more, on average, than children who were AD36-negative. Within the group of obese children, those with evidence of AD36 infection weighed an average of 35 pounds more than obese children who were AD36-negative.

"This amount of extra weight is a major concern at any age, but is especially so for a child," said Schwimmer, who is also director of weight and wellness at Rady Children's Hospital in San Diego. "Obesity can be a marker for future health problems like heart disease, liver disease, and diabetes. An extra 35 to 50 pounds is more than enough to greatly increase those risks."

Schwimmer said he hopes this research will help shift some of the burden that falls so heavily upon obese people, in particular children.

"Many people believe that obesity is one's own fault or the fault of one's parents or family. This work helps point out that body weight is more complicated than it's made out to be. And it is time that we move away from assigning blame in favor of developing a level of understanding that will better support efforts at both prevention and treatment. These data add credence to the concept that an infection can be a cause or contributor to obesity."

While an association between AD36 and obesity in both animals and human adults has been previously described, the particulars remain poorly understood. For example, it is not known how often or under what circumstances AD36 infects, why the virus affects people differently, and whether weight gain is the result of an active infection or a lasting change in a person's metabolism.

In cell cultures, Schwimmer said, the virus infects pre-adipocytes or immature fat cells, prompting them to develop more quickly and proliferate in greater numbers than normal. "This might be the mechanism for obesity," Schwimmer said, "but more work needs to be done."

Co-authors of the paper are Charles Gabbert of the department of Pediatrics and Medicine at the UC San Diego School of Medicine; Michael Donohue of the Division of Biostatistics and Bioinformatics, Department of Family and Preventive Medicine, UC San Diego; and John Arnold (CDR, USN) of the Division of Infectious Diseases, Department of Pediatrics, Naval Medical Center, San Diego.

Funding for this study came, in part, from grants from the National Institutes of Health. The opinions stated do not necessarily reflect those of the NIH or the U.S. Navy.

About Childhood Obesity

Obesity is defined by body mass index (BMI), a calculation based on a person's weight and height. For children and adolescents (ages 2–19), the BMI value is plotted on the Centers for Disease Control and Prevention (CDC)'s growth charts to determine a corresponding BMI-for-age percentile. Overweight is defined as a BMI at or above the 85th percentile, but lower than the 95th percentile. Obesity is at or above the 95th percentile for children of the same age and sex.

An estimated 17% of American children and adolescents are obese. Obese children have a 70% to 80% chance of becoming obese adults.

Many risk factors for childhood obesity have been identified: poor eating habits or overeating, lack of exercise, family history, ethnicity, psychological problems such as stress or depression, family circumstances, or socioeconomic status. Overall, obesity is linked to more than 300,000 deaths in the United States each year, with an annual estimated total economic cost of nearly $100 billion, according to the CDC.

Chapter 39

Healthy Weight Loss

Chapter Contents

Section 39.1

Eating for a Healthy Weight

This section excerpted from "Healthy Eating for a Healthy Weight" and "Improving Your Eating Habits," Centers for Disease Control and Prevention (www.cdc.gov), February 15, 2011. Text under the heading "If You Need to Lose Weight" is from "Better Health and You: Tips for Adults," Weight-Control Information Network, National Institute of Diabetes and Digestive and Kidney Diseases (win.niddk.nih.gov), March 2008.

Healthy Eating for a Healthy Weight

A healthy lifestyle involves many choices. Among them is choosing a balanced diet or eating plan. So how do you choose a healthy eating plan? According to the *Dietary Guidelines for Americans*, a healthy eating plan follows these guidelines:

- Emphasizes fruits, vegetables, whole grains, and fat-free or low-fat milk and milk products

- Includes lean meats, poultry, fish, beans, eggs, and nuts

- Is low in saturated fats, trans fats, cholesterol, salt (sodium), and added sugars

- Stays within your daily calorie needs

Eat Healthfully and Enjoy It

A healthy eating plan that helps you manage your weight includes a variety of foods you may not have considered. Try refocusing on all the new foods you can eat:

- **Fresh fruits:** Don't think just apples or bananas. Try some "exotic" fruits, too. How about a mango? Or a juicy pineapple or kiwifruit? When your favorite fresh fruits aren't in season, try a frozen, canned, or dried variety of a fresh fruit you enjoy. Be sure and choose canned fruit packed in water or in their own juice.

- **Fresh vegetables:** Try something new. You may find that you love grilled vegetables or steamed vegetables with an herb you

464

haven't tried, like rosemary. You can sauté vegetables in a non-stick pan with a small amount of cooking spray. When trying canned vegetables, look for vegetables without added salt, butter, or cream sauces.

- **Calcium-rich foods:** You may automatically think of a glass of low-fat or fat-free milk when someone says "eat more dairy products." But low-fat and fat-free yogurts without added sugars come in a wide variety of flavors and can be a great dessert substitute for those with a sweet tooth.

- **A new twist on an old favorite:** If your favorite recipe calls for frying fish or breaded chicken, try healthier variations using baking or grilling. Maybe even try a recipe that uses dry beans in place of higher-fat meats.

Take a look at these healthy meal plans and see what you can have:

- The ChooseMyPlate.gov eating plan is based upon the approximate number of calories your body needs according to your age, sex, height, weight, and activity level. The plan gives you the amounts of foods from the various food groups you should eat each day to meet that calorie goal.

- The DASH eating plan (at www.nhlbi.nih.gov/health/public/ heart/hbp/dash/introduction.html) was originally developed as an eating plan to reduce hypertension. (DASH stands for Dietary Approaches to Stop Hypertension.) However, the plan also represents a healthy approach to eating for those who do not have a problem with hypertension.

Do I Have to Give Up My Favorite Comfort Food?

No! Healthy eating is all about balance. You can enjoy your favorite foods even if they are high in calories, fat, or added sugars. The key is eating them only once in a while and balancing them with healthier foods and more physical activity.

Some general tips for comfort foods:

- Consume them less often. If you normally eat these foods every day, cut back to once a week or once a month.

- Eat smaller amounts. If your favorite higher-calorie food is an afternoon chocolate bar, have a smaller size or only half a bar.

- Try a lower-calorie version. Use lower-calorie ingredients or prepare it differently. For example, if your macaroni and cheese recipe uses whole milk, butter, and full-fat cheese, try remaking it with nonfat milk, less butter, light cream cheese, fresh spinach, and tomatoes.

You can figure out how to include almost any food in your healthy eating plan in a way that still helps you lose weight or maintain a healthy weight.

Being consistently healthy is the key. Making the same healthy eating choices over time can lead to better eating habits.

If You Need to Lose Weight

A weight loss of as little as 5% to 15% of your body weight over six months or longer has been shown to improve health. A safe rate of weight loss is one-half to two pounds per week.

Try some of these ideas to support your weight-loss efforts:

- Keep a food diary.

- Shop from a list and shop when you are not hungry.

- Store foods out of sight, or do not keep many high-fat, high-sugar foods in your home.

- Dish up smaller servings. At restaurants, eat only half your meal and take the rest home.

- Eat at the table and turn off the TV.

- Be realistic about weight-loss goals. Aim for a slow, modest weight loss.

- Seek support from family and friends.

- Expect setbacks and forgive yourself if you regain a few pounds.

- Add moderate-to-vigorous intensity physical activity to your weight-loss plan. Doing regular physical activity may help you control your weight.

Improving Your Eating Habits

When it comes to eating, we have strong habits. Some are good ("I always eat breakfast"), and some are not so good ("I always clean my plate"). Making sudden, radical changes to eating habits such as eating nothing but cabbage soup can lead to short-term weight loss. However, such radical changes are neither healthy nor a good idea and won't be successful in the long run. Permanently improving your eating habits requires a thoughtful approach in which you reflect, replace, and reinforce.

- **Reflect** on all of your specific eating habits, both bad and good, and your common triggers for unhealthy eating.

- **Replace** your unhealthy eating habits with healthier ones.

- **Reinforce** your new, healthier eating habits.

Reflect, Replace, Reinforce: A Process for Improving Your Eating Habits

1. Create a list of your eating habits. Keeping a food diary for a few days, in which you write down everything you eat and the time of day you ate it, will help you uncover your habits. It's good to note how you were feeling when you decided to eat.

2. Highlight the habits on your list that may be leading you to overeat. Common eating habits that can lead to weight gain are the following:

    - Eating too fast

    - Always cleaning your plate

    - Eating when not hungry

    - Eating while standing up (may lead to eating mindlessly or too quickly)

    - Always eating dessert

    - Skipping meals (or maybe just breakfast)

3. Look at the unhealthy eating habits you've highlighted. Be sure you've identified all the triggers that cause you to engage in those habits. Identify a few you'd like to work on improving first.

4. Create a list of cues by reviewing your food diary to become more aware of when and where you're "triggered" to eat for reasons other than hunger. Often an environmental cue, or a particular emotional state, is what encourages eating for non-hunger reasons. Common triggers for eating when not hungry are the following:

- Opening up the cabinet and seeing your favorite snack food
- Sitting at home watching television
- Before or after a stressful meeting or situation at work
- Coming home after work and having no idea what's for dinner
- Walking past a candy dish on the counter
- Sitting in the break room beside the vending machine
- Seeing a plate of doughnuts at the morning staff meeting
- Swinging through your favorite drive-through every morning
- Feeling bored or tired and thinking food might offer a pick-me-up

5. Circle the cues on your list that you face on a daily or weekly basis. But for now, focus on the ones you face more often.

6. Ask yourself these questions for each cue you've circled:

    - Is there anything I can do to avoid the cue or situation? This option works best for cues that don't involve others.

    - For things I can't avoid, can I do something differently that would be healthier? Obviously, you can't avoid all situations that trigger your unhealthy eating habits, like staff meetings at work. In these situations, evaluate your options.

7. Replace unhealthy habits with new, healthy ones. For example, in reflecting upon your eating habits, you may realize that you eat too fast when you eat alone. So, make a commitment to share a lunch each week with a colleague, or have a neighbor over for dinner one night a week. Here are more ideas to help you replace unhealthy habits:

    - Eat more slowly. If you eat too quickly, you may "clean your plate" instead of paying attention to whether your hunger is satisfied.

    - Eat only when you're truly hungry instead of when you are tired, anxious, or feeling an emotion besides hunger. If you find yourself eating when you are experiencing an emotion besides hunger, try to find a non-eating activity to do instead.

    - Plan meals ahead of time to ensure that you eat a healthy, well-balanced meal.

8.   Reinforce your new, healthy habits and be patient with yourself. Habits take time to develop. You can do it! It just takes one day at a time.

Section 39.2

Eating Mindfully

"Weight Reduction Tips," by Nancy Clark, MS, R.D., FACSM. Reprinted with permission of the American College of Sports Medicine, ACSM Fit Society ® Page, Spring 2008, pp 6–7. © 2008 American College of Sports Medicine (www.acsm.org).

As an athlete, you are likely lean and fit. But with more than 60% of Americans being overweight or obese, you undoubtedly know someone who struggles with how to shed undesired body fat. At the American Dietetic Association's annual convention last fall [2008], nutrition researchers presented alternatives to the standard "eat less and exercise more" diet advice. Here's some food for thought on nondieting ways to tackle weight problems.

Curbing the Obesity Epidemic

James Hill, PhD, believes we need to focus on stopping weight gain, as opposed to advocating for weight loss. One simple way to limit weight gain is to eat 100 to 200 fewer calories at the end of the day. This small calorie deficit contrasts to standard diets that severely restrict calories and are no fun. People on strict diets tend to stop losing weight after six months. Hill believes they dislike the drudgery of always being on a diet.

Yet, during the first six months of dieting, most dieters create new health habits—such as regular exercise—that they maintain. Exercise helps prevent (or reduce) weight regain. Surveys with "successful losers" indicate they include exercise as a part of their daily routine. For some, exercise offers spiritual benefits. For others, it provides a handy opportunity to socialize with friends. Some diet-and-exercisers even become "athletes." (Sound familiar to anyone you know?)

Dr. Hill also recommends we address the obesity epidemic by changing the way people think about weight. For example, Denver wants to become known as "America's Healthiest City." City leaders are working to create a culture where healthy eating and daily activity are the sustainable norm. Healthier employees will hopefully attract businesses to Denver because of lower health care costs. For health-promoting strategies, visit aom.americaonthemove.org.

Curbing Mindless Eating

Brian Wansink, PhD, of Cornell University's Food and Brand Lab, is campaigning to end mindless eating. You know, munching entire tubs of popcorn without even being hungry; nibbling on M&Ms while waiting for someone; unknowingly finishing the kid's leftovers. Just 100 extra mindless calories a day can contribute to gaining 10 pounds of undesired body fat a year.

Dr. Wansink recommends we curb weight gain by making mindful decisions about the calories that end up in our mouths. He reported we make about 250 food decisions a day. We decide not only what we eat (turkey or tuna sandwich? Low-fat or regular mayo?), but also how much (half or whole sandwich?). He has determined that we eat 92% of what we serve ourselves. We generally stop eating when our plate is empty. That means we eat with our eyes, not with our stomachs! Think about it: When do you stop eating? Chances are you stop eating when your plate is empty (or when the TV show ends). We don't always stop when our stomach signals it is full.

To prove this point, Wansink masterminded an interesting experiment with a refillable soup bowl that never emptied. (It was refilled via hidden tubing connected to a big soup pot.) Compared to the group who ate from standard bowls, the 30 adults who (unknowingly) ate from the refillable bowls consumed about 73% more soup. And believe it or not, they did not rate themselves as feeling any fuller than normal. (How can you be full if the bowl still has half the soup in it?) Only two people realized the bowl refilled—one dropped his napkin (and noticed the tubing); the other tried to pick up the bowl (surprise!).

Wansink created another experiment to determine if serving size influences the amount of food a person eats. He arranged for a movie theater to announce that all customers would receive free popcorn and soda on a certain day in honor of "Illinois History Month." The moviegoers were given five-day-old popcorn (yucky). Yet, even though the popcorn tasted bad, the people still ate 35% more when they were given a big bucket of popcorn compared to a smaller bucket. They mindlessly ate the stale popcorn slowly (in contrast to a previous experiment in which the moviegoers quickly devoured fresh popcorn).

Based on these and other experiments, Wansink believes a simple way to cut calories (and control weight) is to buy smaller bowls, plates, and also glasses. He reports you'll drink less if you pour your beverage into a tall, thin glass compared to a short, fat glass. And you'll eat less pasta if it's served from a small dish rather than a large platter.

Wansink has noticed that mindless eaters fall into categories of those who:

- eat too much at meals;

- graze mindlessly throughout the day;

- overeat at restaurants or on special occasions;

- mindlessly eat at their desks or in their cars.

If you relate to one or more these areas (and if you want to lose body fat), your goal should be to focus on that bad eating habit. You don't have to change your whole lifestyle. You just might need to cook less dinner so there are no leftovers, or take the candy jar off your desk.

Wansink recommends mindless eaters commit to 28 days of changing their fattening eating habit. Then, after 28 days, they can go on to improve another bad habit (such as drinking less soda, or crunching on baby carrots instead of chips). On www.mindlesseating.org, Wansink offers a free chart to help monitor daily success. You might also want to read his book, *Mindless Eating: Why We Eat More Than We Think*. Perhaps it can help you fight fat with less effort than a harder workout.

Section 39.3

How to Cut Calories from Your Diet

This section excerpted from "Eat More, Weigh Less?" and
"Cutting Calories," February 15, 2011, Centers for Disease Control
and Prevention (www.cdc.gov).

Have you tried to lose weight by cutting down the amount of food
you eat? Do you still feel hungry and not satisfied after eating? Or
have you avoided trying to lose weight because you're afraid of feeling
hungry all the time? Many people throw in the towel on weight loss
because they feel deprived and hungry when they eat less. But there
is another way. Aim for a slow, steady weight loss by decreasing calorie
intake while maintaining an adequate nutrient intake and increasing
physical activity. The key is to eat foods that will fill you up without
eating a large amount of calories.

If I Cut Calories, Won't I Be Hungry?

Research shows that people get full by the amount of food they eat,
not the number of calories they take in. You can cut calories in your
favorite foods by lowering the amount of fat and/or increasing the
amount of fiber-rich ingredients, such as vegetables or fruit.

Let's take macaroni and cheese as an example. The original recipe
uses whole milk, butter, and full-fat cheese. This recipe has about 540
calories in one serving (one cup).

Here's how to remake this recipe with fewer calories and less fat:

- Use 2 cups nonfat milk instead of 2 cups whole milk.

- Use 8 ounces light cream cheese instead of 2 1/4 cups full-fat
  cheddar cheese.

- Use 1 tablespoon butter instead of 2 or use 2 tablespoons of soft,
  trans fat–free margarine.

- Add about 2 cups of fresh spinach and 1 cup diced tomatoes (or
  any other veggie you like).

Your redesigned mac and cheese now has 315 calories in one serving (one cup).

What Foods Will Fill Me Up?

To be able to cut calories without eating less and feeling hungry, you need to replace some higher-calorie foods with foods that are lower in calories and fat and will fill you up. In general, this means foods with lots of water and fiber.

Less calories: These foods will fill you up with less calories. Choose them more often.

- Fruits and vegetables (prepared without added fat)
- Low-fat and fat-free milk products
- Broth-based soup
- Whole grains
- Lean meat, poultry, and fish
- Legumes (beans and peas)

More calories: These foods can pack more calories into each bite. Choose them less often.

- Fried foods
- Full-fat milk products
- Dry snack foods
- Higher-fat and higher-sugar foods
- Fatty cuts of meat

The number of calories in a particular amount or weight of food is called "calorie density" or "energy density." Low-calorie-dense foods are ones that don't pack a lot of calories into each bite. Foods that have a lot of water or fiber and little fat are usually low in calorie density. They will help you feel full without an unnecessary amount of calories.

Good Things Can Come in Big Packages!

People eat more than they realize when faced with large portion sizes. This usually means eating too many calories. But not all large portions are created equal. Larger portions of water- and fiber-rich foods, like fruits, vegetables, and broth-based soups, can fill you up with fewer calories. Start your meals with a broth-based soup or a green salad without a large amount of cheese or croutons. Research shows that if you eat a low-calorie appetizer before a meal, you will eat fewer total calories during the meal.

473

Fruits and Veggies: Keep It Simple!

Most fruits and veggies are low calorie and will fill you up, but the way you prepare them can change that. Breading and frying, and using high-fat creams or butter with vegetables and fruit, will add extra calories. Try steaming vegetables and using spices and low-fat sauces for flavor.

What about Beverages?

While drinking beverages is important to good health, they don't help you feel full and satisfied the way food does. Choose drinks without calories, like water, sparkling water, or unsweetened iced tea. Drink fat-free or low-fat milk instead of 2% or whole milk.

Section 39.4

Maintaining a Healthy Weight

"Maintaining a Healthy Weight," © 2010 The Cleveland Clinic Foundation, 9500 Euclid Avenue, Cleveland, OH 44195, http://my.clevelandclinic .org. Additional information is available from the Cleveland Clinic Health Information Center, 216-444-3771, toll-free 800-223-2273 extension 43771, or at http://my.clevelandclinic.org/health.

You have worked hard to lose your excess body fat and developed some new eating and exercise methods that now need to become habit.

Once you have achieved a desired weight, a positive attitude is very important in your efforts to successfully manage it. To lose weight permanently, you must make a commitment to gradually adopt a healthier way of life. Maintaining your new weight is not an easy task, but it will become easier over time once your choices become new habits. This will take time and perseverance.

Maintaining your new weight is not an impossible task. It simply means burning the same amount of calories that you eat. Eating smaller portions and choosing foods that are low in total fat and added sugar are essential to maintaining your desired weight. Establishing a regular exercise routine is equally important.

Tips to Help Maintain Your New Weight

- Motivation is a key to maintaining a healthy weight. Remind yourself of your motivation daily.

- Build support from family members, friends, or join a support group

- With the help of your dietitian, determine a calorie goal for weight maintenance. This can be more accurately determined with a simple breathing test.

- Set a maximum weight for yourself—a weight which you will not let yourself go above. Then weigh yourself weekly or monthly. If you are nearing your maximum weight, increase your focus on portion sizes, food choices, exercise, and attitude.

- Eat fewer calories by cutting down on portions and/or decreasing the total amount of fat and sugar in your diet.

- Limit added fats such as fried foods, margarine/butter, salad dressing, rich sauces, gravy, and mayonnaise. Season instead with herbs, lemon, vinegar, wine, and low-calorie marinades.

- Do not skip meals; four to five "mini-meals" may help to satisfy your hunger while keeping your weight under control

- Do not "starve" yourself. That can leave you feeling deprived and increase the temptation to binge (eat an uncontrolled, excessive amount). Rather, apply the techniques that helped you meet your goal weight.

- Keep low-calorie, low-fat snacks on hand such as popcorn, raw vegetables with low-calorie dips, or fruit.

- Choose foods high in fiber such as whole-grain breads, high-fiber cereals, brown rice, whole wheat pasta, and fruits and vegetables.

- Keep a food and exercise journal. Write down everything you eat or drink including portion sizes. Be honest and accurate, otherwise the journal is not as helpful. The food journal will help you learn about your eating habits and help you assess the food choices you are making. Try web-based journals for easy calorie counting.

- Limit the variety of foods available to you to only the healthiest options. Avoid buffets and stuffed refrigerators.

- Keep trigger foods out of the house and/or office.

- Aim for a minimum of 30 minutes of aerobic exercise most days of the week and a minimum of 20 minutes of strength training twice a week. You may need 45–90 minutes of exercise per day; try breaking up sessions into 3–15 minute periods. Look for small chunks of time that you can get in some exercise.

- Try using a pedometer and aim for 10,000–15,000 steps daily.

Foods to Choose for Weight Management

Breads and grains: Four or more servings/day; focus on whole grains

- Breads, rolls, buns
- Bagels
- English muffins
- Rice cakes
- Low-fat crackers (such as matzo, bread sticks, rye crisps, saltines)
- Hot and cold cereals
- Spaghetti, macaroni, noodles, rice
- Plain baked potato

Fruits and vegetables: Five or more servings/day

- Fresh, frozen, dried, or canned fruits (in own juice)
- Fresh, frozen, or canned vegetables

Meat, fish, poultry: Two to three servings per day

- Lean cuts of meat with fat trimmed*
- Chicken and turkey without skin*
- Fish*
- Eggs
- Dried beans

* Bake, boil, broil, roast, grill, or poach

Dairy: Two or more servings/day (three to four servings for pregnant or breastfeeding women)

- Low-fat milk
- Low-fat yogurt
- Low-fat cottage cheese
- Low-fat cheese with no more than three grams of fat per ounce

Fats and oils: In limited amounts

- Olive, canola, or peanut oils
- Margarine
- Nuts, seeds, salad dressing

Sweets and snacks: In limited amounts

- Baked goods
- Frozen desserts
- Jelly
- Pudding
- Gelatin

Chapter 40

Weight Loss and Nutrition Myths

Myth: Fad diets work for permanent weight loss.

Fact: Fad diets are not the best way to lose weight and keep it off. Fad diets often promise quick weight loss or tell you to cut certain foods out of your diet. You may lose weight at first on one of these diets. But diets that strictly limit calories or food choices are hard to follow. Most people quickly get tired of them and regain any lost weight.

Fad diets may be unhealthy because they may not provide all of the nutrients your body needs. Also, losing weight at a very rapid rate (more than three pounds a week after the first couple of weeks) may increase your risk for developing gallstones (clusters of solid material in the gallbladder that can be painful). Diets that provide less than 800 calories per day also could result in heart rhythm abnormalities, which can be fatal.

Tip: Research suggests that losing one-half to two pounds a week by making healthy food choices, eating moderate portions, and building physical activity into your daily life is the best way to lose weight and keep it off. By adopting healthy eating and physical activity habits, you may also lower your risk for developing type 2 diabetes, heart disease, and high blood pressure.

This section excerpted from "Weight-Loss and Nutrition Myths," Weight-Control Information Network, National Institute of Diabetes and Digestive and Kidney Diseases (win.niddk.nih.gov), March 2009.

Myth: High-protein/low-carbohydrate diets are a healthy way to lose weight.

Fact: The long-term health effects of a high-protein/low-carbohydrate diet are unknown. But getting most of your daily calories from high-protein foods like meat, eggs, and cheese is not a balanced eating plan. You may be eating too much fat and cholesterol, which may raise heart disease risk. You may be eating too few fruits, vegetables, and whole grains, which may lead to constipation due to lack of dietary fiber. Following a high-protein/low-carbohydrate diet may also make you feel nauseous, tired, and weak.

Eating fewer than 130 grams of carbohydrate a day can lead to the buildup of ketones in your blood. Ketones are partially broken-down fats. A buildup of these in your blood (called ketosis) can cause your body to produce high levels of uric acid, which is a risk factor for gout (a painful swelling of the joints) and kidney stones. Ketosis may be especially risky for pregnant women and people with diabetes or kidney disease. Be sure to discuss any changes in your diet with a health care professional, especially if you have health conditions such as cardiovascular disease, kidney disease, or type 2 diabetes.

Tip: High-protein/low-carbohydrate diets are often low in calories because food choices are strictly limited, so they may cause short-term weight loss. But a reduced-calorie eating plan that includes recommended amounts of carbohydrate, protein, and fat will also allow you to lose weight. By following a balanced eating plan, you will not have to stop eating whole classes of foods, such as whole grains, fruits, and vegetables—and miss the key nutrients they contain. You may also find it easier to stick with a diet or eating plan that includes a greater variety of foods.

Myth: Starches are fattening and should be limited when trying to lose weight.

Fact: Many foods high in starch, like bread, rice, pasta, cereals, beans, fruits, and some vegetables (like potatoes and yams), are low in fat and calories. They become high in fat and calories when eaten in large portion sizes or when covered with high-fat toppings like butter, sour cream, or mayonnaise. Foods high in starch (also called complex carbohydrates) are an important source of energy for your body.

Tip: A healthy eating plan is one that does the following:

1. Emphasizes fruits, vegetables, whole grains, and fat-free or low-fat milk and milk products

2. Includes lean meats, poultry, fish, beans, eggs, and nuts

3. Is low in saturated fats, trans fat, cholesterol, salt (sodium), and added sugars

Myth: Certain foods, like grapefruit, celery, or cabbage soup, can burn fat and make you lose weight.

Fact: No foods can burn fat. Some foods with caffeine may speed up your metabolism (the way your body uses energy, or calories) for a short time, but they do not cause weight loss.

Tip: The best way to lose weight is to cut back on the number of calories you eat and be more physically active.

Myth: Natural or herbal weight-loss products are safe and effective.

Fact: A weight-loss product that claims to be "natural" or "herbal" is not necessarily safe. These products are not usually scientifically tested to prove that they are safe or that they work. For example, herbal products containing ephedra (now banned by the U.S. government) have caused serious health problems and even death. Newer products that claim to be ephedra free are not necessarily danger free, because they may contain ingredients similar to ephedra.

Tip: Talk with your health care provider before using any weight-loss product. Some natural or herbal weight-loss products can be harmful.

Myth: "I can lose weight while eating whatever I want."

Fact: To lose weight, you need to use more calories than you eat. It is possible to eat any kind of food you want and lose weight. You need to limit the number of calories you eat every day and/or increase your daily physical activity. Portion control is the key. Try eating smaller amounts of food and choosing foods that are low in calories.

Tip: When trying to lose weight, you can still eat your favorite foods—as long as you pay attention to the total number of calories that you eat.

Myth: "Low fat" or "fat free" means no calories.

Fact: A low-fat or fat-free food is often lower in calories than the same size portion of the full-fat product. But many processed low-fat or fat-free foods have just as many calories as the full-fat versions of the same foods—or even more calories. They may contain added sugar, flour, or starch thickeners to improve flavor and texture after fat is removed. These ingredients add calories.

Tip: Read the Nutrition Facts on a food package to find out how many calories are in a serving. Check the serving size, too—it may be less than you are used to eating.

Myth: Fast foods are always an unhealthy choice and you should not eat them when dieting.

Fact: Fast foods can be part of a healthy weight-loss program with a little bit of know-how.

Tip: Avoid supersized combo meals, or split one with a friend. Sip on water or fat-free milk instead of soda. Choose salads and grilled foods, like a grilled chicken breast sandwich or small hamburger. Try a "fresco" taco (with salsa instead of cheese or sauce) at taco stands. Fried foods, like french fries and fried chicken, are high in fat and calories, so order them only once in a while, order a small portion, or split an order with a friend. Also, use only small amounts of high-fat, high-calorie toppings, like regular mayonnaise, salad dressings, bacon, and cheese.

Myth: Skipping meals is a good way to lose weight.

Fact: Studies show that people who skip breakfast and eat fewer times during the day tend to be heavier than people who eat a healthy breakfast and eat four or five times a day. This may be because people who skip meals tend to feel hungrier later on and eat more than they normally would. It may also be that eating many small meals through-out the day helps people control their appetites.

Tip: Eat small meals throughout the day that include a variety of healthy, low-fat, low-calorie foods.

Myth: Eating after 8 p.m. causes weight gain.

Fact: It does not matter what time of day you eat. It is what and how much you eat and how much physical activity you do during the whole day that determines whether you gain, lose, or maintain your weight. No matter when you eat, your body will store extra calories as fat.

Tip: If you want to have a snack before bedtime, think first about how many calories you have eaten that day. And try to avoid snacking in front of the TV at night—it may be easier to overeat when you are distracted by the television.

Myth: Nuts are fattening and you should not eat them if you want to lose weight.

Fact: In small amounts, nuts can be part of a healthy weight-loss program. Nuts are high in calories and fat. However, most nuts contain healthy fats that do not clog arteries. Nuts are also good sources of protein, dietary fiber, and minerals, including magnesium and copper.

Tip: Enjoy small portions of nuts. One-half ounce of mixed nuts has about 84 calories.

Myth: Eating red meat is bad for your health and makes it harder to lose weight.

Fact: Eating lean meat in small amounts can be part of a healthy weight-loss plan. Red meat, pork, chicken, and fish contain some cholesterol and saturated fat (the least healthy kind of fat). They also contain healthy nutrients like protein, iron, and zinc.

Tip: Choose cuts of meat that are lower in fat and trim all visible fat. Lower-fat meats include pork tenderloin and beef round steak, tenderloin, sirloin tip, flank steak, and extra lean ground beef. Also, pay attention to portion size. Three ounces of meat or poultry is the size of a deck of cards.

Myth: Dairy products are fattening and unhealthy.

Fact: Low-fat and fat-free milk, yogurt, and cheese are just as nutritious as whole-milk dairy products, but they are lower in fat and calories. Dairy products have many nutrients your body needs. They offer protein to build muscles and help organs work properly and calcium to strengthen bones. Most milk and some yogurt are fortified with vitamin D to help your body use calcium.

Tip: The 2005 *Dietary Guidelines for Americans* recommends consuming three cups per day of fat-free/low-fat milk or equivalent milk products.

If you cannot digest lactose (the sugar found in dairy products), choose low-lactose or lactose-free dairy products or other foods and beverages that offer calcium and vitamin D:

- **Calcium:** Soy-based beverage or tofu made with calcium sulfate; canned salmon; dark leafy greens like collards or kale

- **Vitamin D:** Soy-based beverage or cereal (getting some sunlight on your skin also gives you a small amount of vitamin D)

Myth: "Going vegetarian" means you are sure to lose weight and be healthier.

Fact: Research shows that people who follow a vegetarian eating plan, on average, eat fewer calories and less fat than nonvegetarians. They also tend to have lower body weights relative to their heights than nonvegetarians. Choosing a vegetarian eating plan with a low fat content may be helpful for weight loss. But vegetarians—like nonvegetarians—can make food choices that contribute to weight gain, like eating large amounts of high-fat, high-calorie foods or foods with little or no nutritional value.

Vegetarian diets should be as carefully planned as nonvegetarian diets to make sure they are balanced. Nutrients that nonvegetarians normally get from animal products, but that are not always found in a vegetarian eating plan, are iron, calcium, vitamin D, vitamin B12, zinc, and protein.

Tip: Choose a vegetarian eating plan that is low in fat and that provides all of the nutrients your body needs. Food and beverage sources of nutrients that may be lacking in a vegetarian diet are listed here:

- **Iron:** Cashews, spinach, lentils, garbanzo beans, fortified bread or cereal

- **Calcium:** Dairy products, fortified soy-based beverages, tofu made with calcium sulfate, collard greens, kale, broccoli

- **Vitamin D:** Fortified foods and beverages including milk, soy-based beverages, and cereal

- **Vitamin B12:** Eggs, dairy products, fortified cereal or soy-based beverages, tempeh, miso (tempeh and miso are foods made from soybeans)

- **Zinc:** Whole grains (especially the germ and bran of the grain), nuts, tofu, leafy vegetables (spinach, cabbage, lettuce)

- **Protein:** Eggs, dairy products, beans, peas, nuts, seeds, tofu, tempeh, soy-based burgers

If you do not know whether or not to believe a weight-loss or nutrition claim, check it out! The Federal Trade Commission has information on deceptive weight-loss advertising claims. You can find this online at www.ftc.com or by calling 877-FTC-HELP (382-4357). You can also find out more about nutrition and weight loss by talking with a registered dietitian. To find a registered dietitian in your area, visit the American Dietetic Association online (www.eatright.org) or call 800-877-1600.

Chapter 41

Diet Medications and Supplements

At any given time, half of the U.S. adult population is attempting to lose weight, and in today's busy world, many Americans looking for a quick-fix are turning to diet pills. As a result, the diet medication and supplement industry has exploded in recent years, and there are currently nearly 200 different dietary aids on the market. While a few of these weight-loss aids have scientific merit and can be incorporated into a healthy weight loss program, most are no more than gimmicks that can have potentially dangerous health consequences.

Medications

Medications differ from supplements in that they must be approved for use by the Food and Drug Administration (FDA), must undergo effectiveness and safety testing, and can only be obtained by a prescription. Currently there are only two medications approved by the FDA for the long-term treatment of obesity: orlistat and sibutramine. In early 2007, an orlistat-based product became the first weight-loss medication approved by the FDA for over-the-counter use.

"Diet Medications and Supplements," by Bryan K. Smith, Ph.D., CSCS, and Emily L. Van Walleghen, Ph.D. Reprinted with permission of the American College of Sports Medicine, ACSM Fit Society ® Page, Winter 2007, p 3. © 2007 American College of Sports Medicine (www.acsm.org).

Orlistat

Orlistat promotes weight loss by preventing the absorption of fat during the digestion of food, effectively reducing caloric intake. A recent review reported that individuals randomized to orlistat lost an additional 5.9 lbs, or 2.9% of their body weight, when compared to a placebo group. Long-term studies indicate that weight regain is similar between those using orlistat and the placebo group. When compared to a control group, orlistat users report between 16% to 40% more side effects. Most of these side effects are gastrointestinal in nature and include fatty/oily stool, fecal urgency, and oily spotting.

Sibutramine

Sibutramine promotes weight loss by suppressing appetite or enhancing satiety. A recent review reported that individuals using sibutramine lost an additional 9.5 lbs, or 4.6% of their body weight, when compared to a placebo group. Sibutramine appears to be effective during weight maintenance. A recent study reported that 27% more individuals using sibutramine were able to maintain 80% or more of their original weight loss when compared to the placebo group. The most reported side effect of sibutramine is an increase in blood pressure and heart rate. Other side effects include insomnia, dry mouth, nausea, and constipation.

Dietary Supplements

Unlike medications, dietary supplements are not required to undergo testing and approval by the FDA. Because they are not FDA regulated, dietary supplements are more likely to not work as claimed and to have potentially dangerous side effects. Although there are many different categories of dietary supplements, two of the most popular types are stimulants and appetite suppressants. Other types of supplements are advertised to decrease body fat, block nutrient absorption, and increase fullness.

Stimulants

Stimulants are intended to work by increasing metabolic rate and caloric expenditure. While one of the most popular stimulants, ephedra, was banned by the FDA in 2004 due to cardiovascular-related deaths resulting from its use, a number of other weight-loss stimulants are still available. These supplements, such as green tea, bitter orange, and guarana, contain ephedra-like compounds or caffeine, which increase energy expenditure. When taken at the recommended doses, however, these supplements do not consistently affect body weight in human studies. Further, when taken at higher doses, these supplements may have dangerous side effects, including heart palpitations and tremors.

Appetite Suppressants

By lessening the desire to eat, appetite suppressants are purported to decrease caloric intake. There are a number of appetite suppressants available, either individually or in combination with stimulants or other types of weight-loss supplements. One appetite suppressant that has recently become popular is *Hoodia gordonii*, a plant native to Africa. Although it is claimed that pills containing compounds extracted from this plant can suppress appetite, the effectiveness of *Hoodia* is unproven, and it may have unintended side effects, including liver damage.

Other Dietary Supplements

There is no definitive scientific evidence that any type of dietary supplement on the market today is beneficial for body weight management, and more research is necessary before recommendations regarding the effectiveness and safety of these supplements can be made to consumers.

Conclusions and Recommendations

There is more research-based evidence supporting the use of diet medications for weight management when compared to dietary supplements. However, this evidence does not imply that one can just take a pill and expect to lose weight or maintain weight loss. In research studies, these medications and supplements were used in conjunction with a low-calorie, low-fat diet and an exercise program. In addition, one must consider if the additional weight loss due to the diet aids is worth the potential side effects they may cause. Although many individuals would prefer to just take a pill, in most cases, we are better off following a healthy diet, practicing portion control, and exercising on a daily basis to manage our weight.

Chapter 42

Popular Diets Evaluated

Chapter Contents

Section 42.1

Review of Popular Low-Carb/ High-Protein Diets

"Lose weight! Increase energy! Look great! This book will...show you how to change your life once and for all."

"I'm not exaggerating when I say that this diet can, as a fringe benefit, save your life."

"...Learn to live a healthier, fuller life from this point forward."

Guess which of those promises come from which of the three top-selling diet books, *Dr. Atkins' New Diet Revolution, The South Beach Diet,* and Dr. Phil's *The Ultimate Weight Solution.* (Answer: they're in order.) Most diet books follow a formula. Amid the dispelled myths, tips, and personal success stories, nearly all promise that:

- it's not a diet but a way of life;

- the food is delicious and you won't be hungry;

- you're overweight because you ate the wrong (not too much) food;

- you'll lose weight because you'll eat the right (not less) food; and

- the diet will prevent either the major—or virtually all—diseases.

If you believe all that, we've got some old Enron stock for you.

After all these years, publishers know what sells. And, with a few exceptions, what's selling now are books about "good carbs."

Books like *The South Beach Diet, The Zone,* and *Good Carbs, Bad Carbs* argue that "bad" carbs are making us fat. Even the Atkins diet, which has urged dieters to limit *all* carbs since the 1970s, has modeled its recent advice (especially for Phase 2) after the "good-carb" books. In a nutshell, here's what they claim:

1. Bad carbs cause a quick rise in blood sugar.

2. High blood sugar raises blood insulin levels.

3. Insulin leads to weight gain (either by making the body store fat or by lowering blood sugar levels so much that it causes hunger).

The solution? Simple, say the books. All dieters have to do is eat "good" carbs (like whole grains, vegetables, and beans) instead of "bad" carbs (like sugar, white bread, and potatoes).

Yet most obesity experts, including those who believe in that advice, agree that the research cupboard is bare. "It's amazing how few good studies have looked at how different carbohydrates affect weight loss," says Walter Willett, chair of the nutrition department at the Harvard School of Public Health in Boston, Massachusetts.

"So far, the long-term evidence on weight loss is meager. We need bigger and longer randomized trials."

Glycemic Confusion

The South Beach Diet calls them "slow sugar" and "fast sugar." To *Good Carbs, Bad Carbs*, they're "tricklers" and "gushers."

But the message is the same: "As far as obesity is concerned," says *South Beach*, "fast sugar is worse for you; slower is better." How do you know which foods are which?

"In the early 1980s, Dr. David Jenkins led a team of Canadian researchers who devised a scale to measure the rapidity and degree with which a fixed quantity of food increases your blood sugar," writes *South Beach* author Arthur Agatston. "They called it the glycemic index."

In fact, the index is much more complicated than most books pretend.

"People think that a food has a definitive glycemic index, but it depends on how the food is processed, stored, ripened, cut, and cooked," says Xavier Pi-Sunyer, an obesity expert at Columbia University College of Physicians and Surgeons in New York.

Furthermore, diet books imply that "good" carbs like whole grains have a low glycemic index (GI, for short), while "bad" carbs like sugars, white flour, and other refined grains have a high GI. In fact:

- **Bread** is typically high-GI, whether whole wheat or white, because it's made from finely ground flour.

- **Pasta** is low-GI, whether whole wheat or white, but there are variations. "Thin linguine has a higher GI than thick linguine," notes Pi-Sunyer. "How would we advise the public about this major difference?"

- **Rice** ranges from high-GI (instant white) to low-GI (Uncle Ben's converted white), with brown and long-grain white rice in the middle. "Are we going to specify for the public which kind of rice they should eat and which kind they shouldn't?" asks Pi-Sunyer.

- **Sugars** range from high-GI (glucose) to low-GI (fructose). Sucrose (table sugar) is smack in the middle. What's more, "researchers have found no relation between the sugar content of foods and their glycemic index," says Pi-Sunyer.

And it's not even clear that the rise in blood sugar that comes from eating high-GI foods leads to high blood insulin levels, or that higher insulin leads people to overeat, says Pi-Sunyer.[1]

"The glycemic index may account for less than a quarter of the insulin response to a food," he suggests. "And there is no evidence that the typical post-meal levels of insulin increase food intake or body weight."

Which leads to the question: how good is the evidence that low-glycemic-index foods promote weight loss?

No Magic Bullet

You'll find a glycemic-index ranking of foods in *The Zone*; *Dr. Atkins*; *Good Carbs, Bad Carbs*; and *The New Glucose Revolution*.

But unlike the other books, *The New Glucose Revolution* was written by scientists who have actually studied the glycemic index. In fact, one of its authors, Thomas Wolever of the University of Toronto, was one of the researchers who helped devise the scale.

The glycemic index is no magic bullet for dieters, says Wolever.

"I've yet to see evidence that a low-GI diet aids weight loss," he explains. "One or two studies show it and a number of others don't."

Despite the "Lose Weight" claim on the cover of Wolever's *The New Glucose Revolution*, "it's not really a diet book," he says. "It's information about the glycemic index and how to use it for health." Wolever's research uses a low-glycemic-index diet to lower the risk of heart disease and to control diabetes.

"The chapter on weight says that a low-GI diet may be helpful for people who want to lose weight," he says. "But the best way to do that is to reduce calorie intake and increase activity level."

When Wolever put people on low-GI diets to control their diabetes, the pounds didn't melt away. "People tended to lose a little weight, but it wasn't significant," he explains. "And we found no differences in how full they felt on low-GI foods."

In fact, in one study of 35 people with diabetes, those who were given high-GI cereals (Corn Flakes, puffed rice, or crispy rice) lost two pounds after six weeks, while those who got low-GI cereals (Bran Buds or a Cheerios-type cereal, plus an added fiber called psyllium) lost no weight.[2]

Others agree that the research is in its infancy.

"A low-GI diet may suppress hunger. But until there is research over the long term, we just don't know," says Susan Roberts of the Jean Mayer U.S. Department of Agriculture Human Nutrition Research Center on Aging at Tufts University in Boston.

A recent review of the evidence reached this conclusion:[3] "The ideal human intervention study on low-GI vs. high-GI diets has not yet been conducted."

For example, in many studies, the diets differ in fiber or protein content, not just in the glycemic index of their foods. "A lot of articles hypothesize about the glycemic index, but there are not a lot of controlled studies to see whether a low-GI diet works," says Bonnie Brehm, an obesity researcher at the University of Cincinnati in Ohio.

The Atkins' Low-Evidence Revolution

Robert Atkins died last spring [2004] after falling on the icy pavement outside his New York City office. A few months later, his clinic closed its doors for good.

But his work lives on, not only in the diet books that continue to sell like (low-carb) hotcakes, but in his more than 100 snack bars, frozen dinners, muffin mixes, ice creams, and other foods and supplements that carry his name.

The pitch: Atkins-brand foods have fewer "net" carbohydrates than conventional foods. What are net carbs? They're what's left after Atkins Nutritionals replaces some of the foods' carbs with protein from soy and wheat, and after it deducts other carbs that, according to the company, have "a minimal impact on blood sugar." (The list includes fiber, glycerine, sugar alcohols, and polydextrose.)

The remaining carbohydrates appear in the "Net Atkins Count" circle on the package. Creative accounting? You bet. Good science? Hardly.

- Atkins Nutritionals won't say whether it has tested its foods to make sure that they don't raise blood sugar. Just because a food is sweetened with glycerine, sugar alcohols, or other sugar substitutes doesn't necessarily mean that it's gentler on your blood sugar. For example, a sugar-free apple muffin or banana cake raises blood sugar as much as its sugar-sweetened counterpart.[a]

- Atkins' books claim that only carbs that raise blood sugar cause weight gain, but the evidence is scanty.

What's more, low-carb foods aren't cheap. A 12-ounce box of pasta costs $5.99. Four cups of instant soup run $12. Fifteen brownies will set you back $32.

Supplements: Atkins Nutritionals also sells pills to "help break up a weight loss logjam." Among the ones Atkins recommends:

- **Coenzyme Q10:** Take 100 mg a day, since an "exploratory" study two decades ago found that people who took CoQ10 lost more weight than people who didn't. Reality check: The study, which was never published in a peer-reviewed scientific journal, was never followed up.

- **Carnitine:** Take 1,500 mg a day, just in case you have a deficiency of the amino-acid derivative. Reality check: No good research shows that overweight people are deficient in carnitine, or that taking 1,500 mg a day helps people lose weight.[b]

- **Chromium:** Take up to 1,000 micrograms a day, because preliminary research 15 years ago suggested that it helped build muscle and burn fat. Reality check: Better studies since then have come up empty.

—David Schardt
a. *Amer. J. Clin. Nutr.* 76: 5, 2002.
b. *Int. J. Sport Nutr. Exer. Metab.* 10: 199, 2000.

Dr. Phil's Pills

If you hit it right, a popular diet book can be a gold mine. But the big players know how to dig even deeper. Dr. Phil—who at 6'4" and 240 pounds is clearly overweight—wants fans to pay $120 for his vitamins and up to $90 for his bars and drink mixes every month. Here's the scoop:

Weight Management Supplements: If you've got a waist smaller than 35 inches (women) or 40 inches (men), Dr. Phil wants you to buy his Weight Management Supplement and Complete Multivitamin for Pear Body Types. If you have a larger waist, you need his supplement for Apple Body Types. Either way, it's 12 pills a day, 60 bucks a month.

What's the difference? Very little. Both contain the same 23 vitamins and minerals, plus carnitine (an amino-acid derivative) and four herbs. The "pear" pills also have a speck of soy isoflavones, green tea, and *Rhodiola rosea* root. In contrast, the "apple" pills contain *Gymnema sylvestre* leaves, vanadium, and white kidney bean extract.

Never mind that there are no studies showing that the supplements promote weight loss in anyone, pear or apple. No matter what fruit your body looks like, Dr. Phil thinks you need to "take your weight management efforts to the next level" by plunking down an additional $60 a month on 10 "Intensifier" pills a day. The Intensifiers contain:

- **Coenzyme Q10:** "Required for the production of energy in the body." Reality check: May help with congestive heart failure, not excess weight.

- **Conjugated linoleic acid (CLA):** "May reduce the deposit of excess body fat and increase the ratio of lean body mass to fat, when combined with a low-calorie diet and exercise." Reality check: May also cause liver damage and worsen insulin resistance.

- **EPA and DHA [eicosapentaenoic acid and docosahexaenoic acid]:** "Support healthy body membranes and heart health." Reality check: These omega-3 fats, which are found in fish oil, may help prevent sudden cardiac death, but have nothing to do with weight loss.

- **Tyrosine and L-theanine:** "May help reduce every day stress." Reality check: No good studies back up the benefits of theanine or the trivial amount of tyrosine in Dr. Phil's Intensifier pills.

- **Vitamin C:** "Protects your body against the damaging effects of free radicals." Reality check: There is no evidence that vitamin C has any impact on weight.

Nutrition Shakes: You're nobody in the weight-loss game unless you sell a meal replacement shake. Shape Up! shakes contain "scientifically researched levels of ingredients that can help you change your behavior to take control of your weight," says Dr. Phil. In fact, they're just a run-of-the-mill powder made from milk, eight kinds of fiber, and added vitamins (which you don't need if you're already taking his 22 pills a day...or your own inexpensive multi).

Nutrition Bars: Dr. Phil's Shape Up! bars are concoctions of sugars, oil, soy protein, fiber, and still more added vitamins. So much for his advice to keep sugars and fats "off-limits if you want to successfully control your weight."

—David Schardt

Beyond the Index

If a low-GI diet is no guarantee that we'll all look like Demi Moore and what's-his-name, so what? Maybe it's not a low glycemic index, but more whole grains or fiber, that can keep us slim.

"It's hard to draw conclusions because the studies on fiber are all too different—some use supplements, some use real food, some have a small fiber increase, some have a modestly big increase," says Tufts' Susan Roberts.

Studies on whole grains and weight are even scarcer. "Our study found that diets higher in whole grains and fiber slow weight gain compared to diets high in refined carbohydrates," says Eric Rimm of the Harvard School of Public Health.

But the difference in weight was small—only a few pounds over 12 years—and it's impossible to know whether whole-grain eaters did other things to avoid obesity.[4]

"Would I like to see trials that randomly assign people to eat whole grains or refined grains for a year?" asks Rimm. "Sure." In the meantime, he recommends whole grains for everyone, overweight or not.

"There's a growing body of evidence that whole grains are more beneficial than refined grains to reduce the risk of heart disease, diabetes, and obesity."

Diet vs. Diet

After years of ignoring popular diet books, researchers recently started testing Dr. Atkins head-to-head against "conventional diets," which cut calories mostly from fat. Three research teams released preliminary results last year.[5-7]

"Our study, as well as the two others, were all relatively small and short-term, but the results of all three were consistent," says the University of Cincinnati's Bonnie Brehm. "The healthy obese women in our study lost more weight on the Atkins diet than on the American Heart Association's diet."

Brehm's study lasted only six months. In another study, the Atkins dieters also lost more weight, but the difference between the two groups disappeared after a year. Still, what dieter wouldn't jump at the chance to lose extra weight for six months?

What's more, "we don't have as much reservation as we used to about the cardiovascular risk factors of an Atkins diet," adds Brehm. "The weight loss seems to override the high saturated fat content of the diet."

But what happens to LDL [low-density lipoprotein] ("bad") cholesterol and other risk factors for heart disease once weight stabilizes is an open question, she adds. Also, her study tested women with normal, not high, cholesterol.

"Is the Atkins diet effective?" asks Brehm. "Yes. But I still wouldn't recommend it until we have more research on its safety."

Others are also hesitant to endorse a diet that's loaded with red meat.

"The Atkins diet is potentially related to a long-term risk of cancer" if people stay on it long enough, says Harvard's Eric Rimm.

A few months on Atkins may not cause problems. "But two years on a red meat diet could initiate a cancer," he adds. "It could show up as a polyp in 7 years and as colon cancer in 10."

And Brehm worries about too little fiber, fruits, and vegetables on an Atkins-type low-carb diet.

"The women in our study averaged only five grams of fiber a day," she notes. (That's one-fifth of what experts recommend.) And despite what Atkins claims, "they did have constipation problems."

Phase 2 of the Atkins diet allows more fruits and vegetables, she acknowledges. "But if you don't lose enough weight in Phase 2, you have to move back to Phase 1, so you're on that restricted diet longer than the book says."

"I don't see the medical community recommending Atkins as a healthy diet because it's so restricted," says Brehm. "You miss out on fiber and any phytochemicals in fruits and vegetables that we may not even know about yet."

The Bottom Line

Where does that leave the ever-expanding legions of dieters?

According to media reports last November [2003], a new study found no difference in weight loss on four diets—Atkins, The Zone, Dean Ornish, and Weight Watchers. But until the study has been vetted and published, it's too early to weigh its conclusions.

Ornish's book, *Eat More, Weigh Less,* resurrects an old question: should dieters eat a very-low-fat diet, which gets 70% to 75% of its calories from carbohydrates?

Carbs shouldn't exceed 60% or 65% of calories, say the U.S. National Heart, Lung, and Blood Institute, American Heart Association, and National Academy of Sciences.

"Too many carbs may raise triglycerides and lower HDL [good] cholesterol," says Alice Lichtenstein of Tufts' Human Nutrition Research

Table 42.1. Battle of the Diet Books

Name	Claim	What You Eat	Is the Science Solid?	Is the Diet Healthy?	Worst Feature	Most Preposterous Claim
The South Beach Diet by Arthur Agatston	Switching to good carbs stops insulin resistance, cures cravings, and causes weight loss. Good fats protect the heart and prevent hunger.	**Yes:** Seafood, chicken breast, lean meat, low-fat cheese, most veggies, nuts, oils; (later) whole grains, most fruits, low-fat milk or yogurt, beans. **Less:** Fatty meats, full-fat cheese, refined grains, sweets, juice, potatoes.	Healthy version of Atkins diet that's backed by solid evidence on fats and heart disease.	**Good:** Mostly healthy foods.	Restricts carrots, bananas, pineapple, and watermelon.	You won't ever be hungry (despite menus that average just 1,200 calories a day).
The Ultimate Weight Solution by Phil McGraw	Foods that take time to prepare and chew lead to weight loss. Other "Keys to Weight Loss Freedom" include "no-fail environment," "right thinking," "healing feelings," and "circle of support."	**Yes:** Seafood, poultry, meat, low-fat dairy, whole grains, most veggies, fruits, (limited) oils. **Less:** Fatty meats, sweets, refined grains, full-fat dairy, microwaveable entrees, fried foods.	Tough-love manual that relies more on Dr. Phil's opinion than on science.	**Good:** Mostly healthy foods. **Bad:** Gives no menus, recipes, or advice on how much of what to eat.	Readers may buy Dr. Phil's expensive, questionable supplements, bars, and shakes (see "Dr. Phil's Pills" section).	"Each of these nutrients [in his supplements] has solid clinical evidence (and a record of safety) behind it."
Dr. Atkins' New Diet Revolution by Robert C. Atkins	A low-carb diet is the key to weight loss (and good health) because carbs cause high insulin levels.	**Yes:** Seafood, poultry, meat, eggs, cheese, salad veggies, oils, butter, cream; (later) limited amounts of nuts, fruits, wine, beans, veggies, whole grains. **Less:** Sweets, refined grains, milk, yogurt.	Low-carb "bible" overstates the results of weak studies and the evidence on supplements. (However, in recent small studies, people lost more weight after 6—but not 12—months on Atkins than on a typical diet.)	**Bad:** Too much red meat may raise risk of colon or prostate cancer. **Bad:** Lack of fiber, vegetables, and fruits may raise risk of heart disease, stroke, cancer, diverticulosis, and constipation.	Long-term safety not established.	"Only by doing Atkins can you lose weight eating the same number of calories on which you used to gain weight."

Table 42.1. *continued*

Diet	Claim	Yes / Less	Science	Good / Bad	Comment	Quote
Good Carbs, Bad Carbs by Johanna Burani and Linda Rao	Switching from high-glycemic-index foods ("gushers") to low-glycemic-index foods ("tricklers") aids weight loss.	**Yes:** Sourdough bread, beans, most fruits, low-fat dairy, most veggies, chips, pasta, Special K, pudding, pound cake. **Less:** White bread, sweets, Raisin Bran, potatoes, watermelon.	Dumbed-down, sloppy version of *The New Glucose Revolution* that inflates the importance of the glycemic index.	**Good:** Mostly healthy foods. **Bad:** Few recipes, menus, or specifics. **Bad:** Some low-glycemic-index foods are unhealthy (e.g., sponge cake, chips, chocolate bars).	Dieters may assume that they can eat as many "tricklers" as they want and not gain weight.	"…in spite of the title *Good Carbs, Bad Carbs*, there are no bad carbs."
Eat Right 4 Your Type by Peter J. D'Adamo and Catherine Whitney	Your blood type determines your diet, supplements, and personality because it is "the key to your body's entire immune system."	**Yes:** *Type O:* Meat, seafood, fruits, veggies (**Less:** Wheat, beans). *Type A:* Fruits, veggies, beans, most seafood (**Less:** Meat, dairy, wheat). *Type B:* Meat, beans, fruits, veggies (**Less:** Chicken, wheat). *Type AB:* Seafood, dairy, fruits, veggies (**Less:** Red meat).	About as scientific as a horoscope.	Not applicable (diet varies according to blood type, ancestry, etc.).	May convince people to use these diets to treat cancer, asthma, infections, diabetes, arthritis, hypertension, and infertility.	"If you are a Type A woman with a family history of breast cancer, consider introducing snails into your diet."
Weight Watchers New Complete Cookbook	Following a point system helps dieters cut calories and lose weight.	**Yes:** Fruits, veggies, low-fat dairy, poultry, seafood, lean meats, grains. **Less:** None.	No science cited, but its sensible advice is used by millions.	**Good:** Mostly healthy foods.	Some packaged Weight Watchers foods (none are mentioned in the cookbook) aren't exactly nutritious.	Not applicable (cookbook).
The New Glucose Revolution by Jennie Brand-Miller, Thomas Wolever, Kaye Foster-Powell, and Stephen Colagiuri	Low-glycemic-index foods keep you satisfied longer and help you burn more body fat and less muscle.	**Yes:** Beans, pasta, most fruits, veggies, low-fat dairy, poultry, lean meat, seafood. **Less:** Potatoes, white bread, fatty meats, full-fat dairy, watermelon.	Reasonable interpretation of the science, though stronger for heart disease and diabetes than for weight loss.	**Good:** Mostly healthy foods. **Bad:** Fuzzy limits on low-glycemic-index foods, including pasta, sourdough bread, honey, some sugary cereals, and some dried fruits.	Advice is difficult to follow because glycemic index varies so much for each food (e.g., bananas range from 30 to 70).	Low-glycemic-index diets are easy to teach and easy to learn.

499

Table 42.1. *continued*

Name	Claim	What You Eat	Is the Science Solid?	Is the Diet Healthy?	Worst Feature	Most Preposterous Claim
Enter the Zone by Barry Sears	Eating the right mix of the right fats, carbs, and protein keeps you trim and healthy by lowering insulin.	**Yes:** Seafood, poultry, lean meat, fruits, most veggies, low-fat dairy, nuts. **Less:** Fatty meats, full-fat dairy, butter, shortening, (limited) grains, sweets, potatoes, carrots, bananas.	Exaggerates evidence that the Zone diet is the key to weight loss and implies that the diet can cure virtually every disease.	**Good:** Mostly healthy foods. **Bad:** Few recipes or menus.	May convince people to use the diet to treat cancer, AIDS, chronic pain, impotence, alcoholism, depression, and arthritis.	"I believe that the hormonal benefits gained from a Zone-favorable diet will be considered the primary treatment for all chronic disease states, with drugs being used as secondary backup."
The Fat Flush Plan by Ann Louise Gittleman	Detoxifying the liver and lymph system, taking omega-3 fats that burn calories, and avoiding insulin-raising carbs promote weight loss.	**Yes:** Eggs, meat, poultry, seafood, most veggies, fruits, organic coffee, nuts, cranberry juice; (later) beans, whole grains, cheese. **Less:** Sweets, butter, margarine, refined grains, caffeine, milk, yogurt, yeast.	Kooky mishmash of old detox lore and new good-carb theory.	**Good:** Mostly healthy foods. **Bad:** Too much red meat and eggs.	Useless fat-flush kit costs $68 per month for vitamins, omega-3 fats, etc., that "trigger fat burning…and nourish our tired and overworked livers."	"The best way to give those fatty deposits [in your thighs and arms] the old heave-ho is by cleansing your lymphatic system with a bouncing action or by moving your arms while walking briskly."
Eat More, Weigh Less by Dean Ornish	Slashing fat is the key to weight loss.	**Yes:** Beans, fruits, veggies, grains, (limited) non-fat dairy. **Less:** Meat, seafood, poultry, oils, nuts, butter, dairy (except non-fat), sweets, alcohol.	Diet worked (when combined with exercise and stress reduction) in a small-but-long-term study.	**Good:** Mostly healthy foods. **Bad:** Too many carbs may raise triglycerides and lower HDL [high-density lipoprotein] ("good") cholesterol if people don't exercise, lose weight, and reduce stress.	Unnecessarily restricts seafood, turkey and chicken breast, oils, nuts, and fat-free dairy.	Eating a very-low-fat vegetarian diet is easy.

Center on Aging, who co-authored the American Heart Association's guidelines on very-low-fat diets.

That didn't happen when Ornish put 35 people with heart disease in his Lifestyle Heart Trial for five years. (Their arteries became less clogged.) Was it all the fiber they were eating? Possibly.

"It's also possible that other parts of Ornish's program—vigorous exercise, stress reduction, and weight loss—protected them," says Lichtenstein. "If people don't follow his diet and other advice closely, too many carbs could cause trouble."

Ornish aside, people who think they can eat any and all carbs without consequences are wrong.

"When the pendulum swung as far as it could to low-fat diets in the 1980s, we may have gone too far recommending higher carbs," says Brehm. "People may have lost sight of the fact that carbs have calories."

Now they know better.

"We're saying that you need to cut back on carbs, and you can eat more unsaturated fat," Brehm explains. "People may be ready for a more refined tool that separates good carbs and fats from bad." Sound familiar?

"The South Beach Diet teaches you to rely on the right carbs and the right fats," says the book's first page.

1. *Amer. J. Clin. Nutr.* 76: 290S, 2002.
2. *Amer. J. Clin. Nutr.* 72: 439, 2000.
3. *Obesity Reviews* 3: 245, 2002.
4. *Amer. J. Clin. Nutr.* 78: 920, 2003.
5. *J. Clin. Endocrinol. Metab.* 88: 1617, 2003.
6. *New Eng. J. Med.* 348: 2074, 2003.
7. *New Eng. J. Med.* 348: 2082, 2003.

Battle of the Diet Books

Is it the title? Is it the promises? Is it word of mouth? It's not clear how people pick a diet book, but one thing's for sure: the decision is rarely based on good science. Here's our take on the most popular diet books. Since no large long-term studies have pitted them head-to-head, we can't evaluate the diets' ability to make you skinnier. Instead, we've graded each book's scientific credibility ("Is the Science Solid?") and whether the diet it recommends is healthy. (In "What You Eat," *Yes* means frequently, *Less* means rarely, if ever.)

501

The books are listed in order according to Amazon.com's top-selling "Diet and Weight Loss" books in mid-November [2003]. We added Dean Ornish's *Eat More, Weigh Less* and the Weight Watchers cookbook because a recent study tested both diets. We excluded other cookbooks and how-to spinoffs of the top-sellers.

Table 42.1 gives only thumbnail sketches. See the books for more details.

Section 42.2

About Quick-Weight-Loss Diets

"Quick-Weight-Loss or Fad Diets," reprinted with permission from www.heart.org. © 2010 American Heart Association, Inc.

AHA Recommendation

Our nutrition experts recommend adopting healthy eating habits permanently, rather than impatiently pursuing crash diets in hopes of losing unwanted pounds in a few days.

Why does the AHA care about these diets?

We want to inform the public about misleading weight-loss claims. Many of these diets—like the infamous Cabbage Soup Diet—can undermine your health, cause physical discomfort (abdominal discomfort and flatulence [gas]), and lead to disappointment when you regain weight soon after you lose it.

- Quick-weight-loss diets usually overemphasize one particular food or type of food. They violate the first principle of good nutrition: eat a balanced diet that includes a variety of foods. If you are able to stay on such a diet for more than a few weeks, you may develop nutritional deficiencies, because no one type of food has all the nutrients you need for good health. The aforementioned Cabbage Soup Diet is an example. This so-called fat-burning soup is eaten mostly with fruits and vegetables. The diet supposedly helps heart patients lose 10–17 pounds in seven days before surgery. There are no "superfoods." That's why you should eat moderate amounts from all food groups, not large amounts of a few special foods.

- These diets also violate a second important principle of good nutrition: eating should be enjoyable. These diets are so monotonous and boring that it's almost impossible to stay on them for long periods.

Let's set the record straight: Many of these diets falsely say they are endorsed by or authored by our association. The public should know that the real American Heart Association diet and lifestyle recommendations emphasize flexibility in food selection and stress the importance of eating more nutrient-rich foods—that have vitamins, minerals, fiber, and other nutrients but are lower in calories—and fewer nutrient-poor foods.

Unlike an incomplete liquid protein diet or other fad diets, a good diet can be eaten for years to maintain desirable body weight and good health. Fad diets fail to provide ways to keep weight off.

- Some major medical centers prescribe extremely low-calorie, high-protein diets for selected patients who are carefully monitored by physicians.

In what other ways are quick-weight-loss diets flawed?

- Many don't encourage physical activity—for example, walking 30 minutes most or all days of the week. Being physically active helps you maintain weight loss over a long time. Physical inactivity is a major risk factor for heart disease and stroke.

- Because most quick-weight-loss diets require drastic changes in eating patterns, you can't stay on them for long. Following a regimen for a few weeks won't give you the chance to learn about how to permanently change your eating patterns.

- In addition, many fad diets are based on "food folklore," some dating back to the early 19th century. They have not been documented to be safe in the long term. Ideas about "fat-burning foods" and "food combining" are also classified by the American Heart Association as unsubstantiated myths.

Despite what quick-weight-loss diet books may say, the only sensible way to lose weight and maintain a healthy weight permanently is to eat less and balance your food intake with physical activity.

What is the best way to lose weight?

A healthy diet rich in fresh fruits and vegetables, whole grains, and fat-free or low-fat dairy products, along with regular physical activity, can help most people manage and maintain weight loss for both cardiovascular health and appearance. The American Heart Association urges people to take a safe and proven route to losing and maintaining weight—by following our guidelines for healthy, nutritionally balanced weight loss for a lifetime of good health.

Section 42.3

Does the Mediterranean Diet Offer Health Benefits?

"Mediterranean Diet," and "Lyon Diet Heart Study," reprinted with permission from www.heart.org. © 2010 American Heart Association, Inc.

Mediterranean Diet

What is the "Mediterranean" diet?

There's no one "Mediterranean" diet. At least 16 countries border the Mediterranean Sea. Diets vary between these countries and also between regions within a country. Many differences in culture, ethnic background, religion, economy, and agricultural production result in different diets. But the common Mediterranean dietary pattern has these characteristics:

- High consumption of fruits, vegetables, bread and other cereals, potatoes, beans, nuts, and seeds

- Olive oil is an important monounsaturated fat source

- Dairy products, fish, and poultry are consumed in low to moderate amounts, and little red meat is eaten

- Eggs are consumed zero to four times a week

- Wine is consumed in low to moderate amounts

Does a Mediterranean-style diet follow American Heart Association dietary recommendations?

Mediterranean-style diets are often close to our dietary recommendations, but they don't follow them exactly. In general, the diets of Mediterranean peoples contain a relatively high percentage of calories from fat. This is thought to contribute to the increasing obesity in these countries, which is becoming a concern.

People who follow the average Mediterranean diet eat less saturated fat than those who eat the average American diet. In fact, saturated fat consumption is well within our dietary guidelines.

More than half the fat calories in a Mediterranean diet come from monounsaturated fats (mainly from olive oil). Monounsaturated fat doesn't raise blood cholesterol levels the way saturated fat does.

The incidence of heart disease in Mediterranean countries is lower than in the United States. Death rates are lower, too. But this may not be entirely due to the diet. Lifestyle factors (such as more physical activity and extended social support systems) may also play a part.

Before advising people to follow a Mediterranean diet, we need more studies to find out whether the diet itself or other lifestyle factors account for the lower deaths from heart disease.

Lyon Diet Heart Study

What is the Lyon Diet Heart Study?

This was a randomized, controlled trial with free-living subjects. Its goal was to test the effectiveness of a Mediterranean-type diet on the rate of coronary events in people who've had a first heart attack. The results suggest that a Mediterranean-style Step I diet may help reduce recurrent events in patients with heart disease.

What were the methods used?

A total of 302 experimental- and 303 control-group subjects were randomized into the study. All were patients who had survived a first heart attack. The two groups had a similar coronary risk factor profile (blood lipids and lipoproteins, systolic and diastolic blood pressure, body mass index, and smoking status). Patients in the experimental group were asked to comply with a specific Mediterranean-type diet. Patients in the control group received no dietary advice from the researchers but were asked by their physicians to follow a prudent diet.

An intermediate analysis was performed after a minimum follow-up of one year for each patient. The study was stopped at that point because of significant beneficial effects noted in the original group. All patients were invited to the research unit for a final exam, where they were informed of the results. 204 of the control group and 219 of the experimental group participated in the final visit. This represented 93% of the patients still alive at the time.

What are the Step I and Step II diets?

The Step I and Step II diet guidelines were developed by the National Cholesterol Education Program and the American Heart Association to treat patients with high blood cholesterol. These diets were replaced in 2001 by the publication of the Adult Treatment Panel III (ATP III) of the National Cholesterol Education Program (NCEP). Step II has been replaced by the Total Lifestyle Change (TLC) diet. It's for all people who are at high risk of heart disease or who have heart disease.

What was the diet in the Lyon Diet Heart Study?

The Mediterranean-style diet used in the Lyon Diet Heart Study was quite comparable to the common pattern but different in a significant way. It was high in alpha-linolenic (lin"o-LEN'ik) acid (a type of polyunsaturated omega-3 fatty acid). It included:

- more bread, more root vegetables and green vegetables, more fish;
- less beef, lamb, and pork (replaced with poultry);
- no day without fruit;
- butter and cream were replaced with margarine high in alpha-linolenic acid.

The diet averaged 30% of calories from fat, 8% from saturated fat, 13% from monounsaturated fat, 5% from polyunsaturated fat, and 203 mg/day of cholesterol. Compared to the control group, people in the experimental group consumed less linoleic acid and more oleic acid, alpha-linolenic acid, and dietary fiber.

What was the diet in the control group?

People in the control group consumed a diet with about 34% of calories from fat, 12% from saturated fat, 11% from monounsaturated fat, 6% polyunsaturated fat, and 312 mg/day of cholesterol. This diet is comparable to what is typically consumed in the United States.

The control group's diet did not meet the association's Eating Plan for Healthy Americans diet guidelines. Nor did it meet the Therapeutic Lifestyle Changes (TLC) diet guidelines, which are recommended for people at high risk of heart disease or who have had a heart attack.

What were the results of the study?

After an average follow-up of 46 months (almost four years), patients following the Mediterranean-style diet had a 50%–70% lower risk of recurrent heart disease. The risk was measured by three combinations of outcome measures:

- Cardiac death and non-fatal heart attacks

- The previous two measures plus major events (unstable angina, stroke, heart failure, and pulmonary or peripheral embolism)

- All of these measures plus minor events that required hospitalization

What were the problems with the study?

These results are quite impressive. However, limitations in study methods raise questions about the true impact of this diet on risk of recurrent heart disease and related measures. Specifically, the baseline diet was only assessed in the experimental group at the start of the study. The control group's diet was only assessed at the conclusion. This was done to avoid influencing the dietary behavior of these subjects. Thus, it's not clear whether there were any dietary changes made by the control group.

Dietary data at the final visit are reported for only 83 out of 303 subjects (30%) in the control group and 144 out of 302 (less than 50%) in the experimental group. The diet of the other subjects who completed the study is unknown. This raises questions about the role of diet in explaining the results reported for recurrent coronary events.

What are the conclusions?

The Lyon Diet Heart Study showed the potential importance of a dietary pattern that emphasizes fruits, vegetables, breads and cereals, and fish as well as alpha-linolenic acid. The findings from this study imply risk factors beyond lipids and lipoproteins (cholesterol) that have been our primary focus in secondary prevention. The fact that omega-3 fatty acids exert cardioprotective effects in several ways suggests that they could have accounted for the results that were observed. The reduction in coronary recurrence rates, even though lipid and lipoprotein risk factors were comparable, clearly points to other important risk factor changes as major influences in the development of CVD [cardiovascular disease]. There's a pressing need to identify these risk factor(s) and find effective treatment strategies.

Chapter 43

Consuming Foods Marketed as Low Fat or Diet

Chapter Contents

Section 43.1

Nutrition Concerns about Diet Foods

"Beware Diet Food Fraud," *Young and Healthy Magazine*, Winter 2005. © 2005 Cincinnati Children's Hospital Medical Center (www.cincinnati childrens.org). All rights reserved. Reviewed by David A. Cooke, MD, FACP, January 2011.

For generations, cakes, cookies, and ice cream have been sending out their seductive siren calls from supermarket shelves. But for a decade or more, dozens of diet foods have been joining the "buy me / try me" chorus.

Do we sometimes trick ourselves into thinking that lower-fat, lower-calorie foods are "free" for the over-indulging? And are our children also falling for these diet food imposters?

"Reduced-fat peanut butter and regular peanut butter have the same number of calories per serving," says Ann Marie Kemer, RD, LD, a dietitian in the Teen Health Center at Cincinnati Children's Hospital Medical Center. "The fat has been replaced by sugar."

"One brand of sugar-free oatmeal cookie has 110 calories—the same as the brand's regular oatmeal cookie. It might not have table sugar, but it's packed with carbohydrates, and you're back to square one."

When "Diet Foods" Substitute for Real Food

Ideally, children and teens would be eating such a balanced diet of whole grains, vegetables, fruit, and dairy, supplemented by smaller amounts of protein and fat, that they'd never look at a diet food or drink. But in the real world, with many parents dieting and society emphasizing thinness, the pantry is often stocked with low-fat, low-sugar options.

"With less fat, there's usually more sugar," says Ms. Kemer, "and with less sugar, there's usually more fat. They have to add other things to give these foods a palatable taste and feel."

"The more children eat 'diet' foods, the more likely they are not to be consuming the essential nutrients. These foods usually don't affect weight management: That's based on the total number of calories coming in."

An Unsatisfying Solution

Although Ms. Kemer acknowledges that a 50-calorie cookie might be preferable to a 110-calorie cookie as a snack, she warns about the rebound effect that can happen with diet foods.

"These foods might not be as exciting and acceptable to a child and can lead to over-indulgence of regular foods later. It's better to teach children how to eat every type of non-'diet' food in moderation."

There's also the danger of eating so much "free" diet food that children consume more calories than they would with one serving of the original form of the food.

"A lot of diet foods are junk foods that are marketed as supposedly better for us now," she cautions. "Regular forms of cookies and candies are all right in moderation. Peanut butter and trail mix are still good for us if they're balanced with the calories for the rest of the day."

Rethinking Snack Time

Snacking is often prime time for diet food imposters. "Many adolescents don't see fruit, vegetables, cheese, or yogurt as a snack. They think a snack is a bag of chips and a can of pop. Parents can present all types of snacks as important and healthful, so children see a wider range of foods as alternatives," Ms. Kemer says.

Instead of low-fat chips, for instance, parents can offer crunchy popcorn, pretzels, and carrot sticks. Peanut butter, apples, and bananas can replace sugarfree candy or cookies.

Reading labels is crucial to discerning real food from diet imposters. "A food might have 15 grams of combined sugars, but it's important to read the label to identify the types of sugars used. The natural sugars in raw or basic foods are preferable to added sugars. Fructose, natural fruit sugar, and lactose, natural milk sugar, for instance, are better than added sucrose and corn syrup," she notes.

A careful look at the label can unmask diet food imposters nearly every time.

Section 43.2

Fat-Free versus Regular Calorie Consumption

"Fat-Free versus Regular Calorie Comparison," National Heart, Lung, and Blood Institute (www.nhlbi.nih.gov), August 2005. Reviewed by David A. Cooke, MD, FACP, January 2011.

A calorie is a calorie is a calorie, whether it comes from fat or carbohydrate. Anything eaten in excess can lead to weight gain. You can lose weight by eating fewer calories and by increasing your physical activity. Reducing the amount of fat and saturated fat that you eat is one easy way to limit your overall calorie intake. However, eating fat-free or reduced-fat foods isn't always the answer to weight loss. This

Table 43.1. Calories in Regular and Reduced-Fat Foods

Fat Free or Reduced Fat	Calories	Regular	Calories
Reduced-fat peanut butter, 2 Tbsp	187	Regular peanut butter, 2 Tbsp	191
Reduced-fat chocolate chip cookies, 3 cookies (30 g)	118	Regular chocolate chip cookies, 3 cookies (30 g)	142
Fat-free fig cookies, 2 cookies (30 g)	102	Regular fig cookies, 2 cookies (30 g)	111
Fat-free vanilla frozen yogurt (<1% fat), 1/2 cup	100	Regular whole milk vanilla frozen yogurt (3%–4% fat), 1/2 cup	104
Light vanilla ice cream (7% fat), 1/2 cup	111	Regular vanilla ice cream, (11% fat), 1/2 cup	133
Fat-free caramel topping, 2 Tbsp	103	Caramel topping, homemade with butter, 2 Tbsp	103
Low-fat granola cereal, approx. 1/2 cup (55 g)	213	Regular granola cereal, approx. 1/2 cup (55 g)	257
Low-fat blueberry muffin, 1 small (2 1/2 inch)	131	Regular blueberry muffin, 1 small (2 1/2 inch)	138
Baked tortilla chips, 1 oz	113	Regular tortilla chips, 1 oz	143
Low-fat cereal bar, 1 bar (1.3 oz)	130	Regular cereal bar, 1 bar (1.3 oz)	140

is especially true when you eat more of the reduced-fat food than you would of the regular item. The list of foods and their reduced-fat varieties in Table 43.1 will show you that just because a product is fat free, it doesn't mean that it is "calorie free." And calories do count!

Nutrient data taken from Nutrient Data System for Research, Version v4.02/30, Nutrition Coordinating Center, University of Minnesota.

Section 43.3

Questions and Answers about Fat Replacers

In recent years, low-fat, reduced-fat, and fat-free foods have become a staple in the diets of Americans seeking to lead healthier lifestyles. Lower fat foods not only can help reduce fat intake, but calories as well. How are lower fat foods made? The following list of commonly asked questions and their answers provides insight into the challenges faced in reducing the fat in foods and the solutions food manufacturers have discovered to provide satisfying foods that make it easier for many people to stay with a plan for healthy eating.

What are fat reduction ingredients?

Fat reduction ingredients are ingredients used, often in combination, to replace specific attributes of fat in low-fat, reduced-fat, and fat-free foods. Two calorie-free substances—water and air—can be incorporated into some foods to reduce fat, but they will not always produce an acceptable product. Thus, other fat reduction ingredients are necessary to reduce the fat in a wide variety of foods.

Why are fat reduction ingredients necessary—why can't the fat in foods simply be removed?

Reducing the fat in foods while maintaining taste and texture is a major challenge and often requires the innovative use of both common

513

and more recently developed ingredients. That's because the fat in foods plays a key role in determining texture and taste. For example, fat provides the smooth texture of a salad dressing, the creamy mouth feel of ice cream, the moist, tender texture of cake, and the rich flavor of cheese. Fat is also used as a cooking medium to produce the pleasingly crisp texture of some foods.

What are fat reduction ingredients made of?

Carbohydrates, proteins, and fats are the building blocks from which fat reduction ingredients are made (see Table 43.2). Many of these ingredients are common food components such as gelatin, starches, and water. Several ingredients as well as special processing techniques are often used in combination to produce acceptable food products that are lower in fat.

How do carbohydrate-based fat reduction ingredients reduce the fat in foods?

Carbohydrate-based fat reducers work in a variety of ways to simulate the texture and mouth feel of fat and retain moisture in foods. These fat reducers include ingredients such as cellulose, gums, fiber, dextrins, maltodextrins, modified food starch, modified dietary fibers, and polydextrose. Modified food starches, maltodextrins, and dextrins absorb water to form gels that mimic the texture and mouth feel of fat. Polydextrose acts as a bulking agent to replace volume lost when fat is removed from a food. Gums provide a creamy mouth feel and help stabilize emulsions. Cellulose gel is a purified form of cellulose ground to tiny particles that supply a mouth feel that is similar to fat. The caloric value of carbohydrate-based fat reduction ingredients ranges from zero to four calories per gram, compared to nine calories per gram in traditional fats. They cannot be used as substitutes for oils and other fats in frying.

How do protein-based fat reduction ingredients work?

Protein-based ingredients simulate the mouth feel of fat and can also help stabilize emulsions in sauces, spreads, and salad dressings. Some protein-based ingredients, such as Simplesse, are made through a process that gives fat-like textural properties to protein. Other proteins are heated and blended at high speed to produce tiny protein particles that feel creamy to the tongue. Like carbohydrate-based ingredients, protein-based fat reducers cannot be used as substitutes for oils and other fats in frying. They contribute from one to four calories per gram, depending on the degree to which they are hydrated.

How do fat-based fat reduction ingredients work?

Fat-based fat reduction ingredients are actually made from fats, and thus have the same physical properties as fat, including taste, texture, and mouth feel. Some fat-based ingredients, such as Caprenin and salatrim, are actually fats tailored to contribute fewer calories and less available fat to foods. Others, such as olestra, are structurally modified to provide no calories or fat.

Fat-based ingredients are highly versatile and can be used in a wide variety of foods. In addition, some may be used to fry foods. Their caloric value varies. Ingredients such as olestra are not absorbed and thus contribute no calories. Others such as Caprenin and salatrim contain fewer calories per gram than fat, contributing approximately five calories per gram to the diet.

Do fat-based reduction ingredients cause digestive problems?

At expected usage levels, fat reduction ingredients are without digestive side effects. However, like fiber and many other foods we eat that are not fully absorbed, consumption of large amounts of fat-based and some carbohydrate-based ingredients may lead to common, temporary digestive effects. These effects result from the added bulk of these ingredients in the digestive system.

Do fat-based fat reduction ingredients interfere with the absorption of vitamins and other important foodstuffs?

Some fat-based fat reduction ingredients may affect the absorption of the fat-soluble vitamins A, D, E, and K. If required, manufacturers make up for potential losses by adding specified amounts of these vitamins to the products.

How can I tell what kind of fat reduction ingredient is used in a food?

The ingredient list featured on the label will tell you which ones have been used in a specific product (see Table 43.2). Combinations of fat-reduction ingredients are often used to provide the best taste and texture in a product.

How are fat reduction ingredients approved for use in foods?

Most of the ingredients currently used to modify the fat content of foods have been part of the food supply for many years. Before new ingredients can be used in food, food companies must follow a specific process to confirm safety: New ingredients must be confirmed as "generally recognized as safe" (GRAS) in keeping with Food and Drug Administration (FDA) guidelines, or after thorough review, approved for such use by the FDA. GRAS substances, such as starch, have an extensive history or existing scientific evidence of their safe use in foods.

What is the role of lower-fat foods in the diet?

Foods that are lower in fat can help people adopt a healthy lifestyle. Indeed, the advice to reduce dietary fat represents a cornerstone of existing dietary guidelines designed to promote health and well-being. Reduced-fat, low-fat, and fat-free foods expand the choices from which consumers may select to achieve a diet moderate in fat while continuing to enjoy their favorite foods.

Data also show that taste often influences food choices more than nutrition, and that the consumption of good-tasting, fat-modified foods is among the most easily adopted and maintained strategies for following a lower-fat diet.

In addition, a reduced intake of dietary fat is recommended to help manage body weight. Reduced-fat, low-fat, and fat-free foods that are lower in calories may help people stay with healthful eating plans that foster healthy weights. Success at weight management, however, also generally requires a healthy lifestyle approach that includes physical activity as well as healthful eating.

What has research shown about the nutritional impact of low-fat foods in the diet?

The majority of clinical studies conducted to date suggest lower-fat foods can help people significantly reduce both the actual amount of fat, calories, and the percentage of calories from fat eaten. In addition, data from the 1995 Continuing Survey of Food Intake of Individuals (CSFII) show that adults who used more fat-modified foods also consumed less energy overall and did not eat more because the foods are fat free. Other research has demonstrated that individuals who consume fat- and calorie-reduced foods have a more nutritious diet than those who do not.

What advice can consumers follow to enjoy and use lower-fat foods to reduce the fat in their diets?

According to the American Dietetic Association, foods that contain fat reduction ingredients may offer a safe, feasible, and effective means to maintain the palatability of diets that are controlled in fat and/or calories. Such foods, however, should be used as substitutions for foods higher in fat and/or calories, not as additions to the diet. Further, fat-reduced foods should be consumed as part of an overall healthy eating plan, such as that outlined in the *Dietary Guidelines for Americans.*

Table 43.2. Looking for Fat Reduction Ingredients on the Food Label

Names on Ingredients List	Foods That May Contain Fat Replacers
Carbohydrate-based: Carrageenan, cellulose, gelatin, gellan gum, gels, guar gum, maltodextrins, polydextrose, starches, xanthum gum, modified dietary fibers	Baked goods, cheeses, frozen desserts, gravies, mayonnaise, processed meats, puddings, salad dressings, sauces, sour cream, yogurt
Protein-based: Whey protein concentrate, microparticulated egg white and milk protein (Simplesse)	Baked goods, butter, cheese, frozen dairy desserts, mayonnaise, salad dressings, sour cream
Fat-based: Caprenin, salatrim (Benefat), mono- and diglycerides, olestra (Olean)	Baked goods, cheese, chocolate, chocolate confections, margarine, salted snacks, sour cream, spreads

Part Seven

Nutrition for People with Other Medical Concerns

Chapter 44

Nutrition and Diabetes

Chapter Contents

Section 44.1

Nutrition Tips to Prevent Type 2 Diabetes

This section excerpted from "More than 50 Ways to Prevent Diabetes," November 2009, and "Grade-A Grocery List: Tips to Prevent Type 2 Diabetes," 2009, U.S. Department of Health and Human Services National Diabetes Education Program (ndep.nih.gov).

More than 50 Ways to Prevent Diabetes

Reduce Portion Sizes

1.   Less on your plate, Nate.

2.   Keep meat, poultry and fish portions to about three ounces (about the size of a deck of cards).

3.   Try not to snack while cooking or cleaning the kitchen.

4.   Try to eat meals and snacks at regular times every day.

5.   Make sure you eat breakfast every day.

6.   Use broth and cured meats (smoked turkey and turkey bacon) in small amounts. They are high in sodium. Low sodium broths are available in cans and in powdered form.

7.   Share a single dessert.

8.   When eating out, have a big vegetable salad, then split an entrée with a friend or have the other half wrapped to go.

9.   Stir-fry, broil, or bake with non-stick spray or low-sodium broth and cook with less oil and butter.

10.   Drink a glass of water 10 minutes before your meal to take the edge off your hunger.

11.   Make healthy choices at fast food restaurants. Try grilled chicken (remove skin) instead of a cheeseburger. Skip the french fries and choose a salad.

12.   Listen to music while you eat instead of watching TV (people tend to eat more while watching TV).

13. Eat slowly. It takes 20 minutes for your stomach to send a signal to your brain that you're full.

14. Eat a small meal, Lucille.

15. Teaspoons, salad forks, or child-size utensils may help you take smaller bites and eat less.

16. You don't have to cut out the foods you love to eat. Just cut down on your portion size and eat it less often.

17. Make less food look like more by serving your meal on a salad or breakfast plate.

Move More Each Day

18. Dance it away, Faye.

19. Show your kids the dances you used to do when you were their age.

20. Turn up the music and jam while doing household chores.

21. Deliver a message in person to a co-worker instead of e-mailing.

22. Take the stairs to your office. Or take the stairs as far as you can, and then take the elevator the rest of the way.

23. Make fewer phone calls. Catch up with friends on a regular basis during a planned walk.

24. March in place while you watch TV.

25. Park as far away as possible from your favorite store at the mall.

26. Select a physical activity video from the store or library.

27. Get off of the bus one stop early and walk the rest of the way home or to work several times a week.

Make Healthy Food Choices

28. Snack on a veggie, Reggie.

29. Try getting one new fruit or vegetable every time you grocery shop.

30. Low-fat macaroni and cheese can be a main dish. Serve it with your favorite vegetable and a salad.

31.   Try eating foods from other countries. Many dishes contain more vegetables, whole grains, and beans and less meat.

32.   Cook with a mix of spices instead of salt.

33.   Find a water bottle you really like (from a church or club event, favorite sports team, etc.) and drink water from it wherever and whenever you can.

34.   Always keep a healthy snack with you, such as fresh fruit, a handful of nuts, or whole-grain crackers.

35.   Choose veggie toppings like spinach, broccoli, and peppers for your pizza.

36.   Try different recipes for baking or broiling meat.

37.   Try to choose foods with little or no added sugar.

38.   Gradually work your way down from whole milk to 2% milk until you're drinking and cooking with fat-free (skim) or low-fat milk and milk products.

39.   Eat foods made from whole grains—such as whole wheat, brown rice, oats, and whole-grain corn—every day. Use whole-grain bread for toast and sandwiches; substitute brown rice for white rice for home-cooked meals and when dining out.

40.   Don't grocery shop on an empty stomach. Make a list before you go to the store.

41.   Read food labels. Choose foods low in saturated fats, trans fats, cholesterol, salt (sodium), and added sugars.

42.   Fruits are colorful and make a welcome centerpiece for any table. Enjoy the company of family and friends while sharing a bowl of fruit.

43.   Slow down at snack time. Eating a bag of low-fat popcorn takes longer than eating a slice of cake. Peel and eat an orange instead of drinking orange juice.

44.   Try keeping a written record of what you eat for a week. It can help you see when you tend to overeat or eat foods high in fat or calories.

Nurture Your Mind, Body, and Soul

45.   You can exhale, Gail.

46. Don't try to change your entire way of eating and increasing your physical activity all at once. Try one new activity or food a week.

47. Find mellow ways to relax—try deep breathing, take an easy-paced walk, or enjoy your favorite easy-listening music.

48. Give yourself daily "pampering time." Honor this time, whether it's reading a book, taking a long bath, or meditating.

49. Try not to eat out of boredom or frustration. If you are not hungry, do something else, such as taking a long walk.

Be Creative

50. Honor your health as your most precious gift.

51. Make up your own, Tyrone or Simone.

Grade-A Grocery List: Tips to Prevent Type 2 Diabetes

If you have a family history of diabetes, or you've been told by a health care professional that you're at risk for type 2 diabetes, it's important to take steps now to reduce your risk. Studies show that people at high risk for type 2 diabetes can prevent or delay the onset of the disease if they lose as little as 10 pounds—by walking 30 minutes a day, five days a week and making healthy food choices. A healthy diet doesn't have to be expensive. Start by planning meals and making a grocery list ahead of time to take charge of what you eat. Follow these tips by the National Diabetes Education Program (NDEP) while grocery shopping to help you and your entire family make healthy food choices:

- Don't go to the store hungry. You may buy food you don't need.

- Read and compare food labels. Choose foods with fewer calories that are lower in saturated fats, trans fats, cholesterol, sodium (salt), and added sugars. Check the serving size and the number of servings. Food labels are based on one serving, but many packages contain more. When you compare calories and nutrients between brands, check to see if the serving size is the same.

- Focus on fruits, vary vegetables. Buy a variety of frozen, canned, or in-season fresh fruits such as melons, berries, and oranges rather than fruit juice for most of your fruit choices. Choose fruit without added sugar or syrup. Buy in-season, leafy dark green vegetables such as broccoli and spinach and orange vegetables such as carrots or squash. Choose vegetables without added salt, butter, or sauces.

- Look for calcium-rich foods. Buy low-fat or skim milk instead of whole milk. If you can't drink milk, choose fat-free or low-fat lactose-reduced milk or try calcium-rich leafy green vegetables such as kale or collard greens.

- Make your grains whole. Buy whole-wheat bread, crackers, cereals, brown rice, oatmeal, and barley.

- Go lean with protein. Buy lean meats. For poultry, remove the skin before cooking. Vary your protein choices with more fish, nuts, seeds, and beans and peas such as pinto beans and split peas.

Section 44.2

What People with Diabetes Need to Know about Eating

This section excerpted from "What I Need to Know about Eating and Diabetes," National Diabetes Information Clearinghouse, National Institute of Diabetes and Digestive and Kidney Diseases (diabetes.niddk.nih.gov), October 2007.

You can take good care of yourself and your diabetes by learning the following:

- What to eat
- How much to eat
- When to eat

Making wise food choices can help you in these ways:

- Feel good every day
- Lose weight if you need to
- Lower your risk for heart disease, stroke, and other problems caused by diabetes

Healthful eating helps keep your blood glucose, also called blood sugar, in your target range. Physical activity and, if needed, diabetes medicines also help. The diabetes target range is the blood glucose level suggested by diabetes experts for good health. You can help prevent health problems by keeping your blood glucose levels on target.

Blood Glucose Levels

Target blood glucose levels for people with diabetes

- Before meals: 70 to 130
- One to two hours after the start of a meal: Less than 180

Talk with your health care provider about your blood glucose target levels. Ask your doctor how often you should check your blood glucose on your own. Also ask your doctor for an A1C test at least twice a year. Your A1C number gives your average blood glucose for the past three months. The results from your blood glucose checks and your A1C test will tell you whether your diabetes care plan is working.

You can keep your blood glucose levels on target by doing the following:

- Making wise food choices
- Being physically active
- Taking medicines if needed

For people taking certain diabetes medicines, following a schedule for meals, snacks, and physical activity is best. However, some diabetes medicines allow for more flexibility. You'll work with your health care team to create a diabetes plan that's best for you. What you eat and when you eat affect how your diabetes medicines work. Talk with your doctor or diabetes teacher about when to take your diabetes medicines.

What you eat and when also depend on how much you exercise. Physical activity is an important part of staying healthy and controlling your blood glucose.

Low Blood Glucose (Hypoglycemia)

Low blood glucose can make you feel shaky, weak, confused, irritable, hungry, or tired. You may sweat a lot or get a headache. If you have these symptoms, check your blood glucose. If it is below 70, have one of the following right away:

- 3 or 4 glucose tablets

- 1 serving of glucose gel—the amount equal to 15 grams of carbohydrate
- 1/2 cup (4 ounces) of any fruit juice
- 1/2 cup (4 ounces) of a regular (not diet) soft drink
- 1 cup (8 ounces) of milk
- 5 or 6 pieces of hard candy
- 1 tablespoon of sugar or honey

After 15 minutes, check your blood glucose again. If it's still too low, have another serving. Repeat these steps until your blood glucose level is 70 or higher. If it will be an hour or more before your next meal, have a snack as well.

The Diabetes Food Pyramid

The diabetes food pyramid can help you make wise food choices. It divides foods into groups, based on what they contain. Eat more from the groups at the bottom of the pyramid (vegetables, fruits, starches) and less from the groups at the top (fats and sweets, milk, and meat and meat substitutes). Foods from the starches, fruits, vegetables, and milk groups are highest in carbohydrate. They affect your blood glucose levels the most.

How much should I eat each day?

Have about 1,200 to 1,600 calories a day if you are the following:

- A small woman who exercises
- A small or medium-sized woman who wants to lose weight
- A medium-sized woman who does not exercise much

Choose this many servings from these food groups to have 1,200 to 1,600 calories a day:

- 6 starches
- 2 milks
- 3 vegetables
- 4 to 6 ounces meat and meat substitutes
- 2 fruits
- Up to 3 fats

Have about 1,600 to 2,000 calories a day if you are the following:

- A large woman who wants to lose weight
- A small man at a healthy weight
- A medium-sized man who does not exercise much
- A medium-sized or large man who wants to lose weight

Choose this many servings from these food groups to have 1,600 to 2,000 calories a day:

- 8 starches
- 2 milks
- 4 vegetables
- 4 to 6 ounces meat and meat substitutes
- 3 fruits
- Up to 4 fats

Have about 2,000 to 2,400 calories a day if you are the following:

- A medium-sized or large man who exercises a lot or has a physically active job
- A large man at a healthy weight
- A medium-sized or large woman who exercises a lot or has a physically active job

Choose this many servings from these food groups to have 2,000 to 2,400 calories a day:

- 10 starches
- 2 milks
- 4 vegetables
- 5 to 7 ounces meat and meat substitutes
- 4 fruits
- Up to 5 fats

Talk with your diabetes teacher about how to make a meal plan that fits the way you usually eat, your daily routine, and your diabetes medicines. Then make your own plan.

Starches

Starches are bread, grains, cereal, pasta, and starchy vegetables like corn and potatoes. They provide carbohydrate, vitamins, minerals, and fiber. Whole-grain starches are healthier because they have more vitamins, minerals, and fiber.

Eat some starches at each meal. Eating starches is healthy for everyone, including people with diabetes.

How much is one serving of starch?

- 1 slice of bread
- 1 small potato
- 1/2 cup cooked cereal or 3/4 cup dry cereal flakes
- 1 six-inch tortilla
- 1/2 cup of peas

If your plan includes more than one serving at a meal, you can choose different starches or have several servings of one starch.

What are healthy ways to eat starches?

- Buy whole-grain breads and cereals.
- Eat fewer fried and high-fat starches such as regular tortilla chips and potato chips, french fries, pastries, or biscuits. Try pretzels, fat-free popcorn, baked tortilla chips or potato chips, baked potatoes, or low-fat muffins.
- Use low-fat or fat-free plain yogurt or fat-free sour cream instead of regular sour cream on a baked potato.
- Use mustard instead of mayonnaise on a sandwich.
- Use low-fat or fat-free substitutes such as low-fat mayonnaise or light margarine on bread, rolls, or toast.
- Eat cereal with fat-free (skim) or low-fat (1%) milk.

Vegetables

Vegetables provide vitamins, minerals, and fiber. They are low in carbohydrate.

How much is a serving of vegetables?

- 1/2 cup cooked carrots
- 1/2 cup cooked green beans
- 1 cup salad

What are healthy ways to eat vegetables?

- Eat raw and cooked vegetables with little or no fat, sauces, or dressings.
- Try low-fat or fat-free salad dressing on raw vegetables or salads.
- Steam vegetables using water or low-fat broth.
- Mix in some chopped onion or garlic.
- Use a little vinegar or some lemon or lime juice.
- Add a small piece of lean ham or smoked turkey instead of fat to vegetables when cooking.
- Sprinkle with herbs and spices.
- If you do use a small amount of fat, use canola oil, olive oil, or soft margarines (liquid or tub types) instead of fat from meat, butter, or shortening.

Fruits

Fruits provide carbohydrate, vitamins, minerals, and fiber.

How much is a serving of fruit?

- 1 small apple
- 1/2 cup juice
- 1/2 grapefruit

What are healthy ways to eat fruits?

- Eat fruits raw or cooked, as juice with no sugar added, canned in their own juice, or dried.
- Buy smaller pieces of fruit.
- Choose pieces of fruit more often than fruit juice. Whole fruit is more filling and has more fiber.

- Save high-sugar and high-fat fruit desserts such as peach cobbler or cherry pie for special occasions.

Milk

Milk provides carbohydrate, protein, calcium, vitamins, and minerals.

How much is a serving of milk?

- 1 cup of fat-free or low-fat yogurt
- 1 cup fat-free (skim) or low-fat (1%) milk

What are healthy ways to have milk?

- Drink fat-free (skim) or low-fat (1%) milk.
- Eat low-fat or fat-free fruit yogurt sweetened with a low-calorie sweetener.
- Use low-fat plain yogurt as a substitute for sour cream.

Meat and Meat Substitutes

The meat and meat substitutes group includes meat, poultry, eggs, cheese, fish, and tofu. Eat small amounts of some of these foods each day. Meat and meat substitutes provide protein, vitamins, and minerals.

How much is a serving of meat and meat substitutes?

Meat and meat substitutes are measured in ounces. Here are examples:

- **1-ounce serving:** 1 egg or 2 tablespoons of peanut butter
- **2-ounce serving:** 1 slice of turkey and 1 slice of low-fat cheese
- **3-ounce serving:** 3 ounces of cooked lean meat, chicken, or fish (3 ounces of meat after cooking is about the size of a deck of cards)

What are healthy ways to eat meat and meat substitutes?

- Buy cuts of beef, pork, ham, and lamb that have only a little fat on them. Trim off the extra fat.
- Eat chicken or turkey without the skin.

- Cook meat and meat substitutes in low-fat ways:
    - Broil
    - Grill
    - Stir-fry
    - Roast
    - Steam
    - Microwave
- To add more flavor, use vinegars, lemon juice, soy sauce, salsa, ketchup, barbecue sauce, herbs, and spices.
- Cook eggs using cooking spray or a non-stick pan.
- Limit the amount of nuts, peanut butter, and fried foods you eat. They are high in fat.
- Check food labels. Choose low-fat or fat-free cheese.

Fats and Sweets

Limit the amount of fats and sweets you eat. Fats and sweets are not as nutritious as other foods. Fats have a lot of calories. Sweets can be high in carbohydrate and fat. Some contain saturated fats, trans fats, and cholesterol that increase your risk of heart disease. Limiting these foods will help you lose weight and keep your blood glucose and blood fats under control.

How much is a serving of sweets?

- 1 3-inch cookie
- 1 plain cake doughnut
- 1 tablespoon maple syrup

How much is a serving of fat?

- 1 strip of bacon
- 1 teaspoon oil

How can I satisfy my sweet tooth?

- Try having sugar-free popsicles, diet soda, fat-free ice cream or frozen yogurt, or sugar-free hot cocoa mix.
- Share desserts in restaurants.
- Order small or child-size servings of ice cream or frozen yogurt.
- Divide homemade desserts into small servings and wrap each individually. Freeze extra servings.

Remember, fat-free and low-sugar foods still have calories. Talk with your diabetes teacher about how to fit sweets into your meal plan.

Alcoholic Drinks

Alcoholic drinks have calories but no nutrients. If you have alcoholic drinks on an empty stomach, they can make your blood glucose level go too low. Alcoholic drinks also can raise your blood fats. If you want to have alcoholic drinks, talk with your doctor or diabetes teacher about how much to have.

Chapter 45

Nutrition and Heart Disease

Chapter Contents

Section 45.1

Eating for a Healthy Heart

This section excerpted from "Eat for a Healthy Heart," U.S. Food and
Drug Administration (www.fda.gov), January 29, 2010.

Making healthy food choices is one of many lifestyle changes that
can help reduce your risk for getting heart disease—the number one
killer in the United States. The Nutrition Facts found on most foods
and health claims allowed on some foods can help you choose wisely.

To help ward off heart disease, choose foods with less fat, sodium
(salt), and cholesterol; fewer calories; and more fiber.

"Making better food choices for your health doesn't mean you will
need to exclude favorite foods," says Barbara Schneeman, PhD, director of the Food and Drug Administration (FDA)'s Office of Nutrition,
Labeling, and Dietary Supplements. "You can use one of the most valuable tools people have—the food label—to make dietary trade-offs. For
example, if you eat a food that is high in saturated fat, you can make
other choices during the day that are low in saturated fat to keep your
total daily intake in balance by using the part of the food label called
Nutrition Facts."

People concerned about their blood pressure who want to limit how
much salt they eat may be faced with five different types of tomato soup
on the shelf, says Schneeman. You can compare the sodium content of
each product by looking at Nutrition Facts to choose the one with the
lowest sodium content.

Nutrient Highs and Lows

Most of the nutrients that must be declared under Nutrition Facts
on the food label are listed with a "percent Daily Value" (%DV), which
shows the percent of the recommended daily intake that's in a serving
of that product. Consumers can use the %DVs to create a balanced diet.
The rule of thumb is 20% DV or more is high and 5% DV or less is low.

Health experts recommend keeping the intake of nutrients that
may increase your risk for heart disease—saturated fat, trans fat, and
cholesterol—as low as possible.

There is no %DV for trans fat. When comparing products, look at the total amount of saturated fat plus trans fat to find the one lowest in both of these types of fat.

You can also use the %DV to choose products that contain higher amounts of heart-healthy nutrients, such as fiber. Eating fiber from fruits, vegetables, and grains may help lower your chances of getting heart disease.

Health Claims

Some food products carry health claims—statements that the product may help reduce the risk of developing a certain disease or condition. FDA authorizes some health claims based on "significant scientific agreement," which means that the claim is supported by strong, scientific evidence based on studies in people and that the claim is unlikely to be reversed by new studies. Only foods that meet the criteria for a claim are allowed to carry the claim on their labels.

Here are claims related to heart disease that you may see on some foods:

- While many factors affect heart disease, diets low in saturated fat and cholesterol may reduce the risk of this disease.

- Diets low in sodium may reduce the risk of high blood pressure, a disease associated with many factors.

- Soluble fiber, as part of a diet low in saturated fat and cholesterol, may reduce the risk of heart disease.

Tips for Healthy Eating

- Choose lean meats and poultry. Bake it, broil it, or grill it.

- Most of the fats you eat should come from polyunsaturated and monounsaturated fats, such as those found in fish, nuts, and vegetable oils.

- Look for foods high in potassium (unless your health care professional has told you to restrict the amount of potassium you eat). Potassium counteracts some of the effects of salt on blood pressure.

- Choose foods and beverages low in added sugars. Read the ingredient list to make sure that added sugars are not one of the first few ingredients.

Section 45.2

Cooking for Lower Cholesterol

"Cooking for Lower Cholesterol," reprinted with permission from
www.heart.org. © 2010 American Heart Association, Inc.

It's not hard to whip up recipes that fit with the low-saturated-fat,
low-cholesterol eating plan recommended by scientists to help you
manage your blood cholesterol level and reduce your risk of heart
disease and stroke.

Our suggestions will help you prepare tasty dishes without over-
doing the salt and sodium. Eating less sodium may help some people
lower their blood pressure—which can also help reduce the risk of
heart disease and stroke.

Aim to eat less than 1,500 mg of sodium per day.

Reduce Saturated Fat in Meat and Poultry

The American Heart Association recommends eating no more than
six ounces of cooked lean meat, poultry, fish, or seafood a day for
people who need 2,000 calories. Most meats have about the same
amount of cholesterol, roughly 70 milligrams in each three-ounce
cooked serving (about the size of a deck of cards). But the amount
of saturated fat in meats can vary widely, depending on the cut and
how it's prepared. Here are some ways to reduce the saturated fat
in meat:

- Select lean cuts of meat with minimal visible fat. Lean beef cuts
  include the round, chuck, sirloin, or loin. Lean pork cuts include
  the tenderloin or loin chop, while lean lamb cuts come from the
  leg, arm, and loin.

- Buy "choice" or "select" grades rather than "prime." Select lean or
  extra lean ground beef.

- Trim all visible fat from meat before cooking.

- Broil rather than pan-fry meats such as hamburger, lamb chops,
  pork chops, and steak.

- Use a rack to drain off fat when broiling, roasting, or baking. Instead of basting with drippings, keep meat moist with wine, fruit juices, or an acceptable oil-based marinade.

- Cook a day ahead of time. Stews, boiled meat, soup stock, or other dishes in which fat cooks into the liquid can be refrigerated. Then the hardened fat can be removed from the top.

- When a recipe calls for browning the meat first, try browning it under the broiler instead of in a pan.

- Eat chicken and turkey rather than duck and goose, which are higher in fat.

- Remove the skin from chicken or turkey, preferably before cooking. If your poultry dries out too much, leave the skin on for cooking but remove before eating.

- Limit processed meats such as sausage, bologna, salami, and hot dogs. Many processed meats—even those with "reduced fat" labels—are high in calories and saturated fat. They are often high in sodium as well. Read labels carefully and choose such meats only now and then.

- Organ meats such as liver, sweetbreads, kidney, and brain are very high in cholesterol. If you're on a cholesterol-lowering diet, eat them only occasionally.

Choose Seafood at Least Twice a Week

Fish can be fatty or lean, but it's still low in saturated fat. Prepare fish baked, broiled, grilled, or boiled rather than breaded and fried. Shrimp and crawfish have more cholesterol than most other types of seafood, but they're lower in total fat and saturated fat than most meats and poultry.

Reduce the Meat in Your Meal

Try meatless meals featuring vegetables or beans—think eggplant lasagna, a big grilled portobello mushroom on a bun in place of a burger, or beans-n-weenies without the weenies. Or think of meat as a condiment in casseroles, stews, soups, and spaghetti—use it sparingly, just for flavor, rather than as a main ingredient.

Cook Fresh Vegetables the Low-Fat, Low-Salt Way

Try cooking vegetables in a tiny bit of vegetable oil, adding a little water during cooking if needed, or use a vegetable oil spray. Just one to two teaspoons of oil is enough for a package of frozen vegetables that serves four. Place in a skillet with a tight cover, season, and cook over a very low heat until vegetables are done.

Add herbs and spices to make vegetables even tastier. For example, these combinations add new and subtle flavors:

- Rosemary with peas, cauliflower, and squash

- Oregano with zucchini

- Dill with green beans

- Marjoram with Brussels sprouts, carrots, and spinach

- Basil with tomatoes

Start with a small quantity (1/8 to 1/2 teaspoon to a package of frozen vegetables), then let your own and your family's taste be your guide. Chopped parsley and chives, sprinkled on just before serving, also enhance the flavor of many vegetables.

Use Liquid Vegetable Oils in Place of Solid Fats

Liquid vegetable oils such as canola, safflower, sunflower, soybean, and olive can often be used instead of solid fats such as butter, lard, or shortening. If you must use margarine, try the soft kind. Use a little liquid oil to:

- pan-fry fish and poultry;

- sauté vegetables;

- make cream sauces and soups using low-fat or fat-free milk;

- add to whipped or scalloped potatoes using low-fat or fat-free milk;

- brown rice for Spanish, curried, or stir-fried rice;

- cook dehydrated potatoes and other prepared foods that call for fat to be added;

- make pancakes or waffles.

Substitute Egg Whites for Whole Eggs

The cholesterol in eggs is all in the yolks—without the yolk, egg whites are a heart-healthy source of protein. Many recipes calling for whole eggs come out just as good when you use egg whites or cholesterol-free egg substitute instead of whole eggs. Replace each whole egg with two egg whites. For baking, you may want to add a tablespoon or less of liquid vegetable oil such as canola, safflower, sunflower, or soybean for a moister consistency.

Puree Fruits and Veggies for Baking

You can replace the oil in muffin, cookie, cake, and snack bar recipes with pureed fruits or veggies to give your treats an extra healthy boost. For many recipes, you just use the specified amount of puree instead of oil. Check the mix's package or your cookbook's substitutions page for other conversions.

- Use applesauce in spice muffins or oatmeal cookies.
- Bananas are great in breads and muffins.
- Try zucchini in brownies.

Lowering Dairy Fats

Low-fat (1%) or fat-free (skim) milk can be used in many recipes in place of whole milk or half-and-half. Some dishes like puddings may result in a softer set. You can also use low-fat cottage cheese, part-skim mozzarella or ricotta, and other low-fat cheeses with little or no change in consistency.

Sauces and Gravies

Let your cooking liquid cool, then remove the hardened fat before making gravy. Or, use a fat separator to pour off the good liquid from cooking stock, leaving the fat behind.

Increasing Fiber and Whole Grains

- Toast and crush or cube whole-grain bread to make bread-crumbs, stuffing, or croutons.
- Replace the breadcrumbs in your meatloaf with uncooked oatmeal.
- Serve whole fruit at breakfast in place of juice.
- Use brown rice instead of white rice and try whole-grain pasta.
- Add lots of colorful veggies to your salad—carrots, broccoli, and cauliflower are high in fiber and give your salad a delicious crunch.

Reducing Sodium

Most of us eat much more sodium than we need. In some people, this can lead to high blood pressure, which increases the risk of stroke, heart disease, and kidney disease. Salt is just once source of the sodium you consume every day. Many foods contain sodium in other forms, too. Some medicines are high in sodium.

About 75% of sodium in the typical American diet comes from processed foods and beverages. Be aware of all your sources of sodium and aim to eat less than 1,500 mg of sodium per day.

- Use less salt or no salt at the table and in cooking.

- Use herbs and spices in place of salt.

- Limit your intake of foods high in added sodium, such as:
  - canned and dried soups;
  - canned vegetables;
  - ketchup and mustard;
  - salty snack foods;
  - olives and pickles;
  - luncheon meats and cold cuts;
  - bacon and other cured meats;
  - cheeses;
  - restaurant and carry-out foods (such as french fries, onion rings, and hamburgers).

- To reduce the salt in canned vegetables, drain the liquid, then rinse the vegetables in water before eating.

- Look for "unsalted" varieties of the aforementioned canned foods and snack foods. Some foods may be labeled "no salt" or "without added salt."

- Ask restaurants not to add salt to your order.

- Read the labels of all foods carefully. Even bakery products and cereals can be major sources of sodium.

- Learn about the DASH (Dietary Approaches to Stop Hypertension) eating plan.

Section 45.3

Lowering Your Blood Pressure with the DASH Eating Plan

This section excerpted from "In Brief: Your Guide to Lowering Your Blood Pressure with DASH," National Heart, Lung, and Blood Institute (www.nhlbi.nih.gov), December 2006.

What you eat affects your chances of developing high blood pressure (hypertension). Research shows that high blood pressure can be prevented—and lowered—by following the Dietary Approaches to Stop Hypertension (DASH) eating plan, which includes eating less salt and sodium.

High blood pressure is dangerous because it makes your heart work too hard, hardens the walls of your arteries, and can cause the brain to hemorrhage or the kidneys to function poorly or not at all. If not controlled, high blood pressure can lead to heart and kidney disease, stroke, and blindness.

But high blood pressure can be prevented—and lowered—if you take these steps: Follow a healthy eating plan, such as DASH, that includes foods lower in salt and sodium. Maintain a healthy weight. Be moderately physically active for at least 30 minutes on most days of the week. Also, if you drink alcoholic beverages, do so in moderation.

The DASH Eating Plan

The DASH eating plan is rich in fruits, vegetables, fat-free or low-fat milk and milk products, whole grains, fish, poultry, beans, seeds, and nuts. It also contains less salt and sodium; sweets, added sugars, and sugar-containing beverages; fats; and red meats than the typical American diet. This heart-healthy way of eating is also lower in saturated fat, trans fat, and cholesterol and rich in nutrients that are associated with lowering blood pressure—mainly potassium, magnesium, and calcium, protein, and fiber.

The DASH eating plan requires no special foods and has no hard-to-follow recipes. It simply calls for a certain number of daily servings from various food groups.

The number of servings depends on the number of calories you're allowed each day. Your calorie level depends on your age and how active you are. Think of this as an energy balance system—if you want to maintain your current weight, you should take in only as many calories as you burn by being physically active. If you need to lose weight, eat fewer calories than you burn or increase your activity level to burn more calories than you eat. [Refer to Table 2.2 on page 24 for information about calorie requirements by gender, age, and physical activity level.]

Now that you know how many calories you're allowed each day, find the closest calorie level to yours in Table 45.1. This shows roughly the number of servings from each food group that you can eat each day.

Because fruits and vegetables are naturally lower in sodium than many other foods, DASH makes it easier to eat less sodium. The less salt you eat, the more you may be able to lower your blood pressure.

Choose and prepare foods with less salt, and don't bring the salt shaker to the table. And, because most of the salt, or sodium, that we eat comes from processed foods, be sure to read food labels to check the amount of sodium in different food products. Aim for foods that contain 5% or less of the Daily Value of sodium.

DASH Tips for Gradual Change

- Add a serving of vegetables at lunch one day and dinner the next, and add fruit at one meal or as a snack.

- Increase your use of fat-free and low-fat milk products to three servings a day.

- Limit lean meats to six ounces a day—three ounces a meal, which is about the size of a deck of cards.

- Include two or more vegetarian-style, or meatless, meals each week.

- Increase servings of vegetables, brown rice, whole-wheat pasta, and cooked dry beans.

- For snacks and desserts, use fruits or other foods low in saturated fat, trans fat, cholesterol, sodium, sugar, and calories—for example, unsalted rice cakes; unsalted nuts or seeds; raisins; graham crackers; fat-free, low-fat, or frozen yogurt; popcorn with no salt or butter added; or raw vegetables.

- Use fresh, frozen, or low-sodium canned vegetables and fruits.

Table 45.1. Following the DASH Eating Plan (continued on next page)

Food Group	Servings per Day			Serving Sizes	Examples and Notes	Significance of Each Food Group to the DASH Eating Plan
	1,600 Calories	2,000 Calories	2,600 Calories			
Grains	6	6–8	10–11	1 slice bread, 1 oz dry cereal, 1/2 cup cooked rice, pasta, or cereal	Whole-wheat bread and rolls, whole-wheat pasta, English muffin, pita bread, bagel, cereals, grits, oatmeal, brown rice, unsalted pretzels and popcorn	Major sources of energy and fiber
Vegetables	3–4	4–5	5–6	1 cup raw leafy vegetable, 1/2 cup cut-up raw or cooked vegetables, 1/2 cup vegetable juice	Broccoli, carrots, collards, green beans, green peas, kale, lima beans, potatoes, spinach, squash, sweet potatoes, tomatoes	Rich sources of potassium, magnesium, and fiber
Fruits	4	4–5	5–6	1 medium fruit; 1/4 cup dried fruit; 1/2 cup fresh, frozen, or canned fruit; 1/2 cup fruit juice	Apples, apricots, bananas, dates, grapes, oranges, grapefruit, grapefruit juice, mangoes, melons, peaches, pineapples, raisins, strawberries, tangerines	Important sources of potassium, magnesium, and fiber
Fat-free or low-fat milk and milk products	2–3	2–3	3	1 cup milk or yogurt, 1 1/2 oz cheese	Fat-free (skim) or low-fat (1%) milk or buttermilk; fat-free, low-fat, or reduced-fat cheese; fat-free or low-fat regular or frozen yogurt	Major sources of calcium and protein

Table 45.1. Following the DASH Eating Plan (continued from previous page)

Food Group	Servings per Day	Serving Sizes	Examples and Notes	Significance of Each Food Group to the DASH Eating Plan
Lean meats, poultry, and fish	3–6 6 or less	1 oz cooked meats, poultry, or fish, 1 egg‡	Select only lean; trim away visible fats; broil, roast, or poach; remove skin from poultry	Rich sources of protein and magnesium
Nuts, seeds, and legumes	3 per week 4–5 per week	1/3 cup or 1 1/2 oz nuts, 2 Tbsp peanut butter, 2 Tbsp or 1/2 oz seeds, 1/2 cup cooked legumes (dry beans and peas)	Almonds, hazelnuts, mixed nuts, peanuts, walnuts, sunflower seeds, peanut butter, kidney beans, lentils, split peas	Rich sources of energy, magnesium, protein, and fiber
Fats and oils§	2 2–3	1 tsp soft margarine, 1 tsp vegetable oil, 1 Tbsp mayonnaise, 2 Tbsp salad dressing	Soft margarine, vegetable oil (such as canola, corn, olive, or safflower), low-fat mayonnaise, light salad dressing	The DASH study had 27% of calories as fat, including fat in or added to foods
Sweets and added sugars	0 5 or less per week	1 Tbsp sugar, 1 Tbsp jelly or jam, 1/2 cup sorbet or gelatin, 1 cup lemonade	Fruit-flavored gelatin, fruit punch, hard candy, jelly, maple syrup, sorbet and ices, sugar	Sweets should be low in fat

‡ Since eggs are high in cholesterol, limit egg yolk intake to no more than four per week; two egg whites have the same protein content as one ounce of meat.

§ Fat content changes serving amount for fats and oils. For example, 1 tablespoon of regular salad dressing equals one serving; 1 tablespoon of a low-fat dressing equals one-half serving; 1 tablespoon of a fat-free dressing equals zero servings.

Chapter 46

Lactose Intolerance

What is lactose intolerance?

Lactose intolerance is the inability or insufficient ability to digest lactose, a sugar found in milk and milk products. Lactose intolerance is caused by a deficiency of the enzyme lactase, which is produced by the cells lining the small intestine. Lactase breaks down lactose into two simpler forms of sugar called glucose and galactose, which are then absorbed into the bloodstream.

Not all people with lactase deficiency have digestive symptoms, but those who do may have lactose intolerance. Most people with lactose intolerance can tolerate some amount of lactose in their diet.

People sometimes confuse lactose intolerance with cow milk allergy. Milk allergy is a reaction by the body's immune system to one or more milk proteins and can be life threatening when just a small amount of milk or milk product is consumed. Milk allergy most commonly appears in the first year of life, while lactose intolerance occurs more often in adulthood.

What causes lactose intolerance?

The cause of lactose intolerance is best explained by describing how a person develops lactase deficiency.

This chapter excerpted from "Lactose Intolerance," National Digestive Diseases Information Clearinghouse, National Institute of Diabetes and Digestive and Kidney Diseases (digestive.niddk.nih.gov), June 2009.

Primary lactase deficiency develops over time and begins after about age two when the body begins to produce less lactase. Most children who have lactase deficiency do not experience symptoms of lactose intolerance until late adolescence or adulthood.

Researchers have identified a possible genetic link to primary lactase deficiency. Some people inherit a gene from their parents that makes it likely they will develop primary lactase deficiency. This discovery may be useful in developing future genetic tests to identify people at risk for lactose intolerance.

Secondary lactase deficiency results from injury to the small intestine that occurs with severe diarrheal illness, celiac disease, Crohn disease, or chemotherapy. This type of lactase deficiency can occur at any age but is more common in infancy.

Who is at risk for lactose intolerance?

Lactose intolerance is a common condition that is more likely to occur in adulthood, with a higher incidence in older adults. Some ethnic and racial populations are more affected than others, including African Americans, Hispanic Americans, American Indians, and Asian Americans. The condition is least common among Americans of northern European descent.

Infants born prematurely are more likely to have lactase deficiency because an infant's lactase levels do not increase until the third trimester of pregnancy.

What are the symptoms of lactose intolerance?

People with lactose intolerance may feel uncomfortable 30 minutes to two hours after consuming milk and milk products. Symptoms range from mild to severe, based on the amount of lactose consumed and the amount a person can tolerate.

Common symptoms include the following:

- Abdominal pain
- Abdominal bloating
- Gas
- Diarrhea
- Nausea

How is lactose intolerance diagnosed?

Lactose intolerance can be hard to diagnose based on symptoms alone. People may think they suffer from lactose intolerance because they have digestive symptoms; however, other conditions such as irritable bowel syndrome can cause similar symptoms. After taking a medical history and performing a physical examination, the doctor may first recommend eliminating all milk and milk products from the person's diet for a short time to see if the symptoms resolve. Tests may be necessary to provide more information.

Two tests are commonly used to measure the digestion of lactose.

Hydrogen breath test: The person drinks a lactose-loaded beverage and then the breath is analyzed at regular intervals to measure the amount of hydrogen. Normally, very little hydrogen is detectable in the breath, but undigested lactose produces high levels of hydrogen. Smoking and some foods and medications may affect the accuracy of the results. People should check with their doctor about foods and medications that may interfere with test results.

Stool acidity test: The stool acidity test is used for infants and young children to measure the amount of acid in the stool. Undigested lactose creates lactic acid and other fatty acids that can be detected in a stool sample. Glucose may also be present in the stool as a result of undigested lactose.

Because lactose intolerance is uncommon in infants and children younger than two, a health professional should take special care in determining the cause of a child's digestive symptoms.

How is lactose intolerance managed?

Although the body's ability to produce lactase cannot be changed, the symptoms of lactose intolerance can be managed with dietary changes. Most people with lactose intolerance can tolerate some amount of lactose in their diet. Gradually introducing small amounts of milk or milk products may help some people adapt to them with fewer symptoms. Often, people can better tolerate milk or milk products by taking them with meals.

The amount of change needed in the diet depends on how much lactose a person can consume without symptoms. For example, one person may have severe symptoms after drinking a small glass of milk, while another can drink a large glass without symptoms. Others can easily consume yogurt and hard cheeses such as cheddar and Swiss but not milk or other milk products.

The 2005 Dietary Guidelines for Americans recommend that people with lactose intolerance choose milk products with lower levels of lactose than regular milk, such as yogurt and hard cheese.

Lactose-free and lactose-reduced milk and milk products, available at most supermarkets, are identical to regular milk except that the lactase enzyme has been added. Lactose-free milk remains fresh for about the same length of time or longer than regular milk if it is ultra-pasteurized. Lactose-free milk may have a slightly sweeter taste than regular milk. Soy milk and other products may be recommended by a health professional.

People who still experience symptoms after dietary changes can take over-the-counter lactase enzyme drops or tablets. Taking the tablets or a few drops of the liquid enzyme when consuming milk or milk products may make these foods more tolerable for people with lactose intolerance.

Parents and caregivers of a child with lactose intolerance should follow the nutrition plan recommended by the child's doctor or dietitian.

Lactose intolerance and calcium intake: Milk and milk products are a major source of calcium and other nutrients. Calcium is essential for the growth and repair of bones at all ages. A shortage of calcium intake in children and adults may lead to fragile bones that can easily fracture later in life, a condition called osteoporosis. The amount of calcium a person needs to maintain good health varies by age. Recommendations are shown in Table 46.1.

Women who are pregnant or breastfeeding need between 1,000 and 1,300 mg of calcium daily.

Getting enough calcium is important for people with lactose intolerance when the intake of milk and milk products is limited. Many foods can provide calcium and other nutrients the body needs. Non-milk products that are high in calcium include fish with soft bones such as salmon and sardines and dark green vegetables such as spinach.

Table 46.2 lists foods that are good sources of dietary calcium.

Table 46.1. Recommended Calcium Intake by Age Group

Age Group	Amount of Calcium to Consume Daily in Milligrams (mg)
0–6 months	210 mg
7–12 months	270 mg
1–3 years	500 mg
4–8 years	800 mg
9–18 years	1,300 mg
19–50 years	1,000 mg
51–70+ years	1,200 mg

Source: Adapted from *Dietary Reference Intakes, 2004,* Institute of Medicine, National Academy of Sciences.

Table 46.2. Calcium Content in Common Foods

Non-Milk Products	Calcium Content
Rhubarb, frozen, cooked, 1 cup	348 mg
Sardines, with bone, 3 oz.	325 mg
Spinach, frozen, cooked, 1 cup	291 mg
Salmon, canned, with bone, 3 oz.	181 mg
Soy milk, unfortified, 1 cup	61 mg
Orange, 1 medium	52 mg
Broccoli, raw, 1 cup	41 mg
Pinto beans, cooked, 1/2 cup	40 mg
Lettuce greens, 1 cup	20 mg
Tuna, white, canned, 3 oz.	12 mg
Milk and Milk Products	**Calcium Content**
Yogurt, with active and live cultures, plain, low-fat, vitamin D–fortified, 1 cup	415 mg
Milk, reduced fat, vitamin D–fortified, 1 cup	285 mg
Swiss cheese, 1 oz.	224 mg
Cottage cheese, 1/2 cup	87 mg
Ice cream, 1/2 cup	84 mg

Source: Adapted from U.S. Department of Agriculture, Agricultural Research Service. 2008. USDA National Nutrient Database for Standard Reference, Release 21.

Yogurt made with active and live bacterial cultures is a good source of calcium for many people with lactose intolerance. When this type of yogurt enters the intestine, the bacterial cultures convert lactose to lactic acid, so the yogurt may be well tolerated due to a lower lactose content than yogurt without live cultures. Frozen yogurt does not contain bacterial cultures, so it may not be well tolerated.

Calcium is absorbed and used in the body only when enough vitamin D is present. Some people with lactose intolerance may not be getting enough vitamin D. Vitamin D comes from food sources such as eggs, liver, and vitamin D–fortified milk and yogurt. Regular exposure to sunlight also helps the body naturally absorb vitamin D. Talking with a doctor or registered dietitian may be helpful in planning a balanced diet that provides an adequate amount of nutrients—including calcium and vitamin D—and minimizes discomfort. A health professional can determine whether calcium and other dietary supplements are needed.

What other products contain lactose?

Milk and milk products are often added to processed foods—foods that have been altered to prolong their shelf life. People with lactose intolerance should be aware of the many food products that may contain even small amounts of lactose, such as the following:

- Bread and other baked goods
- Waffles, pancakes, biscuits, cookies, and mixes to make them
- Processed breakfast foods such as doughnuts, frozen waffles and pancakes, toaster pastries, and sweet rolls
- Processed breakfast cereals
- Instant potatoes, soups, and breakfast drinks
- Potato chips, corn chips, and other processed snacks
- Processed meats, such as bacon, sausage, hot dogs, and lunch meats
- Margarine
- Salad dressings
- Liquid and powdered milk-based meal replacements
- Protein powders and bars
- Candies
- Nondairy liquid and powdered coffee creamers
- Nondairy whipped toppings

Checking the ingredients on food labels is helpful in finding possible sources of lactose in food products. If any of the following words are listed on a food label, the product contains lactose:

- Milk
- Lactose
- Whey
- Curds
- Milk by-products
- Dry milk solids
- Nonfat dry milk powder

Lactose is also used in some prescription medicines, including birth control pills, and over-the-counter medicines like products to treat stomach acid and gas. These medicines most often cause symptoms in people with severe lactose intolerance.

Chapter 47

Food Allergies

Chapter Contents

Section 47.1

About Food Allergies

This section excerpted from "Food Allergy," National Institute of Allergy and Infectious Diseases (www.niaid.nih.gov), November 2010.

What Is Food Allergy?

Food allergy is an abnormal response to a food, triggered by the body's immune system. There are several types of immune responses to food. This chapter focuses on one type of adverse reaction to food, in which the body produces a specific type of antibody, called immunoglobulin E (IgE).

The binding of IgE antibodies to specific molecules in a food triggers the immune response. The response may be mild, or in rare cases it can be associated with the severe and life-threatening reaction called anaphylaxis.

If you have a food allergy, it is extremely important for you to work with your health care professional to learn what foods cause your allergic reaction.

Sometimes, a reaction to food is not an allergy at all but another type of reaction called food intolerance.

What Is an Allergic Reaction to Food?

A food allergy occurs when the immune system responds to a harmless food as if it were a threat. The first time a person with food allergy is exposed to the food, no symptoms occur. But the body has been primed, and when the person eats the food again, an allergic response occurs.

An allergic reaction to food usually takes place within a few minutes to several hours after exposure to the allergen. The process of eating and digesting food and the location of immune cells involved in the allergic reaction process both affect the timing and location of the reaction.

Allergic Reaction Process

Step 1: The first time you are exposed to a food allergen, your immune system makes specific IgE antibodies to that allergen. IgE antibodies circulate through your blood and attach to types of immune cells called mast cells and basophils. Mast cells are found in all body tissues, especially in your nose, throat, lungs, skin, and gastrointestinal (GI) tract. Basophils are found in your blood and also in tissues that have become inflamed because of an allergic reaction.

Step 2: The next time you are exposed to the same food allergen, the allergen binds to the IgE antibodies that are attached to the mast cells and basophils. The binding signals the cells to release massive amounts of chemicals such as histamine.

Depending on the tissue in which they are released, these chemicals will cause you to have various symptoms of food allergy. The symptoms can range from mild to severe. A severe allergic reaction can include a potentially life-threatening reaction called anaphylaxis.

Generally, you are at greater risk for developing a food allergy if you come from a family in which allergies—including food allergies and other allergic diseases such as asthma or eczema—are common. Having two parents who have allergies makes you more likely to develop food allergy than someone with one parent who has allergies.

Symptoms of Food Allergy

If you are allergic to a particular food, you may experience some or all of the following symptoms:

- Itching in your mouth or swelling
- GI symptoms, such as vomiting, diarrhea, or abdominal cramps and pain
- Hives or eczema
- Tightening of the throat and trouble breathing
- Drop in blood pressure

Cross-Reactive Food Allergies

If you have a life-threatening reaction to a certain food, your health care professional will show you how to avoid similar foods that may trigger this reaction. For example, if you have a history of allergy to shrimp, allergy testing may show that you are also allergic to other shellfish, such as crab, lobster, and crayfish. This is called cross-reactivity.

Eosinophilic Esophagitis and Food Allergy

Eosinophilic esophagitis (EoE) is a newly recognized chronic disease that can be associated with food allergies. It is increasingly being diagnosed in children and adults. EoE is characterized by inflammation and accumulation of a specific type of immune cell, called an eosinophil, in the esophagus.

Symptoms of EoE include nausea, vomiting, and abdominal pain after eating. A person may also have symptoms that resemble acid reflux from the stomach. In older children and adults, it can cause more severe symptoms, such as difficulty swallowing solid food or solid food sticking in the esophagus for more than a few minutes. In infants, this disease may be associated with failure to thrive.

If you are diagnosed with EoE, you will probably be tested for allergies. In some situations, avoiding certain food allergens will be an effective treatment for EoE.

Oral Allergy Syndrome

Oral allergy syndrome (OAS) is an allergy to certain raw fruits and vegetables, such as apples, cherries, kiwis, celery, tomatoes, and green peppers. OAS occurs mostly in people with hay fever, especially spring hay fever due to birch pollen and late summer hay fever due to ragweed pollen.

Eating the raw food causes an itchy, tingling sensation in the mouth, lips, and throat. It can also cause swelling of the lips, tongue, and throat; watery, itchy eyes; runny nose; and sneezing. Just handling the raw fruit or vegetable may cause a rash, itching, or swelling where the juice touches the skin.

Cooking or processing easily breaks down the proteins in the fruits and vegetables that cause OAS. Therefore, OAS typically does not occur with cooked or baked fruits and vegetables or processed fruits, such as applesauce.

Exercise-Induced Food Allergy

Exercise-induced food allergy requires more than simply eating food to start a reaction. This type of reaction occurs after someone eats a specific food before exercising. As exercise increases and body temperature rises, itching and light-headedness start, hives may appear, and even anaphylaxis may develop. Some people have this reaction from many foods, and others have it only after eating a specific food.

Treating exercised-induced food allergy is simple—avoid eating for a couple of hours before exercising.

Crustacean shellfish, alcohol, tomatoes, cheese, and celery are common causes of exercise-induced food allergy reactions.

What Is Anaphylaxis?

If you have a food allergy, there is a chance that you may experience a severe form of allergic reaction known as anaphylaxis. Anaphylaxis may begin suddenly and may lead to death if not immediately treated.

Anaphylaxis includes a wide range of symptoms that can occur in many combinations. Some symptoms are not life threatening, but the most severe restrict breathing and blood circulation. Many different parts of your body can be affected:

- **Skin:** Itching, hives, redness, swelling
- **Nose:** Sneezing, stuffy nose, runny nose
- **Mouth:** Itching, swelling of lips or tongue
- **Throat:** Itching, tightness, difficulty swallowing, hoarseness
- **Chest:** Shortness of breath, cough, wheeze, chest pain, tightness
- **Heart:** Weak pulse, passing out, shock
- **GI tract:** Vomiting, diarrhea, cramps
- **Nervous system:** Dizziness or fainting

How soon after exposure will symptoms occur?

Symptoms may begin within several minutes to several hours after exposure to the food. Sometimes the symptoms go away, only to return two to four hours later or even as many as eight hours later. When you begin to experience symptoms, seek immediate medical attention because anaphylaxis can be life threatening.

Can anaphylaxis be predicted?

Anaphylaxis caused by an allergic reaction to a certain food is highly unpredictable. The severity of a given attack does not predict the severity of subsequent attacks. The response will vary depending on several factors, such as the following:

- Your sensitivity to the food
- How much of the food you are exposed to
- How the food entered your body

Any anaphylactic reaction may become dangerous and must be evaluated immediately by a health care professional.

How do you know if a person is having an anaphylactic reaction?

Anaphylaxis is highly likely if at least one of the following three conditions occurs:

1. Within minutes or several hours of the onset of an illness, a person has skin symptoms (redness, itching, hives) or swollen lips and either difficulty breathing or a drop in blood pressure.

2. A person was exposed to an allergen likely to cause an allergic reaction and, within minutes or several hours, two or more of the following symptoms occur:

    -   Skin symptoms or swollen lips
    -   Difficulty breathing
    -   A drop in blood pressure
    -   GI symptoms such as vomiting, diarrhea, or cramping

3. A person exposed to an allergen that is previously known to cause an allergic reaction in that person experiences a drop in blood pressure.

Common Food Allergies in Infants, Children, and Adults

In infants and children, the most common foods that cause allergic reactions are the following:

-   Egg
-   Milk
-   Peanut
-   Tree nuts such as walnuts
-   Soy (primarily in infants)
-   Wheat

In adults, the most common foods that cause allergic reactions are the following:

-   Shellfish such as shrimp, crayfish, lobster, and crab
-   Peanut
-   Tree nuts
-   Fish such as salmon

Food allergies generally develop early in life but can develop at any age. Children usually outgrow their egg, milk, and soy allergies, but people who develop allergies as adults usually have their allergies for life. Children generally do not outgrow their allergy to peanut.

Foods that are eaten routinely increase the likelihood that a person will develop allergies to that food. In Japan, for example, rice allergy is more frequent than in the United States, and in Scandinavia, codfish allergy is more common than in the United States.

Is It Food Allergy or Food Intolerance?

Food allergy is sometimes confused with food intolerance.

Lactose Intolerance

Lactose is a sugar found in milk and most milk products. Lactase is an enzyme in the lining of the gut that breaks down or digests lactose. Lactose intolerance occurs when lactase is missing. Instead of the enzyme breaking down the sugar, bacteria in the gut break it down, which forms gas, which in turn causes symptoms of bloating, abdominal pain, and sometimes diarrhea.

Lactose intolerance is uncommon in babies and young children under the age of five years. Because lactase levels decline as people get older, lactose intolerance becomes more common with age. Lactose intolerance also varies widely based on racial and ethnic background.

Your health care professional can use laboratory tests to find out whether your body can digest lactose.

Food Additives

Another type of food intolerance is a reaction to certain products that are added to food to enhance taste, add color, or protect against the growth of microbes. Compounds such as monosodium glutamate (MSG) and sulfites are tied to reactions that can be confused with food allergy.

MSG is a flavor enhancer. When taken in large amounts, it can cause some of the following:

- Flushing
- Sensations of warmth
- Headache
- Chest discomfort

These passing reactions occur rapidly after eating large amounts of food to which MSG has been added.

Sulfites are found in food for several reasons:

- They have been added to increase crispness or prevent mold growth.
- They occur naturally in the food.
- They have been generated during the wine-making process.

Sulfites can cause breathing problems in people with asthma.
The Food and Drug Administration (FDA) has banned sulfites as spray-on preservatives for fresh fruits and vegetables. When sulfites are present in foods, they are listed on ingredient labels.

Gluten Intolerance

Gluten is a part of wheat, barley, and rye. Gluten intolerance is associated with celiac disease. This disease develops when the immune system responds abnormally to gluten. This abnormal response does not involve IgE antibody and is not considered a food allergy.

Food Poisoning

Some of the symptoms of food allergy, such as abdominal cramping, are common to food poisoning. However, food poisoning is caused by microbes, such as bacteria, and bacterial products, such as toxins, that can contaminate meats and dairy products.

Histamine Toxicity

Fish, such as tuna and mackerel that are not refrigerated properly and become contaminated by bacteria, may contain very high levels of histamine. A person who eats such fish may show symptoms that are similar to food allergy. However, this reaction is not a true allergic reaction. Instead, the reaction is called histamine toxicity or scombroid food poisoning.

Other Conditions

Several other conditions, such as ulcers and cancers of the GI tract, cause some of the same symptoms as food allergy. These symptoms, which include vomiting, diarrhea, and cramping abdominal pain, become worse when you eat.

Diagnosis

Detailed History

Your health care professional will begin by taking a detailed medical history to find out if your symptoms are caused by an allergy to specific foods, food intolerance, or other health problems.

A detailed history is the most valuable tool used for diagnosing food allergy. Your health care professional will ask you several questions, including the following:

- Did your reaction come on quickly, usually within several minutes after eating the food?
- Is your reaction always associated with a certain food?
- How much of this potentially allergenic food did you eat before you had a reaction?
- Have you eaten this food before and had a reaction?
- Did anyone else who ate the same food get sick?
- Did you take allergy medicines, and if so, did they help? (Antihistamines should relieve hives, for example.)

Diet Diary

Sometimes your health care professional cannot make a diagnosis based only on your history. You may be asked to keep a diet diary containing details about the foods you eat and whether you have a reaction. Based on the diary record, you and your health care professional may be able to identify a consistent pattern in your reactions.

Elimination Diet

The next step some health care professionals use is a limited elimination diet, in which the food that is suspected of causing an allergic reaction is removed from your diet to see whether that stops your allergic reactions. For example, if you suspect you are allergic to egg, your health care professional will instruct you to eliminate egg from your diet. The limited elimination diet is done under the direction of your health care professional.

Skin Prick Test

If your history, diet diary, or elimination diet suggests a specific food allergy is likely, then your health care professional will use the skin prick test to confirm the diagnosis.

With a skin prick test, your health care professional uses a needle to place a tiny amount of food extract just below the surface of the skin on your lower arm or back. If you are allergic, there will be swelling or redness at the test site. This is a positive result. It means that there are IgE molecules on the skin's mast cells that are specific to the food being tested.

The skin prick test is simple and relatively safe, and results are ready in minutes.

You can have a positive skin test to a food, however, without having an allergic reaction to that food. A health care professional often makes a diagnosis of food allergy when someone has both a positive skin test to a specific food and a history of reactions that suggests an allergy to the same food.

Blood Test

Instead of the skin prick test, your health care professional can take a blood sample to measure the levels of food-specific IgE antibodies.

As with skin testing, positive blood tests do not necessarily mean that you have a food allergy. Your health care professionals must combine these test results with information about your history of reactions to food to make an accurate diagnosis of food allergy.

Oral Food Challenge

Because oral food challenges can cause a severe allergic reaction, they should always be conducted by a health care professional who has experience performing them.

An oral food challenge is the final method health care professionals use to diagnose food allergy. This method includes the following steps:

- Your health care professional gives you individual doses of various foods (masked so that you do not know what food is present), some of which are suspected of starting an allergic reaction.

    - Initially, the dose of food is very small, but the amount is gradually increased during the challenge.

- You swallow the individual dose.

- Your health care professional watches you to see if a reaction occurs.

To prevent bias, oral food challenges are often double blinded. In a true double-blind challenge, neither you nor your health care professional knows whether the substance you eat contains the likely allergen. Another medical professional has made up the individual doses. In a single-blind challenge, your health care professional knows what you are eating but you do not.

A reaction only to suspected foods and not to the other foods tested confirms the diagnosis of a food allergy.

Preventing and Treating Food Allergy

There is currently no cure for food allergies, and the available treatments only ease the symptoms of a food-induced allergic reaction.

Preventing a Food Allergy Reaction

You can only prevent the symptoms of food allergy by avoiding the allergenic food. After you and your health care professional have identified the food(s) to which you are sensitive, you must remove them from your diet.

Read labels: Read the list of ingredients on the label of each prepared food that you are considering eating. Many allergens, such as peanut, egg, and milk, may appear in prepared foods you normally would not associate them with.

Since 2006, U.S. food manufacturers have been required by law to list the ingredients of prepared foods. In addition, food manufacturers must use plain language to disclose whether their products contain (or may contain) any of the top eight allergenic foods—egg, milk, peanut, tree nuts, soy, wheat, shellfish, and fish.

Keep clean: Simple measures of cleanliness can remove most allergens from the environment of a person with food allergy. For example, simply washing your hands with soap and water will remove peanut allergens, and most household cleaners will remove allergens from surfaces.

Treating a Food Allergy Reaction

Unintentional exposure: When you have food allergies, you must be prepared to treat an unintentional exposure. Talk to your health care professional and develop a plan to protect yourself in case of an unintentional exposure to the food. For example, you should take the following steps:

- Wear a medical alert bracelet or necklace

- Carry an auto-injector device containing epinephrine (adrenaline)

563

• Seek medical help immediately

Mild symptoms: Talk to your health care professional to find out what medicines may relieve mild food allergy symptoms that are not part of an anaphylactic reaction. However, be aware that it is very hard for you to know which reactions are mild and which may lead to anaphylaxis.

Section 47.2

Reading Food Labels for Allergen Content

This section excerpted from "Food Allergies: What You Need to Know," U.S. Food and Drug Administration (www.fda.gov), June 2010.

Each year, millions of Americans have allergic reactions to food. Although most food allergies cause relatively mild and minor symptoms, some food allergies can cause severe reactions, and may even be life-threatening.

There is no cure for food allergies. Strict avoidance of food allergens—and early recognition and management of allergic reactions to food—are important measures to prevent serious health consequences.

FDA's Role: Labeling

To help Americans avoid the health risks posed by food allergens, Congress passed the Food Allergen Labeling and Consumer Protection Act of 2004 (FALCPA). The law applies to all foods whose labeling is regulated by FDA, both domestic and imported. (FDA regulates the labeling of all foods, except for poultry, most meats, certain egg products, and most alcoholic beverages.)

• Before FALCPA, the labels of foods made from two or more ingredients were required to list all ingredients by their common or usual names. The names of some ingredients, however, do not clearly identify their food source.

- Now, the law requires that labels must clearly identify the food source names of all ingredients that are—or contain any protein derived from—the eight most common food allergens, which FALCPA defines as "major food allergens."

As a result, food labels help allergic consumers to identify offending foods or ingredients so they can more easily avoid them.

What Are Major Food Allergens?

While more than 160 foods can cause allergic reactions in people with food allergies, the law identifies the eight most common allergenic foods. These foods account for 90% of food allergic reactions and are the food sources from which many other ingredients are derived.

The eight foods identified by the law are the following:

1. Milk
2. Eggs
3. Fish (e.g., bass, flounder, cod)
4. Crustacean shellfish (e.g. crab, lobster, shrimp)
5. Tree nuts (e.g., almonds, walnuts, pecans)
6. Peanuts
7. Wheat
8. Soybeans

These eight foods, and any ingredient that contains protein derived from one or more of them, are designated as "major food allergens" by FALCPA.

How Major Food Allergens Are Listed

The law requires that food labels identify the food source names of all major food allergens used to make the food. This requirement is met if the common or usual name of an ingredient (e.g., buttermilk) that is a major food allergen already identifies that allergen's food source name (i.e., milk). Otherwise, the allergen's food source name must be declared at least once on the food label in one of two ways.

The name of the food source of a major food allergen must appear in one of the following two ways:

1. In parentheses following the name of the ingredient (examples: "lecithin (soy)," "flour (wheat)," and "whey (milk)").

2. Immediately after or next to the list of ingredients in a "contains" statement (example: "Contains Wheat, Milk, and Soy.").

Food Allergies: What to Do If Symptoms Occur

The appearance of symptoms after eating food may be a sign of a food allergy. The food(s) that caused these symptoms should be avoided, and the affected person should contact a doctor or health care provider for appropriate testing and evaluation.

- Persons found to have a food allergy should be taught to read labels and avoid the offending foods. They should also be taught, in case of accidental ingestion, to recognize the early symptoms of an allergic reaction, and be properly educated on—and armed with—appropriate treatment measures.

- Persons with a known food allergy who begin experiencing symptoms while, or after, eating a food should initiate treatment immediately and go to a nearby emergency room if symptoms progress.

About Other Allergens

Persons may still be allergic to—and have serious reactions to—foods other than the eight foods identified by the law. So, always be sure to read the food label's ingredient list carefully to avoid the food allergens in question.

Food Allergen "Advisory" Labeling

FALCPA's labeling requirements do not apply to the potential or unintentional presence of major food allergens in foods resulting from "cross-contact" situations during manufacturing, e.g., because of shared equipment or processing lines. In the context of food allergens, "cross-contact" occurs when a residue or trace amount of an allergenic food becomes incorporated into another food not intended to contain it. FDA guidance for the food industry states that food allergen advisory statements, e.g., "may contain [allergen]" or "produced in a facility that also uses [allergen]," should not be used as a substitute for adhering to current good manufacturing practices and must be truthful and not misleading. FDA is considering ways to best manage the use of these types of statements by manufacturers to better inform consumers.

Chapter 48

Celiac Disease and a Gluten-Free Diet

What is celiac disease?

Celiac disease is a digestive disease that damages the small intestine and interferes with absorption of nutrients from food. People who have celiac disease cannot tolerate gluten, a protein in wheat, rye, and barley. Gluten is found mainly in foods but may also be found in everyday products such as medicines, vitamins, and lip balms.

When people with celiac disease eat foods or use products containing gluten, their immune system responds by damaging or destroying villi—the tiny, fingerlike protrusions lining the small intestine. Villi normally allow nutrients from food to be absorbed through the walls of the small intestine into the bloodstream. Without healthy villi, a person becomes malnourished, no matter how much food one eats.

Celiac disease is both a disease of malabsorption—meaning nutrients are not absorbed properly—and an abnormal immune reaction to gluten. Celiac disease is also known as celiac sprue, nontropical sprue, and gluten-sensitive enteropathy. Celiac disease is genetic, meaning it runs in families. Sometimes the disease is triggered—or becomes active for the first time—after surgery, pregnancy, childbirth, viral infection, or severe emotional stress.

"Celiac Disease," National Digestive Diseases Information Clearinghouse, National Institute of Diabetes and Digestive and Kidney Diseases (digestive. niddk.nih.gov), September 2008.

What are the symptoms of celiac disease?

Symptoms of celiac disease vary from person to person. Symptoms may occur in the digestive system or in other parts of the body. Digestive symptoms are more common in infants and young children and may include the following:

• Abdominal bloating and pain

• Chronic diarrhea

• Vomiting

• Constipation

• Pale, foul-smelling, or fatty stool

• Weight loss

Irritability is another common symptom in children. Malabsorption of nutrients during the years when nutrition is critical to a child's normal growth and development can result in other problems such as failure to thrive in infants, delayed growth and short stature, delayed puberty, and dental enamel defects of the permanent teeth.

Adults are less likely to have digestive symptoms and may instead have one or more of the following:

• Unexplained iron-deficiency anemia

• Fatigue

• Bone or joint pain

• Arthritis

• Bone loss or osteoporosis

• Depression or anxiety

• Tingling numbness in the hands and feet

• Seizures

• Missed menstrual periods

• Infertility or recurrent miscarriage

• Canker sores inside the mouth

• An itchy skin rash called dermatitis herpetiformis

People with celiac disease may have no symptoms but can still develop complications of the disease over time. Long-term complications include malnutrition—which can lead to anemia, osteoporosis, and miscarriage, among other problems—liver diseases, and cancers of the intestine.

Why are celiac disease symptoms so varied?

Researchers are studying the reasons celiac disease affects people differently. The length of time a person was breast-fed, the age a person started eating gluten-containing foods, and the amount of gluten-containing foods one eats are three factors thought to play a role in when and how celiac disease appears. Some studies have shown, for example, that the longer a person was breast-fed, the later the symptoms of celiac disease appear.

Symptoms also vary depending on a person's age and the degree of damage to the small intestine. Many adults have the disease for a decade or more before they are diagnosed. The longer a person goes undiagnosed and untreated, the greater the chance of developing long-term complications.

What other health problems do people with celiac disease have?

People with celiac disease tend to have other diseases in which the immune system attacks the body's healthy cells and tissues. The connection between celiac disease and these diseases may be genetic. They include the following:

- Type 1 diabetes
- Autoimmune thyroid disease
- Autoimmune liver disease
- Rheumatoid arthritis
- Addison disease, a condition in which the glands that produce critical hormones are damaged
- Sjögren syndrome, a condition in which the glands that produce tears and saliva are destroyed

How common is celiac disease?

Celiac disease affects people in all parts of the world. Originally thought to be a rare childhood syndrome, celiac disease is now known to be a common genetic disorder. More than 2 million people in the United States have the disease, or about 1 in 133 people. Among people who have a first-degree relative—a parent, sibling, or child—diagnosed with celiac disease, as many as 1 in 22 people may have the disease.

Celiac disease is also more common among people with other genetic disorders including Down syndrome and Turner syndrome, a condition that affects girls' development.

How is celiac disease diagnosed?

Recognizing celiac disease can be difficult because some of its symptoms are similar to those of other diseases. Celiac disease can be confused with irritable bowel syndrome, iron-deficiency anemia caused by menstrual blood loss, inflammatory bowel disease, diverticulitis, intestinal infections, and chronic fatigue syndrome. As a result, celiac disease has long been underdiagnosed or misdiagnosed. As doctors become more aware of the many varied symptoms of the disease and reliable blood tests become more available, diagnosis rates are increasing.

Blood tests: People with celiac disease have higher than normal levels of certain autoantibodies—proteins that react against the body's own cells or tissues—in their blood. To diagnose celiac disease, doctors will test blood for high levels of anti-tissue transglutaminase antibodies (tTGA) or anti-endomysium antibodies (EMA). If test results are negative but celiac disease is still suspected, additional blood tests may be needed.

Before being tested, one should continue to eat a diet that includes foods with gluten, such as breads and pastas. If a person stops eating foods with gluten before being tested, the results may be negative for celiac disease even if the disease is present.

Intestinal biopsy: If blood tests and symptoms suggest celiac disease, a biopsy of the small intestine is performed to confirm the diagnosis. During the biopsy, the doctor removes tiny pieces of tissue from the small intestine to check for damage to the villi. To obtain the tissue sample, the doctor eases a long, thin tube called an endoscope through the patient's mouth and stomach into the small intestine. The doctor then takes the samples using instruments passed through the endoscope.

Dermatitis herpetiformis: Dermatitis herpetiformis (DH) is an intensely itchy, blistering skin rash that affects 15% to 25% of people with celiac disease. The rash usually occurs on the elbows, knees, and buttocks. Most people with DH have no digestive symptoms of celiac disease.

DH is diagnosed through blood tests and a skin biopsy. If the antibody tests are positive and the skin biopsy has the typical findings of DH, patients do not need to have an intestinal biopsy. Both the skin disease and the intestinal disease respond to a gluten-free diet and recur if gluten is added back into the diet. The rash symptoms can be controlled with antibiotics such as dapsone. Because dapsone does not treat the intestinal condition, people with DH must maintain a gluten-free diet.

Screening: Screening for celiac disease means testing for the presence of autoantibodies in the blood in people without symptoms. Americans are not routinely screened for celiac disease. However, because celiac disease is hereditary, family members of a person with the disease may wish to be tested: 4% to 12% of an affected person's first-degree relatives will also have the disease.

How is celiac disease treated?

The only treatment for celiac disease is a gluten-free diet. Doctors may ask a newly diagnosed person to work with a dietitian on a gluten-free diet plan. A dietitian is a health care professional who specializes in food and nutrition. Someone with celiac disease can learn from a dietitian how to read ingredient lists and identify foods that contain gluten in order to make informed decisions at the grocery store and when eating out.

For most people, following this diet will stop symptoms, heal existing intestinal damage, and prevent further damage. Improvement begins within days of starting the diet. The small intestine usually heals in three to six months in children but may take several years in adults. A healed intestine means a person now has villi that can absorb nutrients from food into the bloodstream.

To stay well, people with celiac disease must avoid gluten for the rest of their lives. Eating even a small amount of gluten can damage the small intestine. The damage will occur in anyone with the disease, including people without noticeable symptoms. Depending on a person's age at diagnosis, some problems will not improve, such as short stature and dental enamel defects.

Some people with celiac disease show no improvement on the gluten-free diet. The most common reason for poor response to the diet is that small amounts of gluten are still being consumed. Hidden sources of gluten include additives such as modified food starch, preservatives, and stabilizers made with wheat. And because many corn and rice products are produced in factories that also manufacture wheat products, they can be contaminated with wheat gluten.

Rarely, the intestinal injury will continue despite a strictly gluten-free diet. People with this condition, known as refractory celiac disease, have severely damaged intestines that cannot heal. Because their intestines are not absorbing enough nutrients, they may need to receive nutrients directly into their bloodstream through a vein or intravenously. Researchers are evaluating drug treatments for refractory celiac disease.

The gluten-free diet: A gluten-free diet means not eating foods that contain wheat, rye, and barley. The foods and products made from these grains should also be avoided. In other words, a person with celiac disease should not eat most grain, pasta, cereal, and many processed foods.

Despite these restrictions, people with celiac disease can eat a well-balanced diet with a variety of foods. They can use potato, rice, soy, amaranth, quinoa, buckwheat, or bean flour instead of wheat flour. They can buy gluten-free bread, pasta, and other products from stores that carry organic foods or order products from special food companies. Gluten-free products are increasingly available from mainstream stores.

"Plain" meat, fish, rice, fruits, and vegetables do not contain gluten, so people with celiac disease can freely eat these foods. In the past, people with celiac disease were advised not to eat oats. New evidence suggests that most people can safely eat small amounts of oats, as long as the oats are not contaminated with wheat gluten during processing. People with celiac disease should work closely with their health care team when deciding whether to include oats in their diet.

The gluten-free diet requires a completely new approach to eating. Newly diagnosed people and their families may find support groups helpful as they learn to adjust to a new way of life. People with celiac disease must be cautious about what they buy for lunch at school or work, what they purchase at the grocery store, what they eat at restaurants or parties, and what they grab for a snack. Eating out can be a challenge. When in doubt about a menu item, a person with celiac disease should ask the waiter or chef about ingredients and preparation or if a gluten-free menu is available.

Gluten is also used in some medications. People with celiac disease should ask a pharmacist if prescribed medications contain wheat. Because gluten is sometimes used as an additive in unexpected products—such as lipstick and play dough—reading product labels is important. If the ingredients are not listed on the label, the manufacturer should provide a list upon request. With practice, screening for gluten becomes second nature.

New food labeling: The Food Allergen Labeling and Consumer Protection Act (FALCPA), which took effect on January 1, 2006, requires food labels to clearly identify wheat and other common food allergens in the list of ingredients. FALCPA also requires the U.S. Food and Drug Administration to develop and finalize rules for the use of the term "gluten free" on product labels.

What are some examples of the gluten-free diet?

In 2006, the American Dietetic Association updated its recommendations for a gluten-free diet. The following are based on the 2006 recommendations. This list is not complete, so people with celiac disease should discuss gluten-free food choices with a dietitian or physician who specializes in celiac disease. People with celiac disease should always read food ingredient lists carefully to make sure the food does not contain gluten.

Allowed foods

- Amaranth
- Cassava
- Indian rice grass
- Millet
- Quinoa
- Seeds
- Tapioca
- Yucca

- Arrowroot
- Corn
- Job's tears
- Nuts
- Rice
- Sorghum
- Teff

- Buckwheat
- Flax
- Legumes
- Potatoes
- Sago
- Soy
- Wild rice

Foods to avoid

- Wheat, including einkorn, emmer, spelt, kamut
- Wheat starch, wheat bran, wheat germ, cracked wheat, hydrolyzed wheat protein
- Barley
- Rye
- Triticale (a cross between wheat and rye)

Other wheat products to avoid

- Bromated flour
- Enriched flour
- Graham flour
- Plain flour
- Semolina

- Durum flour
- Farina
- Phosphated flour
- Self-rising flour
- White flour

Processed foods that may contain wheat, barley, or rye*

- Bouillon cubes
- Candy
- Cold cuts, hot dogs, salami, sausage
- French fries
- Imitation fish
- Rice mixes
- Seasoned tortilla chips
- Soups
- Vegetables in sauce
- Brown rice syrup
- Chips/potato chips
- Communion wafers
- Gravy
- Matzo
- Sauces
- Self-basting turkey
- Soy sauce

* Most of these foods can be found gluten free. When in doubt, check with the food manufacturer.

Source: Thompson T. *Celiac Disease Nutrition Guide,* 2nd ed. Chicago: American Dietetic Association; 2006. © American Dietetic Association. Adapted with permission. For a complete copy of the *Celiac Disease Nutrition Guide,* please visit www.eatright.org.

Chapter 49

Eating Disorders

What Are Eating Disorders?

An eating disorder is marked by extremes. It is present when a person experiences severe disturbances in eating behavior, such as extreme reduction of food intake or extreme overeating, feelings of extreme distress, or concern about body weight or shape.

A person with an eating disorder may have started out just eating smaller or larger amounts of food than usual, but at some point, the urge to eat less or more spirals out of control. Eating disorders are very complex, and despite scientific research to understand them, the biological, behavioral, and social underpinnings of these illnesses remain elusive.

Eating disorders frequently appear during adolescence or young adulthood, but some reports indicate that they can develop during childhood or later in adulthood. Women and girls are much more likely than males to develop an eating disorder. Men and boys account for an estimated 5% to 15% of patients with anorexia or bulimia and an estimated 35% of those with binge-eating disorder. Eating disorders are real, treatable medical illnesses with complex underlying psychological and biological causes. They frequently coexist with other psychiatric disorders such as depression, substance abuse, or anxiety disorders. People with eating disorders also can suffer from numerous other physical health complications, such as heart conditions or kidney failure, which can lead to death.

This chapter excerpted from "Eating Disorders," National Institute of Mental Health (www.nimh.nih.gov), August 24, 2010.

Eating Disorders Are Treatable Diseases

Psychological and medicinal treatments are effective for many eating disorders. However, in more chronic cases, specific treatments have not yet been identified.

In these cases, treatment plans often are tailored to the patient's individual needs that may include medical care and monitoring; medications; nutritional counseling; and individual, group, and/or family psychotherapy. Some patients may also need to be hospitalized to treat malnutrition or to gain weight, or for other reasons.

Anorexia Nervosa

Anorexia nervosa is characterized by emaciation, a relentless pursuit of thinness and unwillingness to maintain a normal or healthy weight, a distortion of body image and intense fear of gaining weight, a lack of menstruation among girls and women, and extremely disturbed eating behavior. Some people with anorexia lose weight by dieting and exercising excessively; others lose weight by self-induced vomiting or misusing laxatives, diuretics, or enemas.

Many people with anorexia see themselves as overweight, even when they are starved or are clearly malnourished. Eating, food, and weight control become obsessions. A person with anorexia typically weighs herself or himself repeatedly, portions food carefully, and eats only very small quantities of only certain foods. Some who have anorexia recover with treatment after only one episode. Others get well but have relapses. Still others have a more chronic form of anorexia, in which their health deteriorates over many years as they battle the illness.

According to some studies, people with anorexia are up to 10 times more likely to die as a result of their illness compared to those without the disorder. The most common complications that lead to death are cardiac arrest and electrolyte and fluid imbalances. Suicide also can result.

Many people with anorexia also have coexisting psychiatric and physical illnesses, including depression, anxiety, obsessive behavior, substance abuse, cardiovascular and neurological complications, and impaired physical development.

Other symptoms may develop over time, including the following:

- Thinning of the bones (osteopenia or osteoporosis)

- Brittle hair and nails

- Dry and yellowish skin

- Growth of fine hair over body (e.g., lanugo)

- Mild anemia, and muscle weakness and loss
- Severe constipation
- Low blood pressure, slowed breathing and pulse
- Drop in internal body temperature, causing a person to feel cold all the time
- Lethargy

Treating anorexia involves three components:

1. Restoring the person to a healthy weight

2. Treating the psychological issues related to the eating disorder

3. Reducing or eliminating behaviors or thoughts that lead to disordered eating, and preventing relapse

Some research suggests that the use of medications, such as antidepressants, antipsychotics, or mood stabilizers, may be modestly effective in treating patients with anorexia by helping to resolve mood and anxiety symptoms that often coexist with anorexia. Recent studies, however, have suggested that antidepressants may not be effective in preventing some patients with anorexia from relapsing. In addition, no medication has shown to be effective during the critical first phase of restoring a patient to healthy weight. Overall, it is unclear if and how medications can help patients conquer anorexia, but research is ongoing.

Different forms of psychotherapy, including individual, group, and family based, can help address the psychological reasons for the illness. Some studies suggest that family-based therapies in which parents assume responsibility for feeding their afflicted adolescent are the most effective in helping a person with anorexia gain weight and improve eating habits and moods.

Others have noted that a combined approach of medical attention and supportive psychotherapy designed specifically for anorexia patients is more effective than just psychotherapy. But the effectiveness of a treatment depends on the person involved and his or her situation. Unfortunately, no specific psychotherapy appears to be consistently effective for treating adults with anorexia. However, research into novel treatment and prevention approaches is showing some promise.

Bulimia Nervosa

Bulimia nervosa is characterized by recurrent and frequent episodes of eating unusually large amounts of food (e.g., binge eating) and feeling a lack of control over the eating. This binge eating is followed by a type of behavior that compensates for the binge, such as purging (e.g., vomiting, excessive use of laxatives or diuretics), fasting, and/or excessive exercise.

Unlike anorexia, people with bulimia can fall within the normal range for their age and weight. But like people with anorexia, they often fear gaining weight, want desperately to lose weight, and are intensely unhappy with their body size and shape. Usually, bulimic behavior is done secretly because it is often accompanied by feelings of disgust or shame. The binging and purging cycle usually repeats several times a week. Similar to anorexia, people with bulimia often have coexisting psychological illnesses, such as depression, anxiety, and/or substance abuse problems. Many physical conditions result from the purging aspect of the illness, including electrolyte imbalances, gastrointestinal problems, and oral and tooth-related problems.

Other symptoms include the following:

- Chronically inflamed and sore throat

- Swollen glands in the neck and below the jaw

- Worn tooth enamel and increasingly sensitive and decaying teeth as a result of exposure to stomach acids

- Gastroesophageal reflux disorder

- Intestinal distress and irritation from laxative abuse

- Kidney problems from diuretic abuse

- Severe dehydration from purging of fluids

As with anorexia, treatment for bulimia often involves a combination of options and depends on the needs of the individual.

To reduce or eliminate binge and purge behavior, a patient may undergo nutritional counseling and psychotherapy, especially cognitive behavioral therapy (CBT), or be prescribed medication. Some antidepressants, such as fluoxetine (Prozac), which is the only medication approved by the U.S. Food and Drug Administration for treating bulimia, may help patients who also have depression and/or anxiety. It also appears to help reduce binge eating and purging behavior, reduces the chance of relapse, and improves eating attitudes.

CBT that has been tailored to treat bulimia also has shown to be effective in changing binging and purging behavior and eating attitudes. Therapy may be individually oriented or group based.

Binge-Eating Disorder

Binge-eating disorder is characterized by recurrent binge-eating episodes during which a person feels a loss of control over his or her eating. Unlike bulimia, binge-eating episodes are not followed by purging, excessive exercise, or fasting. As a result, people with binge-eating disorder often are overweight or obese. They also experience guilt, shame, and/or distress about the binge eating, which can lead to more binge eating.

Obese people with binge-eating disorder often have coexisting psychological illnesses including anxiety, depression, and personality disorders. In addition, links between obesity and cardiovascular disease and hypertension are well documented.

Treatment options for binge-eating disorder are similar to those used to treat bulimia. Fluoxetine and other antidepressants may reduce binge-eating episodes and help alleviate depression in some patients.

Patients with binge-eating disorder also may be prescribed appetite suppressants. Psychotherapy, especially CBT, is also used to treat the underlying psychological issues associated with binge eating, in an individual or group environment.

How Are Men and Boys Affected?

Although eating disorders primarily affect women and girls, boys and men are also vulnerable. One in four preadolescent cases of anorexia occurs in boys, and binge-eating disorder affects females and males about equally.

Like females who have eating disorders, males with the illness have a warped sense of body image and often have muscle dysmorphia, a type of disorder that is characterized by an extreme concern with becoming more muscular. Some boys with the disorder want to lose weight, while others want to gain weight or "bulk up." Boys who think they are too small are at a greater risk for using steroids or other dangerous drugs to increase muscle mass.

Boys with eating disorders exhibit the same types of emotional, physical, and behavioral signs and symptoms as girls, but, for a variety of reasons, boys are less likely to be diagnosed with what is often considered a stereotypically "female" disorder.

How Are We Working to Better Understand and Treat Eating Disorders?

Researchers are unsure of the underlying causes and nature of eating disorders. Unlike a neurological disorder, which generally can be pinpointed to a specific lesion on the brain, an eating disorder likely involves abnormal activity distributed across brain systems. With increased recognition that mental disorders are brain disorders, more researchers are using tools from both modern neuroscience and modern psychology to better understand eating disorders.

One approach involves the study of the human genes. With the publication of the human genome sequence in 2003, mental health researchers are studying the various combinations of genes to determine if any DNA variations are associated with the risk of developing a mental disorder. Neuroimaging, such as the use of magnetic resonance imaging (MRI), may also lead to a better understanding of eating disorders.

Neuroimaging already is used to identify abnormal brain activity in patients with schizophrenia, obsessive-compulsive disorder, and depression. It may also help researchers better understand how people with eating disorders process information, regardless of whether they have recovered or are still in the throes of their illness.

Conducting behavioral or psychological research on eating disorders is even more complex and challenging. As a result, few studies of treatments for eating disorders have been conducted in the past. New studies currently underway, however, are aiming to remedy the lack of information available about treatment.

Researchers also are working to define the basic processes of the disorders, which should help identify better treatments. For example, is anorexia the result of skewed body image, self-esteem problems, obsessive thoughts, compulsive behavior, or a combination of these? Can it be predicted or identified as a risk factor before drastic weight loss occurs, and therefore avoided?

These and other questions may be answered in the future as scientists and doctors think of eating disorders as medical illnesses with certain biological causes. Researchers are studying behavioral questions, along with genetic and brain systems information, to understand risk factors, identify biological markers, and develop medications that can target specific pathways that control eating behavior. Finally, neuroimaging and genetic studies may also provide clues for how each person may respond to specific treatments.

Chapter 50

Cancer and Nutrition

Chapter Contents

Section 50.1

Nutrition and Cancer Prevention

"Nutrition and Cancer Prevention" by Ruth MacDonald, R.D., Ph.D. Reprinted with permission of the American College of Sports Medicine, ACSM Fit Society ® Page, Spring 2009, pp 1–2. © 2009 American College of Sports Medicine (www.acsm.org).

Cancer is a frightening disease that affects the lives of millions worldwide. Many of us know someone personally who has struggled with cancer or has lost a loved one to this disease—or have suffered from it ourselves.

The good news is that recent National Cancer Institute statistics show a reduction in the incidence of cancer in the United States. This may be due in part to earlier detection and better screening for cancers, or perhaps it reflects a reduction in the number of people who smoke cigarettes. Cancer is a complex disease that can occur in almost all types of cells in our body, and there is no single cause of cancer. Some factors, such as cigarette smoking, have clear links to cancer. Other strongly linked factors include exposure to radiation (including sunlight) and environmental chemicals and pollutants. For centuries, foods have been linked to cancer, in both promotion and protective capacities. More recently, we are learning that physical activity and maintaining a healthy weight are also closely linked to reducing cancer risk.

All foods, from fruits and vegetables to processed cheese and cookies, are complex mixtures of many chemicals. Foods contain known nutrients like carbohydrates, fats, proteins, vitamins and minerals; but also thousands of other chemicals such as polyphenols, tannins, catechins, sterols, and flavonols. Hence, to understand the role of foods in cancer, we must understand the chemical composition of foods and the roles of these specific chemicals in the cancer process. This is a daunting task and one that may never be fully completed because of the number of chemicals and the multitude of possible interactions in a normal diet.

There are several ways to study the associations between foods and cancer. One way is to compare cancer incidence in populations with the foods they consume. This type of epidemiological study provides correlations but cannot prove cause and effect, but it does allow scientists to identify which dietary factors may be most important for further study. Over the past 50 years, many studies have been conducted to clarify the role of foods and ingredients in cancer. Some of these have been popularized in the lay press and have been promoted in the grocery store. For example, higher intakes of dietary fiber were correlated with lower risk of colon cancer. As a result of this finding, food manufacturers rushed to increase the fiber content of foods and promoted high fiber diets to reduce colon cancer risk. Subsequent large human clinical trials, however, have been ambiguous about the protective effects of fiber in colon cancer.

Another dietary component thought to play a significant role in cancer is dietary fat. Some studies found a higher incidence of breast and colon cancer in populations that consumed high amounts of fat. Many studies were done to identify the specific types of fat and the mechanisms through which these components may impact cancer risk, but as with fiber, large human studies of dietary fat related to cancer have not shown a clear relationship. This is frustrating to consumers but reflects the complexity of the disease, the diet, and the interactions between the two that occur in the human body. As we develop better molecular tools, it is likely that we will be able to clarify which genetic factors influence the response to dietary components in individuals. While we wait for science to reach this point, diets high in fiber and low in fat may have many positive health benefits and continue to be recommended to reduce cancer risk.

Food ingredients, including flavors, colors, preservatives, and artificial sweeteners, have been widely publicized as cancer causing. These concerns are largely unfounded. The FDA [Food and Drug Administration] has stringent requirements to demonstrate safety before any component is added to the nation's food supply. While we may never be fully sure that a chemical will never cause cancer given the right environment in a specific individual, the U.S. food supply is very safe. However, we may not assume that the food supply is free of carcinogens, because some edible plants contain naturally occurring mutagenic compounds and environmental pollutants do contaminate plant and animal foods. In general, these are in very low concentrations. To reduce the risk of exposure to these compounds, one should consume a wide variety of foods from reputable sources.

The American Institute for Cancer Research has undertaken an extensive evaluation of the scientific research of the relationships among foods and cancer. They have identified the following foods as being helpful in reducing the risk of the main forms of cancer in the

United States, to include breast, prostate, and colon cancers. These foods should be part of one's everyday diet because they are rich in vitamins, minerals, fiber, and many beneficial compounds such as polyphenols, flavonoids, and catechins, which have a variety of positive effects on the body.

- Citrus fruits, grapes, and berries
- Cruciferous vegetables (broccoli, cauliflower)
- Dark green leafy vegetables (spinach, kale)
- Colorful vegetables (tomatoes, squash, pumpkin)
- Beans
- Whole grains
- Fish and flaxseed
- Dairy foods (yogurt, skim milk)
- Nuts (walnuts, almonds)
- Green and black tea

While a healthy diet is critically important to lowering cancer risk, many other lifestyle features are also important. Here are ways to improve overall health and protect yourself from cancer:

- Avoid smoked, salted, or burnt meats
- Seek a balanced diet, adequate in protein, fat, and carbohydrates
- Maintain a healthy weight
- Perform regular exercise
- Avoid sugary drinks and high-fat foods
- Get routine screenings and checkups
- Don't smoke
- Get enough sleep
- Use household and farm chemicals properly
- Enjoy life and manage stress

Section 50.2

Antioxidants and Cancer Prevention

This section excerpted from "Antioxidants and Cancer Prevention,"
National Cancer Institute (www.cancer.gov), July 28, 2004. Revised by
David A. Cooke, MD, FACP, February 2011.

What are antioxidants?

Antioxidants are substances that may protect cells from the damage caused by unstable molecules known as free radicals. Free radical damage may lead to cancer. Antioxidants interact with and stabilize free radicals and may prevent some of the damage free radicals might otherwise cause. Examples of antioxidants include beta-carotene; lycopene; vitamins C, E, and A; and other substances.

Can antioxidants prevent cancer?

Considerable laboratory evidence from chemical, cell culture, and animal studies indicates that antioxidants may slow or possibly prevent the development of cancer. However, a number of large clinical trials have failed to show anti-cancer benefits from beta-carotene, vitamin C, and vitamin E supplements.

How might antioxidants prevent cancer?

Antioxidants neutralize free radicals as the natural by-product of normal cell processes. Free radicals are molecules with incomplete electron shells, which makes them more chemically reactive than those with complete electron shells. Exposure to various environmental factors, including tobacco smoke and radiation, can also lead to free radical formation. In humans, the most common form of free radicals is oxygen. When an oxygen molecule (O_2) becomes electrically charged, or "radicalized," it tries to steal electrons from other molecules, causing damage to the DNA and other molecules. Over time, such damage may become irreversible and lead to disease, including cancer. Antioxidants are often described as "mopping up" free radicals, meaning they neutralize the electrical charge and prevent the free radical from taking electrons from other molecules.

Which foods are rich in antioxidants?

Antioxidants are abundant in fruits and vegetables, as well as in other foods including nuts, grains, and some meats, poultry, and fish. The following list describes food sources of common antioxidants.

- Beta-carotene is found in many foods that are orange in color, including sweet potatoes, carrots, cantaloupe, squash, apricots, pumpkin, and mangos. Some green, leafy vegetables, including collard greens, spinach, and kale, are also rich in beta-carotene.

- Lutein, best known for its association with healthy eyes, is abundant in green, leafy vegetables such as collard greens, spinach, and kale.

- Lycopene is a potent antioxidant found in tomatoes, watermelon, guava, papaya, apricots, pink grapefruit, blood oranges, and other foods. Estimates suggest 85% of American dietary intake of lycopene comes from tomatoes and tomato products.

- Selenium is a mineral, not an antioxidant nutrient. However, it is a component of antioxidant enzymes. Plant foods like rice and wheat are the major dietary sources of selenium in most countries. The amount of selenium in soil, which varies by region, determines the amount of selenium in the foods grown in that soil. Animals that eat grains or plants grown in selenium-rich soil have higher levels of selenium in their muscle. In the United States, meats and bread are common sources of dietary selenium. Brazil nuts also contain large quantities of selenium.

- Vitamin A is found in three main forms: retinol (Vitamin A1), 3,4-didehydroretinol (Vitamin A2), and 3-hydroxy-retinol (Vitamin A3). Foods rich in vitamin A include liver, sweet potatoes, carrots, milk, egg yolks, and mozzarella cheese.

- Vitamin C is also called ascorbic acid, can be found in high abundance in many fruits and vegetables, and is also found in cereals, beef, poultry, and fish.

- Vitamin E, also known as alpha-tocopherol, is found in almonds; in many oils including wheat germ, safflower, corn, and soybean oils; and in mangos, nuts, broccoli, and other foods.

Section 50.3

Nutrition in Cancer Care

This section excerpted from "What You Should Know about Cancer
Treatment, Eating Well, and Eating Problems," National Cancer
Institute (www.cancer.gov), September 30, 2009.

People with cancer have different diet needs.

People with cancer often need to follow diets that are different from
what they think of as healthy. For most people, a healthy diet includes
the following:

- Lots of fruits and vegetables, and whole grain breads and cereals

- Modest amounts of meat and milk products

- Small amounts of fat, sugar, alcohol, and salt

When you have cancer, though, you need to eat to keep up your
strength to deal with the side effects of treatment. When you are
healthy, eating enough food is often not a problem. But when you are
dealing with cancer and treatment, this can be a real challenge.

When you have cancer, you may need extra protein and calories. At
times, your diet may need to include extra milk, cheese, and eggs. If
you have trouble chewing and swallowing, you may need to add sauces
and gravies. Sometimes, you may need to eat low-fiber foods instead of
those with high fiber. Your dietitian can help you with any diet changes
you may need to make.

Cancer treatment can cause side effects that lead to eating problems.

Cancer treatments are designed to kill cancer cells. But these treatments can also damage healthy cells. Damage to healthy cells can cause
side effects. Some of these side effects can lead to eating problems.

Common eating problems during cancer treatment include the following:

- Appetite loss

- Changes in sense of taste or smell

• Constipation	• Diarrhea
• Dry mouth	• Lactose intolerance
• Nausea	• Sore mouth
• Sore throat and trouble swallowing	• Vomiting
• Weight gain	• Weight loss

Some people have appetite loss or nausea because they are stressed about cancer and treatment. People who react this way almost always feel better once treatment starts and they know what to expect.

Take these steps before you start cancer treatment.

- Until treatment starts you will not know what, if any, side effects or eating problems you may have. If you do have problems, they may be mild. Many side effects can be controlled. Many problems go away when cancer treatment ends.

- Think of your cancer treatment as a time to get well and focus just on yourself.

- Eat a healthy diet before treatment starts. This helps you stay strong during treatment and lowers your risk of infection.

- Go to the dentist. It is important to have a healthy mouth before you start cancer treatment.

- Ask your doctor, nurse, or dietitian about medicine that can help with eating problems.

- Discuss your fears and worries with your doctor, nurse, or social worker. He or she can discuss ways to manage and cope with these feelings.

- Learn about your cancer and its treatment. Many people feel better when they know what to expect.

There are many ways you can get ready to eat well.

- Fill the refrigerator, cupboard, and freezer with healthy foods. Make sure to include items you can eat even when you feel sick.

- Stock up on foods that need little or no cooking, such as frozen dinners and ready-to-eat cooked foods.

- Cook some foods ahead of time and freeze in meal-sized portions.

- Ask friends or family to help you shop and cook during treatment. Maybe a friend can set up a schedule of the tasks that need to be done and the people who will do them.

- Talk with your doctor, nurse, or dietitian about what to expect. See the lists of foods and drinks that can help with many types of eating problems (at www.cancer.gov/cancertopics/coping/eating hints/page7).

Not everyone has eating problems during cancer treatment.

There is no way to know if you will have eating problems and, if so, how bad they will be. You may have just a few problems or none at all. In part, this depends on the type of cancer you have, where it is in your body, what kind of treatment you have, how long treatment lasts, and the doses of treatment you receive.

During treatment, there are many helpful medicines and other ways to manage eating problems. Once treatment ends, many eating problems go away. Your doctor, nurse, or dietitian can tell you more about the types of eating problems you might expect and ways to manage them. If you start to have eating problems, tell your doctor or nurse right away.

Talk with your doctor, nurse, or dietitian about foods to eat.

Talk with your doctor or nurse if you are not sure what to eat during cancer treatment. Ask him or her to refer you to a dietitian. A dietitian is the best person to talk with about your diet. He or she can help choose foods and drinks that are best for you during treatment and after.

Make a list of questions for your meeting with the dietitian. Ask about your favorite foods and recipes and if you can eat them during cancer treatment. You might want to find out how other patients manage their eating problems.

If you are already on a special diet for diabetes, kidney or heart disease, or another health problem, it is even more important to speak with a doctor and dietitian. Your doctor and dietitian can advise you about how to follow your special diet while coping with eating problems caused by cancer treatment.

For more information on how to find a dietitian, contact the American Dietetic Association (at www.eatright.org).

Follow these tips to get the most from foods and drinks.

During treatment, you may have good days and bad days when it comes to food. Here are some ways to manage:

- Eat plenty of protein and calories when you can. This helps you keep up your strength and helps rebuild tissues harmed by cancer treatment.

- Eat when you have the biggest appetite. For many people, this is in the morning. You might want to eat a bigger meal early in the day and drink liquid meal replacements later on.

- Eat those foods that you can, even if it is only one or two items. Stick with these foods until you are able to eat more. You might also drink liquid meal replacements for extra calories and protein.

- Do not worry if you cannot eat at all some days. Spend this time finding other ways to feel better, and start eating when you can. Tell your doctor if you cannot eat for more than two days.

- Drink plenty of liquids. It is even more important to get plenty to drink on days when you cannot eat. Drinking a lot helps your body get the liquid it needs. Most adults should drink 8 to 12 cups of liquid a day. You may find this easier to do if you keep a water bottle nearby.

Take special care with food to avoid infections.

Some cancer treatments can make you more likely to get infections. When this happens, you need to take special care in the way you handle and prepare food.

- Keep hot foods hot and cold foods cold. Put leftovers in the refrigerator as soon as you are done eating.

- Scrub all raw fruits and vegetables before you eat them. Do not eat foods (like raspberries) that cannot be washed well. You should scrub fruits and vegetables that have rough surfaces, such as melons, before you cut them.

- Wash your hands, knives, and counter tops before and after you prepare food. This is most important when preparing raw meat, chicken, turkey, and fish.

- Use one cutting board for meat and one for fruits and vegetables.

- Thaw meat, chicken, turkey, and fish in the refrigerator or defrost them in the microwave. Do not leave them sitting out.

- Cook meat, chicken, turkey, and eggs thoroughly. Meats should not have any pink inside. Eggs should be hard, not runny.

- Do not eat raw fish or shellfish, such as sushi and uncooked oysters.

- Make sure that all of your juices, milk products, and honey are pasteurized.

- Do not use foods or drinks that are past their freshness date.

- Do not buy foods from bulk bins.

- Do not eat at buffets, salad bars, or self-service restaurants.

- Do not eat foods that show signs of mold. This includes moldy cheeses such as bleu cheese and Roquefort.

For more information about infection and cancer treatment, see *Chemotherapy and You: Support for People with Cancer*, a book from the National Cancer Institute. You can get it free by calling 800-4-CAN-CER (800-422-6237) or online at www.cancer.gov/publications.

You may choose to use food, vitamins, and other supplements to fight cancer.

Many people want to know how they can help their body fight cancer by eating certain foods or taking vitamins or supplements. But, there are no studies that prove that any special diet, food, vitamin, mineral, dietary supplement, herb, or combination of these can slow cancer, cure it, or keep it from coming back. In fact, some of these products can cause other problems by changing how your cancer treatment works.

Talk with your doctor, nurse, or dietitian before going on a special diet or taking any supplements. To avoid problems, be sure to follow their advice.

For more information about complementary and alternative therapies, see *Thinking about Complementary & Alternative Medicine: A Guide for People with Cancer*. You can get this book free from the National Cancer Institute. Call 800-4-CANCER (800-422-6237) or order online at www.cancer.gov/publications.

Talk with your doctor before going on a special diet or taking any supplements. Some vitamins and supplements can change how your cancer treatment works.

Caregivers should follow these special tips.

- Do not be surprised or upset if your loved one's tastes change from day to day. There may be days when he or she does not want a favorite food or says it tastes bad now.

591

- Keep food within easy reach. This way, your loved one can have a snack when he or she is ready to eat. You might put a snack-pack of applesauce or pudding (along with a spoon) on the bedside table. Or try keeping a bag of cut-up carrots on the refrigerator shelf.

- Offer gentle support. This is much more helpful than pushing your loved one to eat. Suggest that he or she drinks plenty of clear and full liquids when he or she has no appetite. For ideas, see the lists of clear liquids and full-liquid foods (at www.cancer. gov/cancertopics/coping/eatinghints/page7).

- Talk with your loved one about ways to manage eating problems. Doing this together can help you both feel more in control.

Chapter 51

Nutrition and Oral Health

Diet and nutrition may affect the development and progression of diseases of the oral cavity which, in turn, can affect nutritional status. Throughout life, nutrition and oral health are interdependent and influence individuals' overall health status in numerous ways.

Why does the road to good health begin in the mouth?

Good health begins in the mouth for a very simple reason. The mouth is the beginning of the gastrointestinal tract. It is an important factor in the ability to chew, and thus, to digest nutrients. The links between oral health and nutrition are many.

Why is nutrition important to oral health?

Nutrition plays two quite different roles in oral health—protective and preventive. The protective role is in promoting healthy development and maintenance of the mouth's tissues and their natural protective mechanisms. The role of nutrition is also to prevent oral disease through the influence of the food's properties on plaque development and saliva flow. As in dietary guidance for general health, consuming a variety of foods is important for oral health.

Diet and nutrition may affect the development and progression of diseases of the oral cavity, and oral infectious diseases can affect diet and nutrition.

What has changed in recent years about our approach to dental caries prevention?

For many years, oral health care focused on prevention of dental caries (tooth decay) in children by emphasizing dietary influences on caries formation. Now, the emphasis has shifted to other preventive factors such as fluoride, use of sealants, frequency of eating, the length of time that foods and beverages are retained in the mouth, and, of course, good oral hygiene. With evolving science, specific foods no longer are being singled out as major risk factors for dental caries.

Why is fluoride so important?

In a major review of fluoridation facts, the American Dental Association credited fluoride with being the major factor for the dramatic reduction in dental caries over the past two decades. Since the first two-city experiment in 1945, the practice of fluoridating drinking water has been expanding steadily. The use of fluorides in other ways has also been rising rapidly. Virtually all toothpaste used in the U.S. contains fluoride. Fluoride mouthwashes and tablets are used in schools and homes and topical fluorides are applied in dental offices. Around the world, dental caries reduction is also being seen with the use of fluoride-containing toothpaste alone. In some underdeveloped countries, fluoridation of the water supply may not be realistic.

What causes dental caries?

Poor dental care, eating patterns, and food choices can be important factors in tooth decay. Everything eaten passes through the mouth where it can be used by the bacteria in plaque. Plaque, in turn, produces acids that can destroy tooth enamel. Plaque is an almost invisible deposit of bacteria that constantly forms on teeth. Plaque holds the acids on the teeth. Over time, the acids cause tooth enamel to break down, forming a cavity.

What are the factors involved in plaque build-up or acid production?

- **Frequency of eating:** Each time carbohydrate-containing foods are consumed, acids are released to work on teeth. The more frequently carbohydrates are consumed, the more opportunity there is for acids to damage teeth.

- **Food characteristics:** Some foods tend to cling or stick to the teeth. Not necessarily foods one would consider sticky, "cooked starches" such as chips and crackers rank high on the list of sticky foods as compared to candy bars and toffee.

- **Time that food remains in the mouth:** Foods that are slow to dissolve, such as cookies and granola bars, provide more time for the acids that destroy enamel to work than those that dissolve quickly, such as caramels and jelly beans.

- **Whether or not the food is eaten as part of a meal:** High carbohydrate-containing foods produce less acid when eaten with a meal than when eaten alone because saliva production is increased during a meal to help neutralize acid production and clear food from the mouth. Also, when consumed with beverages, sticky foods may be washed from the teeth more quickly, lessening the opportunity for acid production.

What role does regular dental care play?

Regular dental care is important from as early as six months after birth throughout the life cycle. For children, preventing decay of primary teeth, including baby bottle tooth decay, is critical. This condition can occur when an infant is allowed to nurse continuously from a bottle of milk, formula, sugar water, or fruit juice during naps or at night. Preschool years are an important time to establish good eating habits and good oral hygiene.

For adults, the regular dental exam provides important information on your overall health, and, indeed, on general health. The dentist will check for gum disease as well as precancerous or cancerous lesions, oral sores or irritations, fit of dentures or bridges, and proper bite.

Check-ups are important because some diseases or medical conditions have signs that appear in the mouth. Diabetes, nutrient and vitamin deficiencies, and hormonal irregularities may be detected by oral examination.

What is the role of the dietitian in oral health?

Dietitians working with clients can include assessment of oral health in nutrition assessment protocols (i.e., chewing ability, salivary output, dental status) and, if indicated, request a dental consult.

Those working in community settings can develop nutrition education messages that encourage and promote oral health in school and community nutrition programs. In research settings, dietitians can identify and support oral health issues in appropriate clinical nutrition research.

What can people do to protect and improve dental health?

- Be sensible, flexible, and realistic when making food choices. These are good rules for oral health as well as for nutrition.

- Visit the dentist regularly.

- Limit eating occasions to regular meals and no more than two to three snacking occasions daily.

References

Fluoridation Facts; Caring for Your Teeth and Gums; Why Baby Teeth are Important; Why Do I Need a Dental Exam? American Dental Association.

Mandel, I.D., DDS, Caries Prevention: Current Strategies, New Direction. *Journal of the American Dental Association,* October 1996.

Position of the American Dietetic Association; Oral Health and Nutrition. *Journal of the American Dietetic Association,* February 1996.

Part Eight

Additional Help and Information

Chapter 52

Glossary of Nutrition and Diet Terms

Added sugars: Sugars and syrups that are added to foods during processing or preparation. Added sugars do not include naturally occurring sugars such as lactose in milk or fructose in fruits.[1]

Adequate Intakes (AIs): A recommended average daily nutrient intake level based on observed or experimentally determined approximations or estimates of mean nutrient intake by a group (or groups) of apparently healthy people. This is used when the Recommended Dietary Allowance cannot be determined.[1]

Adipose tissue: Fat tissue in the body.[2]

Body mass index (BMI): A measure of body weight relative to height. BMI is a tool that is often used to determine if a person is at a healthy weight, overweight, or obese, and whether a person's health is at risk due to his or her weight. To figure out BMI, use the following formula: BMI = (weight in pounds x 703) divided by (height in inches squared). A body mass index (BMI) of 18.5 to 24.9 is considered healthy. A person with a BMI of 25 to 29.9 is considered overweight, and a person with a BMI of 30 or more is considered obese.[2]

This glossary contains terms excerpted from glossaries produced by the following government agencies: U.S. Department of Health and Human Services, marked with a superscript 1; and the Weight-Control Information Network, National Institute of Diabetes and Digestive and Kidney Diseases (www.win.niddk .gov), marked with a superscript 2.

Calorie: A unit of energy in food. Foods have carbohydrates, proteins, and/or fats. Some beverages have alcohol. Carbohydrates and proteins have four calories per gram. Fat has nine calories per gram. Alcohol has seven calories per gram.[2]

Carbohydrate: A major source of energy in the diet. There are two kinds of carbohydrates—simple carbohydrates and complex carbohydrates: simple carbohydrates are sugars and complex carbohydrates include both starches and fiber. Carbohydrates have four calories per gram. They are found naturally in foods such as breads, pasta, cereals, fruits, vegetables, and milk and dairy products. Foods such as sugary cereals, soft drinks, fruit drinks, fruit punch, lemonade, cakes, cookies, pies, ice cream, and candy are very high in sugars.[2]

Cholesterol: A fat-like substance that is made by the body and is found naturally in animal foods such as meat, fish, poultry, eggs, and dairy products. Foods high in cholesterol include organ meats, egg yolks, and dairy fats. Cholesterol is needed to carry out functions such as hormone and vitamin production. Cholesterol is carried through the blood in small units called lipoproteins. There are two types of units that carry cholesterol: low-density lipoproteins (LDL) and high-density lipoproteins (HDL). When cholesterol levels are too high, some of the cholesterol is deposited on the walls of the blood vessels. Over time, the deposits can build up and cause the blood vessels to narrow and blood flow to decrease. The cholesterol in food, like saturated fat, tends to raise blood cholesterol, which increases the risk for heart disease. Total blood cholesterol levels above 240 mg/dl are considered high. Levels between 200 and 239 mg/dl are considered borderline high. Levels under 200 mg/dl are considered desirable.[2]

Complex carbohydrates: Large chains of sugar units arranged to form starches and fiber. Complex carbohydrates include vegetables, whole fruits, rice, pasta, potatoes, grains (brown rice, oats, wheat, barley, corn), and legumes (chickpeas, black-eyed peas, lentils, as well as beans such as lima, kidney, pinto, soy, and black beans).[1]

Danger zone: The temperature that allows bacteria to multiply rapidly and produce toxins, between 40° F and 140° F. To keep food out of this "danger zone," keep cold food cold and hot food hot. Keep food cold in the refrigerator, in coolers, or on ice in the service line. Keep hot food in the oven, in heated chafing dishes, or in preheated steam tables, warming trays, and/or slow cookers. Never leave perishable foods, such as meat, poultry, eggs, and casseroles, in the "danger zone" over two hours, one hour in temperatures above 90° F.[1]

Diabetes mellitus: A disease that occurs when the body is not able to use blood glucose (sugar). Blood sugar levels are controlled by insulin, a hormone in the body that helps move glucose (sugar) from the blood to muscles and other tissues. Diabetes occurs when the pancreas does not make enough insulin or the body does not respond to the insulin that is made. There are two main types of diabetes mellitus: type 1 diabetes and type 2 diabetes.[2]

Diet: (1) What a person eats and drinks. (2) Any type of eating plan.[2]

Dietary fiber: Nondigestible carbohydrates and lignin that are intrinsic and intact in plants.[1]

Dietary Reference Intakes (DRIs)—A set of nutrient-based reference values that expand upon and replace the former Recommended Dietary Allowances (RDAs) in the United States and the Recommended Nutrient Intakes (RNIs) in Canada. They are actually a set of four reference values: Estimated Average Requirements (EARs), RDAs, AIs, and Tolerable Upper Intake Levels (ULs).[1]

Empty calories: The balance of calories remaining in a person's "energy allowance" after consuming sufficient nutrient-dense forms of foods to meet all nutrient needs for a day. Discretionary calories may be used in selecting forms of foods that are not the most nutrient dense (e.g., whole milk rather than fat-free milk) or may be additions to foods (e.g., salad dressing, sugar, butter). A person's energy allowance is the calorie intake at which weight maintenance occurs.[1]

Energy density: The calories contained in 100 grams of a particular food defines that food's energy density.[1]

Energy expenditure: The amount of energy, measured in calories, that a person uses. Calories are used by people to breathe, circulate blood, digest food, maintain posture, and be physically active.[2]

Estimated Average Requirements: EAR is the average daily nutrient intake level estimated to meet the requirement of half the healthy individuals in a particular life stage and gender group.[1]

Fat: A major source of energy in the diet. All food fats have nine calories per gram. Fat helps the body absorb fat-soluble vitamins, such as vitamins A, D, E, and K, and carotenoids. Some kinds of fats, especially saturated fats and trans fats, may raise blood cholesterol and increase the risk for heart disease. Other fats, such as unsaturated fats, do not raise blood cholesterol. Fats that are in foods are combinations of monounsaturated, polyunsaturated, and saturated fatty acids.[2]

601

Foodborne disease: Disease caused by consuming contaminated foods or beverages. Many different disease-causing microbes, or pathogens, can contaminate foods, so there are many different foodborne infections. In addition, poisonous chemicals, or other harmful substances, can cause foodborne diseases if they are present in food. The most commonly recognized foodborne infections are those caused by the bacteria *Campylobacter, Salmonella,* and *E. coli* O157:H7, and by a group of viruses called calicivirus, also known as the Norwalk and Norwalk-like viruses.[1]

Glucose: A building block for most carbohydrates. Digestion causes some carbohydrates to break down into glucose. After digestion, glucose is carried in the blood and goes to body cells where it is used for energy or stored.[2]

Glycemic index: A classification proposed to quantify the relative blood glucose response to carbohydrate-containing foods. Operationally, it is the area under the curve for the increase in blood glucose after the ingestion of a set amount of carbohydrate in a food (e.g., 50 grams) during the two-hour postprandial period relative to the same amount of carbohydrate from a reference food (white bread or glucose) tested in the same individual under the same conditions using the initial blood glucose concentration as a baseline.[1]

High blood pressure: Another word for "hypertension." Blood pressure rises and falls throughout the day. An optimal blood pressure is less than 120/80 mmHg (millimeters of mercury). When blood pressure stays high—greater than or equal to 140/90 mmHg—you have high blood pressure. With high blood pressure, the heart works harder, your arteries take a beating, and your chances of a stroke, heart attack, and kidney problems are greater. Prehypertension is blood pressure between 120 and 139 for the top number, or between 80 and 89 for the bottom number. If your blood pressure is in the prehypertension range, it is more likely that you will develop high blood pressure unless you take action to prevent it.[2]

High-density lipoprotein: A unit made up of proteins and fats that carry cholesterol to the liver. The liver removes cholesterol from the body. HDL is commonly called "good" cholesterol. High levels of HDL cholesterol lower the risk of heart disease. An HDL level of 60 mg/dl or greater is considered high and is protective against heart disease. An HDL level less than 40 mg/dl is considered low and increases the risk for developing heart disease.[2]

High fructose corn syrup (HFCS): A corn sweetener derived from the wet milling of corn. Cornstarch is converted to a syrup that is nearly all dextrose. Enzymes isomerize the dextrose to produce a 42% fructose syrup called HFCS-42. By passing HFCS-42 through an ion-exchange column that retains fructose, corn refiners draw off 90% HFCS and blend it with HFCS-42 to make a third syrup, HFCS-55. HFCS is found in numerous foods and beverages on the grocery store shelves. HFCS-90 is used in natural and "light" foods in which very little is needed to provide sweetness.

Hydrogenation: A chemical way to turn liquid fat (oil) into solid fat. This process creates a new fat called trans fatty acids. Trans fatty acids are found in margarine, shortening, and some commercial baked foods like cookies, crackers, muffins, and cereals. Eating trans fatty acids may raise heart disease risk.[2]

Low-density lipoprotein: A unit made up of proteins and fats that carry cholesterol in the body. High levels of LDL cholesterol cause a buildup of cholesterol in the arteries. Commonly called "bad" cholesterol. High levels of LDL increase the risk of heart disease. An LDL level less than 100 mg/dl is considered optimal, 100 to 129 mg/dl is considered near or above optimal, 130 to 159 mg/dl is considered borderline high, 160 to 189 mg/dl is considered high, and 190 mg/dl or greater is considered very high.[2]

Metabolic syndrome: A collection of metabolic risk factors in one individual. The root causes of metabolic syndrome are overweight/obesity, physical activity, and genetic factors. Various risk factors have been included in metabolic syndrome. Factors generally accepted as being characteristic of this syndrome include abdominal obesity, atherogenic dyslipidemia, raised blood pressure, insulin resistance with or without glucose intolerance, prothrombotic state, and proinflammatory state.[1]

Micronutrient: An essential nutrient, as a trace mineral or vitamin, that is required by an organism in minute amounts.[1]

Monounsaturated fat: Fats that are in foods are combinations of monounsaturated, polyunsaturated, and saturated fatty acids. Monounsaturated fat is found in canola oil, olives and olive oil, nuts, seeds, and avocados. Eating food that has more monounsaturated fat instead of saturated fat may help lower cholesterol and reduce heart disease risk. However, monounsaturated fat has the same number of calories as other types of fat and may still contribute to weight gain if eaten in excess.[2]

Nutrient adequacy: A goal based on the RDA or AI set by the Institute of Medicine (IOM) in recent Dietary Reference Intake reports.

Goals include targets for vitamins, minerals, and macronutrients and acceptable intake ranges for macronutrients for various age/gender groups. Adequacy of intake relates to meeting the individual's requirement for that nutrient.[1]

Nutrient density: Nutrient-dense foods are those that provide substantial amounts of vitamins and minerals and relatively fewer calories. Foods that are low in nutrient density are foods that supply calories but relatively small amounts of micronutrients (sometimes none at all).[1]

Nutrition: (1) The process of the body using food to sustain life. (2) The study of food and diet.[2]

Obesity: Obesity is excess body fat. Because body fat is usually not measured, a ratio of body weight to height is often used instead. It is defined as BMI. An adult who has a BMI of 30 or higher is considered obese.[2]

Overweight: It is defined as a BMI of 25 to 29.9. Body weight comes from fat, muscle, bone, and body water. It is important to remember that although BMI correlates with the amount of body fat, BMI does not directly measure body fat. As a result, some people, such as athletes, may have a BMI that identifies them as overweight even though they do not have excess body fat.[2]

Phytochemicals: Substances found in edible fruits and vegetables that may be ingested by humans daily in gram quantities and that exhibit a potential for modulating the human metabolism in a manner favorable for reducing the risk of cancer.[1]

Polyunsaturated fat: A highly unsaturated fat that is liquid at room temperature. Fats that are in foods are combinations of monounsaturated, polyunsaturated, and saturated fatty acids. Polyunsaturated fats are found in greatest amounts in corn, soybean, and safflower oils, and many types of nuts. They have the same number of calories as other types of fat and may still contribute to weight gain if eaten in excess.[2]

Portion size: The amount of a food served in one eating occasion.[1]

Protein: One of the three nutrients that provides calories to the body. Protein is an essential nutrient that helps build many parts of the body, including muscle, bone, skin, and blood. Protein provides four calories per gram and is found in foods like meat, fish, poultry, eggs, dairy products, beans, nuts, and tofu.[2]

Recommended Dietary Allowance: The dietary intake level that is sufficient to meet the nutrient requirement of nearly all (97% to 98%) healthy individuals in a particular life stage and gender group.[1]

Saturated fat: A fat that is solid at room temperature. Fats that are in foods are combinations of monounsaturated, polyunsaturated, and saturated fatty acids. Saturated fat is found in high-fat dairy products (like cheese, whole milk, cream, butter, and regular ice cream), ready-to-eat meats, the skin and fat of chicken and turkey, lard, palm oil, and coconut oil. They have the same number of calories as other types of fat and may contribute to weight gain if eaten in excess. Eating a diet high in saturated fat also raises blood cholesterol and risk of heart disease.[2]

Serving size: A standardized amount of a food, such as a cup or an ounce, used in providing dietary guidance or in making comparisons among similar foods.[1]

Simple carbohydrates: Sugars composed of a single sugar molecule (monosaccharide) or two joined sugar molecules (a disaccharide), such as glucose, fructose, lactose, and sucrose. Simple carbohydrates include white and brown sugar, fruit sugar, corn syrup, molasses, honey, and candy.[1]

Tolerable Upper Intake Level: The highest average daily nutrient intake level likely to pose no risk of adverse health affects for nearly all individuals in a particular life stage and gender group. As intake increases above the UL, the potential risk of adverse health affects increases.[1]

Trans fatty acids: A fat that is produced when liquid fat (oil) is turned into solid fat through a chemical process called hydrogenation. Eating a large amount of trans fatty acids also raises blood cholesterol and risk of heart disease.[2]

Type 2 diabetes: Previously known as "noninsulin-dependent diabetes mellitus" or "adult-onset diabetes." Type 2 diabetes is the most common form of diabetes mellitus. About 90% to 95% of people who have diabetes have type 2 diabetes. People with type 2 diabetes produce insulin, but either do not make enough insulin or their bodies do not efficiently use the insulin they make. Most of the people who have this type of diabetes are overweight. Therefore, people with type 2 diabetes may be able to control their condition by losing weight through diet and exercise. They may also need to inject insulin or take medicine along with continuing to follow a healthy program of diet and exercise. Although type 2 diabetes commonly occurs in adults, an increasing number of children and adolescents who are overweight are also developing type 2 diabetes.[2]

Unsaturated fat: A fat that is liquid at room temperature. Vegetable oils are unsaturated fats. Unsaturated fats include polyunsaturated fats and monounsaturated fats. They include most nuts, olives, avocados, and fatty fish, like salmon.[2]

Waist circumference: A measurement of the waist. Fat around the waist increases the risk of obesity-related health problems. Women with a waist measurement of more than 35 inches or men with a waist measurement of more than 40 inches have a higher risk of developing obesity-related health problems, such as diabetes, high blood pressure, and heart disease.[2]

Weight control: Achieving and maintaining a healthy weight by eating nutritious foods and being physically active.[2]

Weight cycling: Losing and gaining weight over and over again. Commonly called "yo-yo" dieting.[2]

Whole-grain foods: Foods made from the entire grain seed, usually called the kernel, which consists of the bran, germ, and endosperm. If the kernel has been cracked, crushed, or flaked, it must retain nearly the same relative proportions of bran, germ, and endosperm as the original grain in order to be called whole grain.[1]

Chapter 53

Government Nutrition Support Programs

Chapter Contents

Section 53.1

Supplemental Nutrition Assistance Program (SNAP)

This section excerpted from "Supplemental Nutrition Assistance Program," U.S. Department of Agriculture Food and Nutrition Service (www.fns.usda.gov), November 2010.

Supplemental Nutrition Assistance Program (SNAP) helps put food on the table for some 31 million people per month in Fiscal Year (FY) 2009. It provides low-income households with electronic benefits they can use like cash at most grocery stores.

Who is SNAP for?

Households must meet eligibility requirements and provide information—and verification—about their household circumstances. Local SNAP offices can provide information about eligibility, and USDA operates a toll-free number (800-221-5689) for people to receive information about SNAP.

- Households may have no more than $2,000 in countable resources, such as a bank account ($3,000 if at least one person in the household is age 60 or older or is disabled). Certain resources are not counted, such as a home and lot.

- The gross monthly income of most households must be 130% or less of the federal poverty guidelines.

- Net monthly income must be 100% or less of federal poverty guidelines.

- Most able-bodied adult applicants must meet certain work requirements.

- All household members must provide a Social Security number or apply for one.

Certain non-citizens, such as those admitted for humanitarian reasons, those admitted for permanent residence, many children, elderly immigrants, and individuals who have been working in the United States for certain periods of time, are eligible for SNAP.

How do I obtain SNAP benefits?

Go to the local SNAP office and fill out an application. The local office will give you an appointment for an interview.

Our pre-screening tool (www.snap-step1.usda.gov/fns/) will tell you whether you might be eligible for SNAP benefits.

How is each household's SNAP allotment determined?

Eligible households are issued a monthly allotment of SNAP benefits based on the Thrifty Food Plan (TFP), a low-cost model diet plan.

An individual household's SNAP allotment is equal to the maximum allotment for that household's size, less 30% of the household's net income.

What foods are eligible for purchase with SNAP benefits?

Households CAN use SNAP benefits to buy foods for the household to eat and seeds and plants that produce food for the household to eat. Households CANNOT use SNAP benefits to buy beer, wine, liquor, cigarettes, or tobacco; any nonfood items, such as pet foods, soaps, paper products, and household supplies; vitamins and medicines; food that will be eaten in the store; or hot foods.

How many people get SNAP benefits, and at what cost?

In 2008, SNAP served 28.4 million people a month at an annual cost of $34.6 billion. In February 2009, SNAP served 32.6 million people, an all-time record. SNAP participation fluctuates with the economy and with the pattern of poverty in America.

Section 53.2

Women, Infants, and Children (WIC) Supplemental Nutrition Program

This section excerpted from "WIC," U.S. Department of Agriculture Food and Nutrition Service (www.fns.usda.gov), November 2009.

The Women, Infants, and Children (WIC) Supplemental Nutrition Program provides nutritious foods, nutrition education, and referrals to health and other social services. WIC serves low-income pregnant, postpartum, and breastfeeding women, and infants and children up to age five who are at nutrition risk. Congress does not set aside funds to allow every eligible individual to participate. Instead, WIC is a federal grant program for which Congress authorizes a specific amount of funding each year for program operations. The Food and Nutrition Sercies and provides these funds to WIC state agencies to provide foods, nutrition education, breastfeeding promotion and support, and administrative costs.

Who is eligible?

Pregnant or postpartum women, infants, and children up to age five are eligible. They must meet income guidelines, a state residency requirement, and be individually determined to be at "nutrition risk" by a health professional.

To be eligible on the basis of income, applicants' income must fall at or below 185% of the U.S. Poverty Income Guidelines.

Nutrition risk is determined by a health professional. This health screening is free to program applicants.

How many people does WIC serve?

During the final quarter of FY 2009, the number of women, infants, and children receiving WIC benefits each month reached approximately 9.3 million. Of the 8.7 million people who received WIC benefits each month in FY 2008, approximately 4.33 million were children, 2.22 million were infants, and 2.15 million were women.

What food benefits do WIC participants receive?

WIC foods include infant cereal, iron-fortified adult cereal, vitamin C–rich fruit or vegetable juice, eggs, milk, cheese, peanut butter, dried and canned beans/peas, and canned fish. Soy-based beverages, tofu, fruits and vegetables, baby foods, whole-wheat bread, and other whole-grain options were recently added to better meet the nutritional needs of WIC participants.

For women who do not fully breastfeed, WIC provides iron-fortified infant formula.

How does WIC support breastfeeding?

Since a major goal of WIC is to improve the nutritional status of infants, WIC mothers are encouraged to breastfeed their infants, unless medically contraindicated.

- WIC mothers who breastfeed their infants are provided information and support.

- Breastfeeding mothers receive a greater quantity and variety of foods than mothers who fully formula feed their infants.

- Breastfeeding mothers are eligible to participate in WIC longer than nonbreastfeeding mothers.

- Breastfeeding mothers may receive follow-up support.

- Breastfeeding mothers may receive breast pumps and other aides to help support breastfeeding.

What is the WIC infant formula rebate system?

Mothers participating in WIC are encouraged to breastfeed their infants if possible, but WIC state agencies provide infant formula for mothers who choose to use this feeding method. For FY 2008, rebate savings were $2.0 billion, supporting an average of 2.14 million participants each month, or 25% of the estimated average monthly caseload.

What is WIC's current funding level?

Congress appropriated $7.252 billion for WIC in FY 2010.

Section 53.3

School Nutrition Programs

This section excerpted from "National School Lunch Program" and
"The School Breakfast Program," September 2010, U.S. Department
of Agriculture Food and Nutrition Service (www.fns.usda.gov).

National School Lunch Program

The National School Lunch Program is a federally assisted meal
program operating in over 101,000 public and nonprofit private schools
and residential child care institutions. It provides nutritionally balanced, low-cost or free lunches to more than 30.5 million children each
school day in 2008.

How does the National School Lunch Program work?

School districts and independent schools that choose to take part in
the lunch program get cash subsidies and donated commodities from
the USDA for each meal they serve. In return, they must serve lunches
that meet federal requirements, and they must offer free or reduced
price lunches to eligible children.

What are the nutritional requirements for school lunches?

School lunches must meet the applicable recommendations of
the *1995 Dietary Guidelines for Americans,* which recommend that
no more than 30% of an individual's calories come from fat, and less
than 10% from saturated fat. Regulations also establish a standard
for school lunches to provide one-third of the Recommended Dietary
Allowances of protein, Vitamin A, Vitamin C, iron, calcium, and calories.

How do children qualify for free and reduced-price meals?

Any child at a participating school may purchase a meal through the
program. Children from families with incomes at or below 130% of the
poverty level are eligible for free meals. Those with incomes between
130% and 185% of the poverty level are eligible for reduced-price meals.

Children from families with incomes over 185% of poverty pay a full price, though their meals are still subsidized to some extent.

After-school snacks are provided to children on the same income eligibility basis as school meals. However, programs that operate in areas where at least 50% of students are eligible for free or reduced-price meals may serve all their snacks for free.

How much does the program cost?

The National School Lunch Program cost $9.3 billion in FY 2008.

For More Information

A listing of all the state agencies responsible for the administration of the programs may be found on FNS website at www.fns.usda.gov/cnd, select "Contact Us", then select "Child Nutrition Programs."

The School Breakfast Program

The School Breakfast Program is a federally assisted meal program operating in public and nonprofit private schools and residential child care institutions.

How does the School Breakfast Program work?

School districts and independent schools that choose to take part in the breakfast program receive cash subsidies from the USDA for each meal they serve. In return, they must serve breakfasts that meet federal requirements, and they must offer free or reduced-price breakfasts to eligible children.

What are the nutritional requirements for school breakfasts?

School breakfasts must meet the applicable recommendations of the *Dietary Guidelines for Americans*. In addition, breakfasts must provide one-fourth of the Recommended Dietary Allowance for protein, calcium, iron, Vitamin A, Vitamin C, and calories.

How do children qualify for free and reduced-price breakfasts?

Any child at a participating school may purchase a meal through the program. Children from families with incomes at or below 130% of the federal poverty level are eligible for free meals. Those with incomes between 130% and 185% of the poverty level are eligible for reduced-price meals. Children from families over 185% of poverty pay full price, though their meals are still subsidized to some extent.

How many children are served?

In FY 2008, over 10.6 million children participated every day. Of those, 8.5 million received their meals free or at a reduced price.

How much does the program cost?

For FY 2008, the School Breakfast Program cost $2.4 billion.

Section 53.4

Senior Nutrition Programs

This section excerpted from "Elderly Nutrition Program," Administration on Aging (www.aoa.gov), June 16, 2009, and "Senior Farmers' Market Nutrition Program," U.S. Department of Agriculture Food and Nutrition Service (www.fns.usda.gov), April 2010.

The Elderly Nutrition Program

The Administration on Aging's (AoA) Elderly Nutrition Program provides grants to support nutrition services to older people throughout the country. The program is intended to improve the dietary intakes of participants and to offer participants opportunities to form new friendships and to create informal support networks.

The Elderly Nutrition Program provides for congregate and home-delivered meals. These meals and other nutrition services are provided in a variety of group settings, such as senior centers, faith based settings, and schools, as well as in the homes of homebound older adults. Meals served under the program must provide at least one-third of the recommended dietary allowances established by the Institute of Medicine of the National Academy of Sciences, as well as the *Dietary Guidelines for Americans*. In practice, the Elderly Nutrition Program's three million elderly participants are receiving an estimated 40% to 50% of required nutrients from meals provided by the program.

The Elderly Nutrition Program also provides a range of related services through the aging network's estimated 4,000 nutrition service providers. Programs such as nutrition screening, assessment, education, and counseling are available to help older participants meet their health and nutrition needs.

Eligibility

A person must be 60 years of age to be eligible. While there is no means test for participation in the Elderly Nutrition Program, services are targeted to older people with the greatest economic or social need, with special attention given to low-income minorities and rural older people.

The following individuals may also receive service:

- A spouse of any age
- Disabled persons under age 60 who reside in housing facilities occupied primarily by the elderly where congregate meals are served
- Disabled persons who reside at home and accompany older persons to meals
- Nutrition service volunteers

Senior Farmers' Market Nutrition Program (SFMNP)

SFMNP awards grants to states, U.S. territories, and federally recognized Indian tribal governments to provide low-income seniors with coupons that can be exchanged for eligible foods at farmers' markets, roadside stands, and community supported agriculture programs. The majority of grant funds must be used for foods that are provided under the SFMNP; state agencies may use up to 10% of their grants for program administrative costs.

The 2008 Farm Bill provided $20.6 million annually to operate the program through 2012.

In FY 2009, 809,711 people received SFMNP coupons.

What is the purpose of the SFMNP?

1. Provide fresh, nutritious, unprepared, locally grown fruits, vegetables, herbs, and honey from farmers' markets, roadside stands, and community supported agriculture programs to low-income seniors.

2. Increase the consumption of agricultural commodities by expanding, developing, or aiding in the development and

expansion of domestic farmers' markets, roadside stands, and community supported agriculture programs.

How does the SFMNP operate?

In 2009, the latest year for which data are available, 18,714 farmers at 3,684 farmers' markets as well as 3,061 roadside stands and 159 community supported agriculture programs participated in the program.

What foods are available through the SFMNP?

Fresh, nutritious, unprepared fruits, vegetables, herbs, and honey may be purchased with SFMNP benefits. State agencies may limit SFMNP sales to specific foods that are locally grown in order to encourage SFMNP recipients to support the farmers in their own states.

Chapter 54

Directory of Nutrition Information Resources

Government Agencies

Administration on Aging (AOA)
1 Massachusetts Ave.
Washington, DC 20201
Phone: 202-619-0724
Fax: 202-357-3560
Website: http://www.aoa.gov
E-mail: aoainfo@aoa.gov

Center for Nutrition Policy and Promotion (CNPP)
3101 Park Center Dr. 10th Floor
Alexandria, VA 22302-1594
Website: http://www.
choosemyplate.gov
E-mail: support@cnpp.usda.gov

Centers for Disease Control and Prevention (CDC)
1600 Clifton Road
Atlanta, GA 30333
Toll-Free: 800-CDC-INFO
(232-4636)
Toll-Free TTY: 888-232-6348
Website: http://www.cdc.gov
E-mail: cdcinfo@cdc.gov

Food and Drug Administration (FDA)
Consumer Inquiries
10903 New Hampshire Ave.
Silver Spring, MD 20993
Toll-Free: 888-INFO-FDA
(463-6332)
Fax: 301-847-8622
Website: http://www.fda.gov
E-mail:
ConsumerInfo@fda.hhs.gov

The information in this chapter was compiled from sources deemed accurate. Inclusion does not imply endorsement, and the list is not intended to be comprehensive. All contact information was verified and updated in March 2011.

Food and Nutrition Information Center (FNIC)
USDA Agriculture Research Service
10301 Baltimore Ave.
Beltsville, MD 20705-2351
Website:
http://www.nal.usda.gov/fnic
E-mail: fnic@nal.usda.gov

Food Safety and Inspection Service (FSIS)
United States Department of Agriculture
1400 Independence Ave., SW
Room 2932-S
Washington, DC 20250-3700
Website:
http://www.fsis.usda.gov
E-mail: fsis@usda.gov

Milk Matters Calcium Education Campaign
31 Center Dr.
Room 2A32
Bethesda, MD 20892-2425
Toll-Free: 800-370-2943
Phone: 301-496-5133
Fax: 301-496-7101
Website:
http://www.nichd.nih.gov/milk
E-mail: NICHDMilkMatters@
nail.nih.gov

National Cancer Institute (NCI)
NCI Public Inquiries Office
6116 Executive Boulevard
Suite 300
Bethesda, MD 20892-8322
Toll-Free: 800-4-CANCER (422-6237), Monday through Friday
9:00 a.m. to 4:30 p.m., EST
Live chat: http://cissecure.nci
.nih.gov/livehelp/welcome.asp
Website: http://www.cancer.gov

National Center for Complementary and Alternative Medicine (NCCAM)
NCCAM Clearinghouse
P.O. Box 7923
Gaithersburg, MD 20898
Toll-Free: 888-644-6226
TTY: 866-464-3615
Fax: 866-464-3616
Website: http://nccam.nih.gov

National Diabetes Education Program (NDEP)
1 Diabetes Way
Bethesda, MD 20814-9692
Phone: 301-496-3583
Toll-Free: 888-693-6337 (to order materials)
Website:
http://www.ndep.nih.gov
E-mail: ndep@mail.nih.gov

National Diabetes Information Clearinghouse (NDIC)
1 Information Way
Bethesda, MD 20892-3560
Toll-Free: 800-860-8747
Toll-Free TTY: 866-569-1162
Fax: 703-738-4929
Website:
http://diabetes.niddk.nih.gov
E-mail: ndic@info.niddk.nih.gov

National Heart, Lung, and Blood Institute (NHLBI)
NHLBI Health Information Center
P.O. Box 30105
Bethesda, MD 20824-0105
Phone: 301-592-8573
TTY: 240-629-3255
Fax: 240-629-3246
Website:
http://www.nhlbi.nih.gov
E-mail:
nhlbiinfo@rover.nhlbi.nih.gov

National Institute of Child Health and Human Development (NICHD)
P.O. Box 3006
Rockville, MD 20847
Toll-Free: 800-370-2943
Toll-Free TTY: 888-320-6942
Fax: 301-984-1473
Website:
http://www.nichd.nih.gov
E-mail:
NICHDInformation
ResourceCenter@mail.nih.gov

National Institute of Diabetes and Digestive and Kidney Diseases (NIDDK)
Office of Communications and Public Liaison
NIDDK, NIH
Building 31
Room 9A06
31 Center Drive, MSC 2560
Bethesda, MD 20892-2560
Phone: 301-496-3583
Website:
http://www.niddk.nih.gov

National Institute on Aging (NIA)
Building 31, Room 5C27
31 Center Drive, MSC 2292
Bethesda, MD 20892
Phone: 301-496-1752
Toll-Free TTY: 800-222-4225
Fax: 301-496-1072
Website: http://www.nia.nih.gov

National Institutes of Health (NIH)
9000 Rockville Pike
Bethesda, MD 20892
Phone: 301-496-4000
TTY: 301-402-9612
Website: http://www.nih.gov
E-mail: NIHinfo@od.nih.gov

National Library of Medicine (NLM)

Reference and Web Services
8600 Rockville Pike
Bethesda, MD 20894
Toll-Free: 888-FIND-NLM
(346-3656)
Toll-Free TDD: 800-735-2258
(via Maryland Relay Service)
Phone: 301-594-5983
Fax: 301-402-1384
Interlibrary loan fax:
301-496-2809
Website: http://www.nlm.nih.gov
E-mail: custserv@nlm.nih.gov

National Women's Health Information Center

U.S. Department of Health and
Human Services
8270 Willow Oaks Corporate
Drive, Suite 300
Fairfax, VA 22031
Toll-Free: 800-994-9662
Toll-Free TTD: 888-220-5446
Website:
http://www.womenshealth.gov

Office of Dietary Supplements (ODS)

National Institutes of Health
6100 Executive Boulevard
Room 3B01, MSC 7517
Bethesda, MD 20892-7517
Phone: 301-435-2920
Fax: 301-480-1845
Website: http://ods.od.nih.gov
E-mail: ods@nih.gov

President's Council on Physical Fitness and Sports (PCPFS)

1101 Wootton Parkway,
Suite 560
Rockville, MD 20852
Phone: 240-276-9567
Fax: 240-276-9860
Website: http://www.fitness.gov
E-mail: fitness@hhs.gov

U.S. Department of Agriculture (USDA)

1400 Independence Ave., SW
Washington, DC 20250
Phone: 202-720-2791
Website: http://www.usda.gov
E-mail: agsec@usda.gov

USDA Meat and Poultry Hotline

Phone: 888-MPHotline
(888-674-6854)
(10 a.m.–4 p.m. EST)
Recorded messages 24/7
E-mail: MPHotline.fsis@usda
.gov and AskKaren.gov

U.S. Department of Health and Human Services (HHS)

200 Independence Avenue, SW
Washington, DC 20201
Toll-Free: 877-696-6775 (Hotline)
Website: http://www.hhs.gov

Weight-Control Information Network (WIN)
National Institute of Diabetes and Digestive and Kidney Diseases
1 WIN Way
Bethesda, MD 20892-3665
Toll-Free: 877-946-4627
Fax: 202-828-1028
Website: http://win.niddk.nih.gov
E-mail: win@info.niddk.nih.gov

Private and Nonprofit Organizations

American Academy of Pediatrics
National Headquarters
141 Northwest Point Boulevard
Elk Grove Village, IL 60007-1098
Phone: 847-434-4000
Fax: 847-434-8000
Website: http://www.aap.org
E-mail: kidsdocs@aap.org

American Association of Diabetes Educators
200 West Madison Street
Suite 800
Chicago, IL 60606
Toll-Free: 800-338-3633
Fax: 312-424-2427
Website: http://www.aadenet.org
E-mail: aade@aadenet.org

American College of Sports Medicine (ACSM)
P.O. Box 1440
Indianapolis, IN 46206-1440
Phone: 317-637-9200
Fax: 317-634-7817
Website: http://www.acsm.org

American Council on Exercise (ACE)
4851 Paramount Drive
San Diego, CA 92123
Toll-Free: 888-825-3636
Phone: 858-576-6500
Fax: 858-576-6564
Website: http://www.acefitness.org
E-mail: support@acefitness.org

American Diabetes Association
1701 North Beauregard Street
Alexandria, VA 22311
Toll-Free: 800-DIABETES
(342-2383)
Website:
http://www.diabetes.com

American Dietetic Association (ADA)
120 S. Riverside Plaza
Suite 2000
Chicago, IL 60606-6995
Toll-Free: 800-877-1600
Fax: 312-899-4899
Website: http://www.eatright.org
E-mail: hotline@eatright.org

American Heart Association (AHA)
7272 Greenville Avenue
Dallas, TX 75231-4596
Toll-Free: 800-AHA-USA1
(242-8721)
Website:
http://www.americanheart.org

American Institute for Cancer Research
1759 R Street, NW
Washington, DC 20009
Toll-Free: 800-843-8114
Phone: 202-328-7744
Fax: 202-328-7226
Website: http://www.aicr.org
E-mail: aicrweb@aicr.org

American Public Health Association (APHA)
800 I Street, NW
Washington, DC 20001
Phone: 202-777-2742
TTY: 202-777-2500
Fax: 202-777-2534
Website: http://www.apha.org
E-mail: comments@apha.org

American Society for Metabolic and Bariatric Surgery
100 Southwest 75th Street
Suite 201
Gainesville, FL 32607
Phone: 352-331-4900
Fax: 352-331-4975
Website: http://www.asmbs.org
E-mail: info@asmbs.org

Asthma and Allergy Foundation of America (AAFA)
8201 Corporate Drive
Suite 1000
Landover, MD 20785
Toll-Free: 800-7-ASTHMA
(727-8462)
Website: http://www.aafa.org
E-mail: info@aafa.org

Celiac Disease Foundation
13251 Ventura Blvd
Suite 1
Studio City, CA 91604
Phone: 818-990-2354
Fax: 818-990-2379
Website: http://www.celiac.org
E-mail: cdf@celiac.org

*Center for Science in the
Public Interest*
1220 L St. N.W., Suite 300
Washington, DC 20009
Phone: 202-332-9110
Fax: 202-265-4954
Website: http://www.cspinet.org
E-mail: cspi@cspinet.org

Cleveland Clinic
9500 Euclid Avenue
Cleveland, OH 44195
Toll-Free: 800-223-2273
Phone: 216-444-2200
TTY: 216-444-0261
Website:
http://www.clevelandclinic.org

*Eating Disorder Referral
and Information Center*
2923 Sandy Pointe
Suite 6
Del Mar, CA 92014-2052
Phone: 858-792-7463
Fax: 858-220-7417
Website:
http://www.edreferral.com
E-mail: edreferral@aol.com

*Food Allergy and
Anaphylaxis Network
(FAAN)*
11781 Lee Jackson Hwy.
Suite 160
Fairfax, VA 22033
Toll-Free: 800-929-4040
Website:
http://www.foodallergy.org
E-mail: faan@foodallergy.org

*Institute of Food
Technologists*
525 West Van Buren
Suite 1000
Chicago, IL 60607
Toll-Free: 800-IFT-FOOD
(438-3663)
Website: http://www.ift.org

*International Food
Information Council
Foundation (IFIC)*
1100 Connecticut Ave., NW
Suite 430
Washington, DC 20036
Phone: 202-296-6540
Website:
http://www.foodinsight.org
E-mail: foodinfo@ific.org

*International
Foundation for Function
Gastrointestinal Disorders
(IFFGD)*
P.O. Box 170864
Milwaukee, WI 53217-8076
Phone: 414-964-1799
Toll-Free: 888-964-2001
Fax: 414-964-7176
Website: http://www.iffgd.org
E-mail: iffgd@iffgd.org

Kidshealth.org
Nemours Foundation
Website:
http://www.kidshealth.org

*National Association of
Anorexia Nervosa and
Associated Eating Disorders*
Helpline: 630-577-1330
Website: http://www.anad.org
E-mail: anadhelp@anad.org

*National Eating Disorders
Association*
603 Stewart Street
Suite 803
Seattle, WA 98101
Toll-Free: 800-931-2237
Phone: 206-382-3587
Fax: 206-829-8501
Website: http://
www.nationaleatingdisorders.org
E-mail: info@
nationaleatingdisorders.org

The Obesity Society
8757 Georgia Avenue, Suite 1320
Silver Spring, MD 20910
Phone: 301-563-6526
Fax: 301-563-6595
Website: http://www.obesity.org
E-mail: fdea@obesity.org

Shape Up America
Barbara Moore
506 Brackett Creek Road
P.O. Box 149
Clyde Park, MT 59018
Phone: 406-686-4844
Fax: 406-686-4424
Website: http://www.shapeup.org
E-mail:
askshapeup@shapeup.org

Interactive Tools/Online Interactive Resources

*Selected information in this section was compiled from the Food and
Nutrition Information Center's Eating Smart resource list (marked with
a superscript 1) at* http://www.nal.usda.gov/fnic/pubs/bibs/gen/eatsmart
.pdf *and the WIN Resources page at* http://www.win.niddk.nih.gov/
resources/index.htm *(marked with a superscript 2).*

Ask the Dietitian Calculators
Healthy Eating for Life Plan: http://www.dietitian.com/calchelp.php
Healthy Body Calculator: http://www.dietitian.com/calcbody.php
Free online program that helps users create a daily meal plan based
on self-determined calorie goals and eating preferences. For a custom
calorie goal, users should try the Healthy Body Calculator to establish
calorie needs based on whether the goal is to lose, maintain, or gain
weight.[1]

Body Mass Index Calculator
National Heart, Lung, and Blood Institute
http://www.nhlbisupport.com/bmi/bmicalc.htm

Calcium Quiz—What's your Calcium Intake?
Dairy Council of California
http://www.dairycouncilofca.org/Tools/CalciumQuiz
This interactive website allows you to enter your food choices for the day to determine how much calcium you are getting in your diet. Calcium-rich foods are listed and recommended based on your calculated intake.[1]

Eat Local
National Resources Defense Council
http://www.simplesteps.org/eat-local
Search for local produce or farmers markets in your area.

Get Moving! Calculator
Calorie Control Council
http://www.caloriecontrol.org/exercalc.html
This site allows users to calculate the number of calories burned during physical activity.[2]

Farmers Market Search
USDA, Agricultural Marketing Service
http://apps.ams.usda.gov/FarmersMarkets
Search for a farmers market in your state based on specific criteria such as city, county, or zip code.[1]

Fruits and Veggies Matter Interactive Tools
Centers for Disease Control and Prevention
http://www.fruitsandveggiesmatter.gov/activities/index.html
Includes "Analyze My Plate," which allows the user to drag food items onto a plate to get a nutritional analysis of the selections, and "Recipe Remix," which provides helpful tips for reducing fat, calories, and sodium in recipes.[1]

Healthy Dining Finder
http://www.healthydiningfinder.com
Online search tool helps users find healthier menu selections and corresponding nutrition information at restaurants ranging from fast food to fine dining.[1]

Kidnetic
International Food Information Council
http://kidnetic.com
This site promotes healthy eating and physical activity among children and their parents.[2]

National Dairy Council
http://www.nutritionexplorations.org
This site includes curriculums for educators, games, recipes for parents, and a variety of teaching tools to promote good nutrition.[2]

Personal Nutrition Planner from Meals Matter
Dairy Council of California
http://www.mealsmatter.org/EatingForHealth/Tools/PNP/
Helps adults determine recommended amounts of foods from each food group and provides recommendations based on a person's disease risk and other factors. Requires free registration.[1]

PubMed
National Institutes of Health, National Library of Medicine
http://www.ncbi.nlm.nih.gov/entrez
This site is a research database.[2]

Rate Your Restaurant Diet
Center for Science in the Public Interest
http://www.cspinet.org/nah/quiz/index.html
This interactive questionnaire helps users determine whether they make healthy food choices at restaurants.[2]

Online Recipe Resources

Information in this section was compiled from the Food and Nutrition Information Center's Eating Smart resource list at http://www.nal.usda .gov/fnic/pubs/bibs/gen/eatsmart.pdf.

The American Institute for Cancer Research Test Kitchen
http://www.aicr.org/site/PageServer?pagename=reduce_diet_recipes_ test_kitchen
Click on links to recipes as well as meal courses including appetizers, soups, salads, and desserts. Each category has dozens of healthy menu options, each with nutrition facts included.

Consumer Corner: Recipes and Cooking Tips
USDA, National Agricultural Library, Food and Nutrition Information Center
http://fnic.nal.usda.gov/consumer/recipes
Links to recipes and cooking tips from a wide variety of online sources. This page also includes sections on cooking with kids and ingredient substitutions.

Delicious Decisions American Heart Association
http://www.deliciousdecisions.org
Features heart-healthy recipes, including their nutritional content, in an online searchable database. Multiple search features allow users to browse recipes by category, or find recipes by main ingredient, cooking method, cuisine, or a combination of approaches.

Keep the Beat: Deliciously Healthy Eating
U.S. Department of Health and Human Services, National Institutes of Health, National Heart Lung and Blood Institute (NHLBI)
http://hp2010.nhlbihin.net/healthyeating/
Provides heart-healthy recipes created for NHLBI by a chef and registered dietitian that can be accessed by ingredient or category search, or by links on the homepage. Site includes a Food Preparation Glossary, safe cooking rules, healthy eating video clips, and more.

Fruits and Veggies—More Matters
Centers for Disease Control and Prevention
http://apps.nccd.cdc.gov/dnparecipe/recipesearch.aspx
Offers searchable recipes with fruits and vegetables as the main ingredient for every course including beverages and desserts. Nutrition facts per serving are included.

Mayo Clinic Healthy Recipes Center
http://www.mayoclinic.com/health/healthy-recipes/RecipeIndex
Features recipes organized by preparation method, ingredients, number of servings, and special nutrition modifications (such as low sodium). All recipes include a "Dietitian's Tip" on preparation techniques and food safety. Nutrition facts per serving are included.

Meals Matter Dairy Council of California
http://www.mealsmatter.org
Offers recipes and meal planning tools from shopping lists to cookbooks. Also found on this website are various interactive tools, educational materials, and a blog.

Nutrition.gov Cooking Methods and Recipes
USDA, National Agricultural Library, Food and Nutrition Information Center
http://www.nutrition.gov/recipes
Links to cooking and recipe resources from various federal government agencies. Also links to FNIC's Vegetarian Recipes and Meal Planning page.

SNAP-Ed Connection Recipe Finder Database
USDA, National Agricultural Library, SNAP-Ed Connection
http://recipefinder.nal.usda.gov
A searchable database of recipes submitted by Supplemental Nutrition
Assistance Program (SNAP) nutrition educators. Each recipe provides
cost per recipe, cost per serving, nutrition facts, a printable shopping
list, and an option to print a 3"x5" recipe card. The search page also
offers links to food demo and food safety tips, and tips for involving
kids in the kitchen. Recipes are also translated into Spanish.

USA.gov American Recipes
http://www.firstgov.gov/Citizen/Topics/Health/Recipes.shtml
Lists links to different types of recipe pages with topics to include
kids' recipes, cooking for a crowd, and special recipe collections and
publications. This unique government site also lists recipes "From
Famous Americans" for some historical American cooking ideas.

Index

Index

Page numbers followed by 'n' indicate a footnote. Page numbers in *italics* indicate a table or illustration.

Health Reference Series